Pharmacy
in Public
Health

BASICS AND BEYOND

Jean Carter, Pharm.D., Ph.D.
Associate Professor
Department of Pharmacy Practice
Skaggs School of Pharmacy
The University of Montana
Missoula, Montana

Marion Slack, Ph.D.
Professor
Department of Pharmacy Practice and Science
College of Pharmacy
The University of Arizona
Tucson, Arizona

American Society of Health-System Pharmacists®

BETHESDA, MD

Any correspondence regarding this publication should be sent to the publisher, American Society of Health-System Pharmacists, 7272 Wisconsin Avenue, Bethesda, MD 20814, attention: Special Publishing.

The information presented herein reflects the opinions of the contributors and advisors. It should not be interpreted as an official policy of ASHP or as an endorsement of any product. Because of ongoing research and improvements in technology, the information and its applications contained in this text are constantly evolving and are subject to the professional judgment and interpretation of the practitioner due to the uniqueness of a clinical situation. The editors, contributors, and ASHP have made reasonable efforts to ensure the accuracy and appropriateness of the information presented in this document. However, any user of this information is advised that the editors, contributors, advisors, and ASHP are not responsible for the continued currency of the information, for any errors or omissions, and/or for any consequences arising from the use of the information in the document in any and all practice settings. Any reader of this document is cautioned that ASHP makes no representation, guarantee, or warranty, express or implied, as to the accuracy and appropriateness of the information contained in this document and specifically disclaims any liability to any party for the accuracy and/or completeness of the material or for any damages arising out of the use or non-use of any of the information contained in this document.

Director, Special Publishing and Acquisitions: Jack Bruggeman
Acquiring Editor: Rebecca Olson
Senior Editorial Project Manager: Dana Battaglia
Project Editor: Johnna Hershey
Compositor: Yvonne Yirka
Designer: DeVall Advertising
Editorial Assistance: Moyo Myers

Library of Congress Cataloging-in-Publication Data

Carter, Jean.
  Pharmacy in public health : basics and beyond / Jean Carter, Marion Slack.
     p. ; cm.
Includes bibliographical references and indexes.
ISBN 978-1-58528-172-5
  1. Pharmacy. 2. Public health. I. Slack, Marion. II. American Society of Health-System Pharmacists. III. Title.
  [DNLM: 1. Community Pharmacy Services. 2. Public Health. WA 730 C323p 2010]
  RS92.C27 2010
  615'.1--dc22
                              2009033465
ASHP is a service mark of the American Society of Health-System Pharmacists, Inc.; registered in the U.S. Patent and Trademark Office.
ISBN: 978-1-58528-172-5

Dedications

To my parents, Ruth and Richard Carter
Jean Carter

To my family—my husband, Don; my daughters, Jonel and Jennifer;
and my mother, Nona Kimball
Marion Slack

To the memory of Lon Larson, a colleague and role model who inspired us both with his
intelligence, insight, and humanity.

Preface

What comes to mind when you think of pharmacy and public health? Immunizations? Medication safety? Is that everything? The answer is no. Pharmacists have the skills, knowledge, and opportunities to facilitate the public health agenda and improve the health of their patients. We chose to write this book because of the limited resources available to pharmacy students and practitioners who want to participate in activities to improve the health of their community. We wanted members of the pharmacy profession to have knowledge of the basic concepts and tools as well as a framework for recognizing public health problems and opportunities for participation in public health activities. We wanted them to know that, as pharmacists, they can be proactive and become leaders in addressing health issues. Finally, we wanted pharmacists to know that they do not have to wait to intervene until the patient develops a disease, which is treated by medication, but can participate in initiatives to improve health and prevent disease.

Because our goal is to make sure that pharmacy students and practitioners develop the knowledge and skills to participate in and lead public health activities, this book is not a comprehensive encyclopedia of facts and figures in public health or a compendium of every public health issue that involves the use of medication. It is instead focused on teaching pharmacists the basic concepts and tools of public health so that they have the understanding and skills to incorporate public health activities into their practice. Public health concepts and tools can be very different than those that govern the use of medications to treat disease. Public health is more concerned with the promotion of health and the prevention of disease in populations rather than the treatment of disease in individuals. This book is structured to provide the three types of knowledge required for public health: concepts, tools, and models of pharmacist participation in public health activities.

The book is divided into three sections that build on one another. This approach is based on the idea that readers will obtain a basic orientation to public health and what it involves in the first section. The second section introduces basic concepts and tools required for engaging in public health activities. The third section provides descriptions of models of public health programs in which pharmacists have participated.

The basic orientation to public health provided in the first section includes chapters on history, ethics, and laws of public health as well as a description of the public health system. The second section provides the underlying concepts of public health using an ecological model of health to describe those factors in the environment related to health and prevention of disease. The ecological model was chosen because it is oriented toward health and because it is useful at any population level from a neighborhood to the global level. The remaining chapters in this section delineate a framework to guide public health activities and provide specific tools, for example, basic epidemiological and statistical concepts. The third section of the book provides models of public health practice that involve pharmacists. We hope pharmacists can use the models to recognize opportunities for becoming involved so they can improve the health of their communities or their world.

When developing each chapter, we decided to use an integrated case study approach. Each chapter is built around a case study. The case study is first introduced at the beginning of the chapter, and is then revisited throughout the chapter to illustrate concepts and applications of public health tools as well as provide a model for how pharmacists can address similar public health issues. Chapter questions are used to help readers focus on the learning outcomes. In the third section of the book, the chapters are entirely based on cases used to illustrate models of pharmacist involvement in various public health services. Additionally, an "Applying Your Knowledge" section provides thought-provoking questions for discussion or suggestions for activities that are intended to move learning from the textbook to the real world of public health. Throughout the book, an effort is made to provide suggestions for actively engaging in activities that will help students learn and enable them to become involved in public health. This book supports the belief that all health care professionals, because of their knowledge and position in the community, have a responsibility to improve health and prevent disease.

This book is designed primarily as a textbook but can be useful in numerous situations, including:

The classroom. The most obvious use of the book is in the classroom. Professors can use the book to introduce students to the basic concepts and tools of public health through the text and the suggested learner activities. (See the Note to Instructors below.)

Student experiential rotations. Students can take the book with them on rotations so that they get to know the community they serve—to understand the context of health and disease in which they practice pharmacy. By understanding the context of their practice, they can better meet the pharmacy-related needs of community residents as well as participate in local efforts to address health issues.

Pharmacy practice. Established practitioners who are interested in tailoring pharmacy services to the needs of community residents or participating in activities to improve health in their service area can use the book to learn the basic concepts and tools of public health.

In the community. In addition to pharmacy education and practice, pharmacists may use the information to become more involved in local, state, national, or international public health efforts that they find are personally or professionally rewarding.

Note to Instructors

This textbook and its supplemental materials can be used in several ways within a pharmacy curriculum. We recognize that some schools may have a single course dedicated to public health topics, while others may have the topics integrated into the curriculum through several courses. To help identify which chapters may be best used in different situations, several tracks have been created.

Track A: All topics covered in one course

If the text is used entirely within one course, then the three sections of the book are best presented in their current order. Within a single section, chapters may be moved around to accommodate the flow of the syllabus. The topics in the first section (chapters 1–5) should be used first, followed by the topics in chapters 6–12. These chapters can serve as the topic areas for lectures. The models in the third section (chapters 13–18) are probably best used as a basis for classroom discussions.

Track B: All or some topics covered in two or more courses

For programs where the topics must be integrated into the curriculum via two or more courses, it will probably be most helpful to present the information in several contiguous lectures. This approach is suggested because students will have to consider issues from a public health perspective rather than a pharmacy perspective. The first course in the curriculum, to include one or more chapters, should begin with the introductory chapter. If there is not sufficient time to use each chapter, the instructor could use the models in the last section (chapters 13–18) as cases or examples.

> *Ethics course.* In addition to the introductory chapter, the instructor should use chapters 2 (history), 5 (ethics), and 7 (culture) to provide a historical context and introductions to public health ethical principles and cultural influences. These chapters set the stage for debates about inherent conflicts between public health and pharmacy ethics, including personal autonomy versus public welfare and privacy versus the public's right to know.
>
> *Drug literature course.* The introductory chapter should set the tone, then chapters 10 (epidemiology), 11 (describing populations), and 12 (community health) should be included. The model chapters in the third section all include statistics and epidemiological data and results that can serve as examples.
>
> *Communication course.* The introductory chapter is the logical place to begin before using chapters 6 (determinants of health) and 7 (culture). Although these chapters do not focus on communication per se, they provide background information about the many forces that shape human behavior and understanding of the world. If not covered elsewhere, chapters 8 (health promotion) and 9 (disease prevention) provide fine examples of how communication is used.
>
> *Introduction to pharmacy practice course.* The introductory chapter and the models in the last chapters (13–18) can provide students with another avenue of practice to consider and provide the instructor with a valuable comparison of health care practice and public health practice.
>
> *Health systems course.* The introductory chapter should be used first and then chapters 2 (history), 3 (public health systems), and 4 (public health law). Chapters 8 (health promotion) and chapter 9 (disease prevention) can be used to compare and contrast similar or different perspectives between health care and public health practices.
>
> *Pharmacy law course.* The law chapter (chapter 4) by itself is not sufficient for teaching pharmacy law; however, it is a good way to introduce the students to why we need pharmacy laws and regulations. Complementary information about government roles and police power are found in chapters 2 (history) and 3 (public health systems), respectively.

Use of supplemental materials

In addition to the textbook, we have created instructional materials. Short slide sets that focus on major topic areas can be mixed and matched or incorporated into existing classroom lectures. These short sets of slides give the instructor more flexibility in arranging the order and allowing time for discussion. We included key figures and tables from the book in the slides. Additional and often more advanced cases are also provided to encourage deeper thinking and discussion of key concepts and applications. Cases may be adapted to the local community or used to illustrate cultural and health issues of other populations. Because new knowledge about health and disease emerge each year, the cases can be updated as needed and re-used for many years. Both the slide sets and cases will be available online to students and instructors.

Acknowlegments

The great fear in writing the acknowledgments is that we won't adequately represent everything the significant people in our professional and personal lives have contributed to this book.

Marion Slack:

I worked in an environment that provided lots of room for creativity but also supported me—the College of Pharmacy at the University of Arizona. Then I was lucky enough to be associated with Dr. Lon Larson in the days just after I received my Ph.D. and was looking for employment. Lon suggested that I participate in the federal grant for interdisciplinary training in rural areas that had just been awarded to the University of Arizona. It happened that the training program was focused on community health, so I learned about rural and community health as well as public or population health. I also began to work with Marylyn McEwen, Ph.D., from nursing and learned about Anderson and McFarlane and their "Community as Partner" model of public health. When the first grant cycle ended on the interdisciplinary training project, Marylyn and I decided that we would become the PIs and work with Nogales, Arizona as our collaborating community. Fortunately, Karen Halverson, the Executive Director of the Southeast Area Health Education Center, and her staff and Gail Randolph, the Director of Nursing at Mariposa Community Health Center, became our collaborators in the community. Joyce Latura and the promotoras (Spanish word for community health workers) taught us so much about the local culture and the issues of trying to be healthy on a low income.

Jean Carter:

As your co-author, I would like to thank you (Marion) for saying "Yes" when I asked if you wanted to write a book about pharmacy and public health. It has been a pleasure working with you. I want to recognize the public health professionals in the Missoula City/County Health Department, especially Ellen Leahy, for their ongoing involvement in our school's "Pharmacy in Public Health" course. I also received great support from the Montana Department of Health and Human Services, which came primarily from Dr. Todd Damrow who was serving as the state's epidemiologist at the time. Another important group of people who provided support for this textbook are my colleagues at The University of Montana. A special thanks goes to my department chair, Mike Rivey, who ensured that I had the time I needed to write; my dean, Dave Forbes, for having a vision for pharmacy involvement in public health; and my colleague, Donna Beall, for her various activities. Her campus TB clinic for students and a rural outreach screening program inspired several cases used in the chapters and provided sources for photographs. I would also like to acknowledge one of my nursing colleagues from Montana State University, Dr. Sandra Kuntz, whose enthusiasm for community and public health is downright infectious!

We would like to acknowledge our three reviewers for their hard work, insightful feedback, and ideas for the chapters, which they provided throughout the writing process. Finally, we both want to acknowledge our guides and editors at the American Society of Health-System Pharmacists. Dana Battaglia and Rebecca Olson provided a structure of support and guidance that helped us take our vision to a reality captured by words. Then Johnna Hershey put the finishing touches on it, so our words became a book of which we can be proud. We hope all those who helped us during this process will be pleased with the results of their influences.

Contents

Reviewers

Leon E. Cosler, R.Ph., Ph.D.

Associate Professor of Pharmacoeconomics
Director, Research Institute for Health Outcomes
Albany College of Pharmacy and Health
    Sciences
Albany, New York

Spencer E. Harpe, Pharm.D., Ph.D., M.P.H.

Assistant Professor
Department of Pharmacy, School of Pharmacy
Department of Epidemiology & Community
    Health, School of Medicine
Virginia Commonwealth University
Richmond, Virginia

Douglas T. Steinke, B.Sc.Pharm., M.Sc., Ph.D.

Department of Pharmacy Practice and Science
University of Kentucky College of Pharmacy
Lexington, Kentucky

PART one

Foundations of Public Health

This section of the book focuses on the key concepts and foundational knowledge that pharmacists need to understand the public health perspective. Chapter 1 provides a framework or map of public health topics for the reader to use throughout the rest of the book. Chapter 2 covers important historical developments in public health to show how it has evolved into its current form and focus. Chapter 3 describes the structure of public health at local, state, national, and international levels. Chapter 4 explores public health law and how it is used to address issues such as faulty medication products and safe medication use. Finally, Chapter 5 compares the ethical foundations of health care practice and research to public health practice and research to provide contrasts and comparisons.

The first two chapters use mini-cases or examples to illustrate the information and ideas. More in-depth cases are used throughout the subsequent chapters to bring the concepts to life. At the end of this section of the book, the reader should have an understanding of the key concepts that guide public health actions and foundational knowledge of public health history, structure, law, and ethics.

Introduction

Learning Outcomes

1. Define public health.
2. Using the framework of the natural history of disease, compare the public health approach to the clinical treatment and clinical prevention approaches.
3. Discuss the population approach to health and the use of epidemiology and statistics in public health.
4. Describe the ecological approach to public health.
5. Identify who is responsible for public health, including whether pharmacy has a responsibility in public health.

Introduction

Public health is more than providing treatment for an illness; it is a concern for health and for the entire population and how to assure that the population is healthy. This chapter provides a framework for understanding the key concepts and tools used in public health, and it also differentiates public health and clinical prevention from clinical treatment. The chapter begins with four short fictitious case studies that involve public health issues. Three definitions are provided, and the role of pharmacy in public health related to medications is described. The definitions reflect the basic concepts of public health: (1) a focus that includes disease prevention and health promotion, (2) a concern that all members of a population have a basic need for health, and (3) knowledge that the environment external to the individual affects health.

The public health approach is differentiated from clinical prevention (focused on individuals) and clinical treatment (focused on treatment of disease in individuals). Because the focus is on the population rather than on the individual, specific tools known as epidemiology and statistics are required for public health. To include all aspects of the environment that are related to health, a public health approach known as ecological is presented and is based on the individual's interactions with his or her external environment. Responsibility for public health is presented by discussing the role of government, health care professionals, and community members in public health. The chapter ends with a discussion of how pharmacists who are already involved with clinical prevention can expand their role in community-based public health. The concepts presented form the basis of the discussion about pharmacists' participation in public health activities described in the remainder of the book.

CASE STUDY 1

Jim's first heart attack

Jim is a 51-year-old male who collapsed while enjoying conversation after dinner with his wife and friends, several of whom smoked. His friends performed CPR, while his wife called the ambulance. At the hospital, his wife was told that Jim had suffered a massive heart attack and his condition was critical. Jim began to respond to therapy after several anxious days and is now expected to recover, although his doctor tells him that he will need quadruple by-pass surgery. Was it necessary for Jim to experience a massive heart attack at age 51 or could it have been prevented? Assuming it could have been prevented, what could be done to prevent heart attacks? When in the disease process would it be best to intervene if the goal is to prevent the heart attack? What could Jim's pharmacist have done related to the prevention of heart attacks?

CASE STUDY 2

Fran experiences vomiting and diarrhea

Fran is a 34-year-old female who works as a pharmacist in a local chain pharmacy. Fran tries to live a healthy lifestyle and makes sure that she eats more than 5 servings of fruits and vegetables every day. Today Fran took a salad for lunch that she had made from fresh baby spinach, avocado, tangerine sections, pecans, and crumbled cheese with an oatmeal cookie for dessert. That evening, Fran became violently ill with vomiting and diarrhea; at 1 a.m., her husband went to the local 24-hour pharmacy to get medicine and fluids for rehydration. The pharmacist told him of one similar case the day before and two more earlier that night. Could this have been an outbreak of disease caused by eating contaminated foods? Whose responsibility is it to assure that foods are safe to eat? Should there be an investigation to see if other cases have been reported? Does the pharmacist have a responsibility beyond providing medication and counseling?

CASE STUDY 3

Daniel has asthma

Daniel is 3 years old and lives in a small apartment with his 22-year-old mother who is a student at the local junior college. Daniel has had asthma since he was 6 months old. After Daniel's most recent hospitalization for an exacerbation of his asthma, Daniel's mother was asked if she had cockroaches in her apartment because asthma can be triggered by cockroach droppings. His mother responded yes, but she didn't think she could do anything about them. She had repeatedly sprayed and tried to make sure no food or other scraps were left lying around. She also had left cockroach traps where she thought they wouldn't be a danger to Daniel. Who is responsible for taking care of the cockroach problem: Daniel's mother or the owner of the apartment house? Would the cockroach problem in the apartment where Daniel lives be considered a public health problem? Could Daniel's mother have gotten advice or other assistance concerning her roach problem from her pharmacist?

CASE STUDY 4

Emily celebrates her 90th birthday

Emily is a 90-year-old female in remarkable health; she has some problem with arthritis and slightly elevated blood pressure, but otherwise has few health issues. Emily spent most of her adult life living on a farm and doing all the work associated with farming. She was famous in the neighborhood for her large vegetable gardens. Currently, Emily is fairly active; she walks the dog twice a day, and likes to go to garage sales with her friend. She also does volunteer work at the local hospital where she is known for her delicious oatmeal cookies. Emily has agreed to participate in a study being conducted by public health researchers from the state university who are studying residents 90 years or older. Why would public health researchers be interested in someone who is not sick? What could the researchers possibly learn from a healthy person? What can pharmacists learn about health and longevity from their patients?

Public Health Defined

Three definitions of public health

Three definitions of public health are shown in the box. These definitions reflect a focus on health and prevention of illness. Two definitions also identify governments (local, state, or national) as the entity primarily responsible for ensuring the health of a population. The definitions hint that the interests of public health are broad—concern with the conditions promoting health and all factors affecting health. These definitions indicate that public health may be concerned with factors such as education or food supply, which are usually considered outside the purview of health care services.

One definition uses the term *population health* rather than *public health.* Generally, population health is a broader concept than public health. Public health implies that government at some level is involved. Population health refers to any effort to address health issues in a population group and may not include a role for government. Community coalitions are examples of attempts to address population health; these coalitions are often formed to address health issues in a neighborhood or community, and typically involve residents who are interested in health but often have no expertise in

Definitions of public health

Public health is a role of local, state, and national governments in assuring conditions in which people can be healthy.[1,2]

Public health is concerned with improving health or preventing illness in a population, and it is usually implemented by a government or a group accountable to a community.[3]

Population health refers to a process of addressing the entire range of factors that determine health and is concerned with the entire population, not just ill or high-risk individuals.[4]

health. Health care professionals also participate in community coalitions even though they have not been trained in public health.

Health care in the context of public health
None of the definitions of public health specifically identify health care services, so how are these services related to public health? Health care services clearly are a necessary component of pubic health; however, these services are viewed from a different perspective. The public health perspective of health care services is a concern with access to services, including financial access and quality of services. From the public health perspective, concern with **primary health care services** is considerable. These services allow individuals to avoid suffering, pain, disability, and death.[5] However, the services must be available to all members of a population if they are to prevent them from having unnecessary illness or injury. Public health also is concerned with the quality of health care. As part of this issue, the licensing requirements of health care practitioners may be within the purview of state health departments.

Pharmacy in Public Health

Like other health care services, pharmacy services are not mentioned specifically in definitions of public health but obviously are an important component of it. The focus of clinical treatment is on identifying the most appropriate medication for a specific disease. In public health, the focus shifts to assuring access to medications; assuring medications are safe and effective; and assuring medications are used in a safe and effective manner, which includes identifying and resolving problems associated with the use of medications.

Assuring access to medications
Access to essential medications is one of the components of primary health care as defined by the World Health Organization (WHO).[5] They are the medications needed to alleviate suffering, for example, pain medications, and to prevent a readily treated disease from resulting in disability or death. A concern with access to essential medications is assuring they are adequately produced and distributed as well as assuring that they are affordable and can be obtained if needed by all members of a population.

Assuring safe and effective medications
Assurance of safe and effective medications probably is the aspect of pharmacy and public health most familiar to the average person. Most people have heard news stories concerning medications being removed from the market because they resulted in deaths or serious side effects. Although the Food and Drug Administration (FDA) is responsible for assuring medications are safe and effective in the United States, many people might not recognize that these assurances are a public health issue.

Assuring medication use is safe

As every pharmacist knows, a large number of effective medications are available. However, these medications must be used in a safe and effective manner or they could result in harm. For example, aspirin is effective for treating headaches and other aches and pains as well as for reducing the risk of myocardial infarction but it is also poisonous, particularly to children, when taken in very high doses. The potential for poisoning is a public health problem. Proper disposal of unused medications is required to prevent poisonings (Figure 1.1). Other medications are effective when used in carefully controlled conditions, but can be harmful if used incorrectly. These are medications that require prescriptions so their use is restricted and the potential for harm reduced.

Figure 1.1—Pharmacy Students Disposing of Medications for Patients at a Health Fair

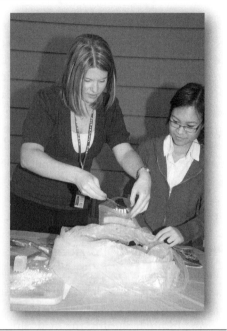

Key Concepts of Public Health

The key concepts of public health differ from those of traditional medical care or clinical treatment. In general, public health is much more focused on health and on maintaining health. Because the focus is on health and disease prevention, the timing of public health interventions will occur much earlier in the disease process than clinical treatment. Additionally, concerns include conditions or the types of environments that result in people being healthy and concerns that all members of the population, not just those seeking clinical treatment, benefit from public health interventions. This section introduces the key concepts of public health and describes how they differ from traditional medical care or clinical treatment.

World Health Organization's definition of health

As noted in the three definitions, public health is concerned with health; none of the definitions include the word "disease," reflecting the difference in focus of public health. Beginning with the World Health Organization (WHO) in 1948, efforts have been made to define health as something more than the absence of disease. WHO defined health as "…a state of complete physical, mental, and social well-being and not merely the absence of disease."[6,7] Therefore, the term "health" is associated with well-being, with the ability to function and to engage in activities for achieving goals. This definition of health implies that improving and maintaining health must involve something more than medical care for sick individuals.[4]

What is health?

- Health is the capacity to function physically, mentally, and socially.
- Health is a resource.
- Health is not just the absence of disease.

Health defined

For the purposes of this discussion, health will be defined as having the capacity to function physically, mentally, and socially. Additionally, a healthy person is not subjected to unnecessary exposure to the causes of disease or unnecessary suffering from preventable disease. Health is a resource to individuals and communities that enables them to achieve their goals. In contrast, illness and suffering require the consumption of resources in an attempt to restore health or to mitigate the consequences of disease.

Health and the Natural History of Disease

The natural history of disease

The natural history of health and disease[4,6] is shown in Figure 1.2. The process begins with a healthy individual who is then exposed to something that is causally related to disease (e.g., smoking or pathogenic bacteria). If the exposure occurs under appropriate conditions, the disease process is initiated, usually without the awareness of the individual. Without treatment to interrupt the disease process, the disease continues to develop until the individual experiences symptoms and seeks clinical treatment. The individual can be treated and restored to health if the health care provider can diagnose the disease and if there is an effective treatment for the disease. If there is no effective treatment, the individual may become disabled or become so ill that the result is death.

Figure 1.2—Health and the Natural History of Disease

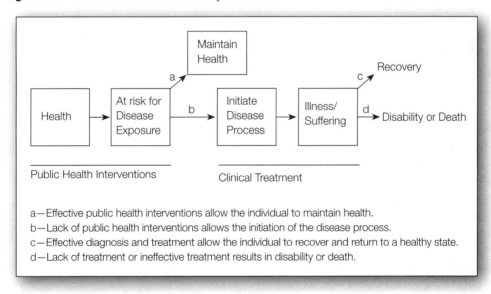

a—Effective public health interventions allow the individual to maintain health.
b—Lack of public health interventions allows the initiation of the disease process.
c—Effective diagnosis and treatment allow the individual to recover and return to a healthy state.
d—Lack of treatment or ineffective treatment results in disability or death.

Clinical Treatment

As shown in Figure 1.2, clinical treatment typically occurs late in the natural history of disease. A person experiences a symptom such as pain; he or she makes an appointment to see the doctor or other health care provider; the provider uses data from the patient's complaint and perhaps from laboratory tests to make a diagnosis; and, based on the diagnosis, a treatment (e.g., medication) is prescribed. The provider can be described as reacting to the patient's illness because the patient is already ill. In the typical patient encounter, there is little concern with how the person developed the disease or with why the person who was healthy is now ill. Therefore, clinical treatment typically does not prevent disease or decrease the number of persons in a population who develop the disease.

Public health

Public health is focused early in the disease process. In the process described in Figure 1.2, public health interventions occur either while the person is healthy or when he or she is at risk for exposure to the disease. Successful public health interventions prevent exposure and allow people to maintain their health; the absence of public health interventions can result in people developing disease. Public health is often described as working upstream rather than downstream.[7] To continue the analogy, imagine if flooding is a frequent occurrence in an area. The downstream approach to the flooding problem is to develop rescue services so that people living in the area can be rescued when a flood occurs. An upstream approach is to identify why floods are occurring and then take steps such as reforestation or construction of a dam to prevent floods. Similarly, the purpose of public health can be described as avoiding the need for clinical treatment by preventing **exposure** to the disease; the person who is not exposed to disease cannot develop the disease with the subsequent need for clinical treatment. Therefore, public health could be described as proactive rather than reactive.

Preventing Disease

Reducing the risk that people will be exposed to a specific disease or exposed to the conditions that produce a specific disease is known as **disease prevention** in public health. Within the framework of the natural history of disease, prevention interventions during the exposure process preclude the development of disease. Disease prevention often is aimed at individuals who are at high risk of developing specific diseases, for example, heart disease or diabetes, with the goal of preventing the disease from developing.

Promoting Health

Health promotion occurs even earlier in the natural history of disease. It occurs before exposure and is aimed at maintaining or improving health in a general sense, not just with preventing a specific disease. Examples of health promotion include public health campaigns focused on convincing people that they should lead healthy lifestyles, which include exercise as well as fruits and vegetables (5 servings a day) in their diet; not smoking or using tobacco products; and not driving while under the influence of alcohol. Health promotion is aimed at everyone, including persons who currently consider themselves healthy. Health screening is an important part of health promotion to prevent disease and monitor health. Health professionals often use health screenings as a way of educating the public in a friendly, casual environment outside of the doctor's office (Figure 1.3).

Figure 1.3—Health Screening at Health Fair

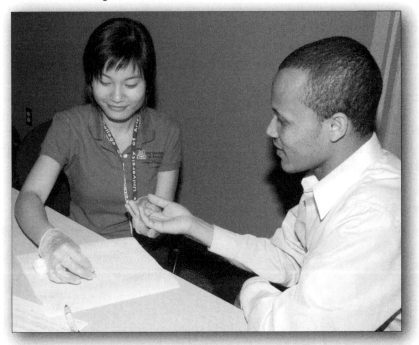

CASE STUDIES (*continued*)

Health prevention: Jim, Fran, Daniel, and Emily

When examined from a public health perspective, the questions related to Jim's heart attack would focus on whether the heart attack could have been prevented and when it would be best to intervene to prevent it. For example, one could consider intervening while Jim was still healthy and had no signs or symptoms of heart disease if the goal is to reduce the likelihood that Jim would experience a heart attack at a relatively young age. The cases involving Fran and Daniel also could be examined from a public health perspective to identify methods of preventing intestinal disease resulting from contaminated foods or asthma from a poor home environment. The case involving Emily might be examined to identify the factors in Emily's life that enabled her to be healthy at age 90. If those factors could be identified, then actions could be taken to assure that others also live in conditions enabling them to be healthy.

Populations

Population concepts

Population Defined

Population usually refers to the number of residents of a specific geographic area or political division (e.g., county, state).[4] Population also can refer to groups of people who share common characteristics, for example, people over the age of 64 or who have American Indian ancestry. From the perspective of health care providers, population can refer to the residents of an area served by their clinic or pharmacy; the population characteristics, for example, average age or ethnicity, can be expected to vary among service areas.

Communities and Broad Populations

Populations can be quite small and refer only to a neighborhood or a small rural community of a few hundred people. Populations can also be quite large when the reference is to the population of a city, county, state, or nation. One could even refer to the global population. Within public health, any of these populations could be included in public health activities or be a group with a public health concern. Public health is concerned with the health of *all* members of the population, regardless of current **health status.** However, population groups with special needs (e.g., women, children, elderly) may be identified and their needs addressed. At the population level, the relative health of different populations is a concern as well as the reasons why one population might be healthier than others (Figure 1.4).

Figure 1.4—Sign Advertising Women's Health Fair

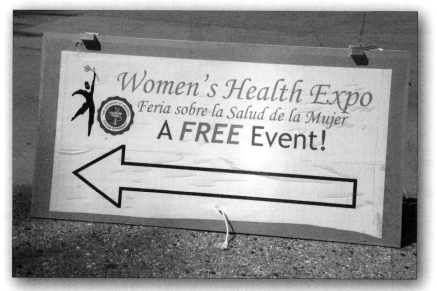

Individual versus population approach

The focus of individual approaches versus a population approach is summarized in Table 1.1. Pharmacists probably are most familiar with the individual approaches in which a single person is usually the target of the intervention. Population approaches are aimed all members of a group or to the health-related conditions of all members of the group.

Individual Approach

The individual approach is characteristic of clinical treatment because the treatment is aimed at a specific disease. In order to identify an appropriate treatment, a disease diagnosis is required before the treatment can begin. Even if a disease is relatively common, for example, high blood pressure, not every member of a population has high blood pressure and, even for those who do, not everyone can be treated with the same medication at the same dose. The treatment needs to be adapted to the individual. The individual approach could use counseling and education to change behaviors, particularly those behaviors that are detrimental to health. Therefore, a basic requirement of most clinical treatment is that it can be adapted to the individual's needs.

Table 1.1

Public Health versus Clinical Prevention and Clinical Treatment

Type of Activity	Focus
Public health	• Health promotion
	• Disease prevention
	• Population—especially the need for all members of a population to be healthy
	• Interventions to create conditions that promote health
Clinical prevention	• Health promotion
	• Disease prevention
	• Individuals—especially those at risk for specific diseases or conditions
	• Interventions with individuals to undertake activities that will promote health or prevent disease
Clinical treatment	• Disease treatment (restoration of health)
	• Individuals—especially those with a specific disease or condition
	• Diagnosis of disease is important so that appropriate treatment can be identified
	• Interventions with individuals to undertake activities that will modify disease process or alleviate pain

Population Approach

The population approach is characteristic of public health because the goal in public health is to create conditions that promote health or, if there is concern with a specific disease, to identify how the disease is spread through a population and how to reduce its spread. Everyone needs to live in conditions that promote health, not just a part of the population with a specific diagnosis. For example, everyone needs access to clean water and nutritious food. In order to assure that everyone has access, a population approach is required.

Treatment with medications also can have a population component. In the example involving the treatment of high blood pressure, access to medications and appropriate treatment is a population issue. Individuals cannot receive appropriate treatment for high blood pressure if they do not have access to medications or physicians. Because a population approach is concerned with factors that might affect health and with entire populations, it is considered the broadest approach to public health.[4] In contrast, some approaches to public health tend to be restricted to factors that are more closely related to health care.[8]

Clinical Prevention Approach

The **clinical prevention** approach combines aspects of clinical treatment and public health. Clinical prevention is provided to individuals, but it is focused on health promotion or disease prevention[9]; these types of interventions typically are under the control of the individual. Clinical prevention often involves identifying individuals who are at risk for a particular disease and then intervening to encourage different behaviors, including taking medications that will lower their risk of disease. Within clinical prevention, health promotion activities would involve intervening with an individual patient to encourage him or her to change a diet and to exercise. Other members of the population might not receive any encouragement to change their lifestyle.

Epidemiology and Statistics

Epidemiology

Epidemiology Defined

Epidemiology is the basic science of public health.[4] As the word indicates, epidemiology was derived from the study of epidemics of communicable disease; it provides tools for describing who became ill and when and where the illness occurred. Knowledge of who, when, and where can help in the identification of methods to avoid the disease, even without knowing how to cure current cases. Epidemiology provides the tools for going beyond the treatment of disease after it has developed to preventing disease and promoting health. In the modern world, communicable disease is only a part of epidemiology. Epidemiology is used to describe the patterns of health and disease within a population and to identify the factors related to any disease, including chronic ones such as diabetes.

Epidemiology describes:

- Who (person)
- When (time)
- Where (place)

of health and disease.

Role of Epidemiology in Public Health

Epidemiology is used throughout the entire public health process. It can be used to determine if a health problem exists by describing who does and does not have the problem. When a problem is identified, epidemiology can be used to determine what factors are related to the problem. If the factors can be modified, epidemiology can be used to determine if the modifications decreased the number of people who experienced the problem. Thus, epidemiology is essential to both research in public health and evaluation of the effects of public health programs.

Statistics

Because epidemiology is concerned with populations, statistics are needed to summarize data. In a single patient, the data from the patient is simply reported as his or her blood pressure, blood sugar, cholesterol level, and so on. However, when a group of people, or a population, is involved, then the data must be summarized by using statistics. For example, the blood pressure in a population could be summarized by reporting the proportion of the population (a statistic) with elevated blood pressure and with normal blood pressure. If the purpose is to determine if a public health intervention reduced the proportion of people in a population with high blood pressure, the readings before and after the intervention could be compared using a statistical test. Thus, statistics are integral to epidemiology and public health.

Population health issues: Jim, Fran, Daniel, and Emily

All of the cases are about individuals, but all of them are associated with population health issues. From a public health perspective, Fran's case is a classic example of when epidemiology and statistics could be used to determine if the problem (an acute episode of vomiting and diarrhea) is likely due to contaminated food or if it is a single, isolated instance. One would want to collect data on everybody who experienced vomiting and diarrhea about the same time as Fran to determine if they consumed similar foods and, if possible, test the foods for bacterial contamination. In Jim's case, one would want to examine the health status statistics for the community to determine if the rate of heart attacks among the residents were high. If so, one could then examine the statistics of factors related to heart disease, for example, smoking, to determine if residents are more likely to smoke. Similar population level questions could be asked in Daniel's case related to whether other residents are having problems with asthma and whether they have cockroaches in their apartment. The perspective for Emily is focused on health. One might want to know if the number of healthy older adults is more than would be expected in a population of similar size.

Environment and the Ecological Approach

Environment

Environment Defined

When a person refers to environment, he or she is likely referring to the *physical* environment; when a person thinks of the environment and health, he or she probably is referring to environmental pollution and its effects on health. Environment in public health is usually used in a broad sense to refer to aspects of the world external to the human body, including social, economic, and cultural factors that affect the individual.[6,10]

Environment as a Source of Disease

The world external to the human body clearly is a source of agents that produce disease in humans. Bacteria-contaminating water or foods are found in the external environment. Air pollutants can produce lung disease. Accidental injuries can occur because of high speed travel on highways, lack of traffic lights for pedestrians to cross the street, or lack of sidewalks that endanger pedestrians trying to avoid oncoming vehicles. Occupational hazards often result from the work environment, for example, farming activities or construction work. Occupations also expose workers to toxins, insecticides in agriculture, or chemical toxins in manufacturing. Thus, the environment external to the human body is a source of many disease-producing agents.

An Ecological Approach

Ecology Defined

Ecology refers to the relationship between an organism and its environment.[3,10] An ecological approach to public health is concerned with the relationship of human populations to any aspect of the environment that may be associated with health, including the relationships of an individual with other members of the population. It is concerned with why one group is healthier than another, even if they live in similar physical environments. It is concerned with what aspects of an environment can be changed to enable residents to lead healthy lives. Within an ecological perspective, you can expect to see topics discussed such as economics, competence of local governments, and cultural aspects of the environment.

Interaction between the Individual and Environment

The ecological approach to public health is based on the premise that the interaction, or the relationship, of the individual with his or her environment affects the individual's health. If the interaction is health enhancing, then the individual's health will be improved; if the interaction is detrimental, health may be compromised and the individual becomes ill or disabled. By studying how interactions vary across populations, insight into aspects of the environment that promote health or prevent disease can be gained.

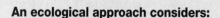

An ecological approach considers:

- All aspects of the environment related to health; and

- The relationship of the person with his or her environment.

Direct and Indirect Interactions with the Environment

In an ecological approach, the individual may interact with the environment either directly or indirectly. Direct interactions are the interactions that occur in the process of living one's daily life such as attending school, going to work, and maintaining a home. Indirect interactions result from more remote aspects of the environment. The aspects of the environment that indirectly affect health include parts of state and national governments or events that occur in other parts of the world. Government actions can affect many areas of health, for example, food supplies, as well as the availability of clinical treatment for persons who are ill. Events in other parts of the world can affect health if resources are diverted to the event (e.g., a natural disaster) or if a disease develops and spreads outside of the originating country.

 CASE STUDIES (continued)

Environmental influences: Jim, Fran, Daniel, and Emily

In an ecological approach to health, one would want to examine the environment in which each person lived for factors that might affect health. With Jim, the most obvious environmental factor is cigarette smoke. Smoking increases the risk of heart disease, and smoky environments appear to precipitate heart attacks.[11] Jim was having dinner with his friends who smoke, which might have precipitated his heart attack. To improve Jim's health, he should not be exposed to smoky environments. Daniel's case also clearly involves his immediate external environment because he lives in an apartment infested with cockroaches, which are known to be associated with asthma. Improvement of Daniel's environment would probably reduce the problems that he has with asthma. The issues with Fran's environment do not appear to be with her home or work environment but with the environment in which the salad greens are grown or processed. Apparently, some type of problem occurred in the growing and processing of the greens that contaminated them with disease-causing bacteria. In Emily's case, the environment appears to be favorable and to promote her health. Emily is able to walk the dog twice a day and attend garage sales so that she remains active even at 90 years of age. Her regular physical activity helps to maintain her health.

The case studies provide examples of interactions with the environment that are conducive to good health as well as detrimental to health and illustrate the types of environmental issues that impact public health.

Responsibility for Public Health

The average person often assumes that someone, without knowing exactly who, is making sure that living conditions are healthy, that there are not unnecessary pollutants, that food and water are safe to consume, and that medications are safe and effective. Although public health is considered a responsibility of government, it does not mean that only government is responsible for all aspects of public health. Health care professionals and community members also share responsibility for the public's health.

Government

Government has a central role in public health, as described in the definition from the Institute of Medicine (IOM). This definition identifies public health as "…a role of local, state, and national governments in assuring conditions in which people can be healthy."[1,2] This role of government is derived from (1) the focus on populations because an individual or a private entity has neither the authority or resources to implement rules and regulations to protect the health of populations; (2) the ability to assure that the conditions, including the ability to enforce rules and regulations, within a geographic area support health; (3) the ability to obtain resources through taxation; and (4) a mandate from a democratic society for assuring that its citizens live in healthy conditions.

Health care professionals

The health care professional responsible for public health is a public health professional—a person with education and experience in public health. However, the IOM Committee on Public Health argues that all health professions schools should include some training in public health; they contend that public health cannot succeed as a niche specialty but must have broad-based participation and support.[1] The Committee made specific recommendations for physicians and nurses. The Committee recognized that physicians have played a large role in public health both historically and in contemporary society; they recommend that all medical students develop an understanding of the ecological model of health and be prepared to participate in population-based prevention interventions through interprofessional approaches. Similar recommendations are made for nursing education, in particular, recognizing the role of nurses in controlling infections, identifying public health issues, and educating patients and families on disease prevention and health promotion.[1]

Community members

Community members also have a responsibility for public health. At a basic level, community members need to understand and support public health interventions. Without community support, public health interventions are, at most, only partially effective. However, community members also need to participate in identifying public health problems; local conditions vary by geographic location, climate, population characteristics, and culture. Local residents know their community and are often in the best position to design a public health intervention that will be successful in the community. Because health care professionals are both members of the community and educated and trained in health, they have additional responsibility for participating in public health.

Expanded Roles for Pharmacy in Public Health

Recognition of pharmacists' current role in public health

Before discussing expanded roles for pharmacists, you should know pharmacists' current roles in public health are often not recognized even by other pharmacists. Pharmacists presently provide education on medications, disease states, and lifestyle issues, all of which is part of clinical prevention. Pharmacists also provide educational programs to groups on issues such as drug abuse or other health issues that are examples of population health activities.[12] Pharmacists provide counseling on a wide range of health promotion products found in the typical retail pharmacy such as sun screens, dental hygiene products, or vitamin and mineral products. Moreover, pharmacists provide immunization services and participate in screening activities. All are examples of public health activities but typically are not recognized as such.

Advocates for an expanded role

The IOM Committee on Public Health advocated in its report that all health professionals receive training in public health, presumably including pharmacists. The American Association of Colleges of Pharmacy included public health outcomes in the document identifying educational outcomes for professional pharmacy programs.[13] The third domain of educational outcomes is public health, "Promote health improvement, wellness, and disease prevention in cooperation with patients, communities, at-risk populations, and other members of an interprofessional team of health care providers." The Accreditation Council for Pharmacy Education[14] has reiterated the importance of public health competencies in their accreditation standards for professional programs in pharmacy. Professional organizations, including the American Society of Health-System Pharmacists and the American Public Health Association, also recognize that pharmacists could have a much greater role in public health.[12,15] Thus, pharmacy students can expect increased emphasis on public health and increased participation in public health activities as pharmacists.

Roles for pharmacy in public health include:

- Assurance of access and safe use of medications;
- Clinical prevention; and
- Participation in population health.

Expanded role in community health

Pharmacists, like other health care professionals, have a responsibility for participating in public health both because they are members of a community and because they are highly trained. Additionally, pharmacists are the most accessible of all health care professionals; many health promotion products are available in a pharmacy; and community pharmacies are located in neighborhoods near where people live. These characteristics of pharmacy make it uniquely suited to participate in community-based public health.[12] Pharmacists are well positioned to collaborate with other community members and other professionals interested in public health to improve the health of their communities as well as to recognize at-risk populations and to develop disease prevention programs. By developing a basic understanding of health, populations, epidemiology, and an ecological perspective, pharmacy students will be ready to join public health activities in their communities to improve health.

Chapter 1 Summary

Public health is concerned with improving health and preventing illness in populations by assuring that people live in healthy conditions. Public health addresses health and illness issues before the disease process is initiated; therefore, public health interventions can be effective even if the disease process in the human body is not understood. While public health interventions can be delivered to individuals through clinical prevention, these interventions often are focused on populations because all members of a population have a basic need for health. In contrast, clinical treatment is usually aimed at those persons with a specific disease diagnosis.

Epidemiology and statistics provide the tools for investigating patterns of health and disease within populations, identifying factors that promote health or prevent disease, and evaluating new interventions. The ecological approach in public health is a broad approach to health promotion and disease prevention, and it incorporates a wide range of medical and non-medical factors into public health. While governments are primarily responsible for assuring conditions in which people can be healthy, health professionals and community members also have critical roles to fill in public health. Because pharmacists already provide clinical preventive services and are the most accessible of all health care professionals, their role could be readily expanded to include public health activities aimed at the community.

References

1. Hernandez L, Gebbie K, Rosenstock L, eds. *Who Will Keep the Public Healthy? Educating Public Health Professionals for the 21st Century.* Washington, DC: The National Academies Press; 2003.
2. Institute of Medicine. *The Future of Public Health.* Washington, DC: The National Academies Press; 1988.
3. Beaglehole R. *Public Health at the Crossroads: Achievements and Prospects,* 2nd ed. West Nyack, NY: Cambridge University Press; 2004.
4. Young TK. *Population Health: Concepts and Methods.* New York, NY: Oxford University Press; 1998.
5. Anderson ET, McFarlane J. *Community as Partner: Theory and Practice in Nursing.* Philadelphia, PA: Lippincott Williams & Wilkins; 2008.
6. Last JM, ed. *A Dictionary of Epidemiology.* New York, NY: Oxford University Press; 2001.
7. Evans RG, Barer ML, Marmor TR, eds. *Why Are Some People Healthy and Others Not? The Determinants of Heath of Populations.* New York, NY: Aldine de Gruyter; 1994.
8. Wallace RB, ed. *Maxcy-Rosenau-Last Public Health & Preventive Medicine.* Stamford, CT: Appleton & Lange; 1998.
9. Allan J, Barwick TA, Cashman S, et al. Clinical prevention and population health: curriculum framework for health professions. *Am J Prev Med.* 2004; 27(5):417–22.
10. Last JM. *Public Health and Human Ecology.* Stamford, CT: Appleton & Lange; 1998.

11. Sargent RP, Shepard RM, Stanton AG. Reduced incidence of admissions for myocardial infarction associated with public smoking ban: before and after study. *BMJ*. 2004; 328:977–80.

12. American Public Health Association. The Role of the Pharmacist in Public Health. Available at: http://www.apha.org/advocacy/policy/policysearch/default.htm?id=1338. Accessed April 29, 2009.

13. American Association of Colleges of Pharmacy. Educational Outcomes 2004. Available at: http://www.aacp.org/resources/education/Pages/CAPEEducationalOutcomes.aspx. Accessed April 26, 2009.

14. Accreditation Council for Pharmacy Education. Accreditation Standards and Guidelines for the Professional Program in Pharmacy Leading to the Doctor of Pharmacy Degree. Available at: http://www.acpe-accredit.org/. Accessed April 26, 2009.

15. American Society of Health-System Pharmacists. ASHP Statement on the Role of Health-System Pharmacists in Public Health. Available at: http://www.ashp.org/DocLibrary/BestPractices/PublicHealth.aspx. Accessed April 29, 2009.

Suggested Readings

Sargent RP, Shepard RM, Stanton AG. Reduced incidence of admissions for myocardial infarction associated with public smoking ban: before and after study. *BMJ*. 2004; 328:977–80.

This is a wonderful little study on what happened in a rural town in Montana when a no-smoking ordinance was passed but then was overturned at the end of 6 months. The outcome was a significant drop in hospital admissions for acute myocardial infarction during the 6 months that the ordinance was in effect with a subsequent rise in admissions when the ordinance was repealed.

Association of Schools of Public Health. What Is Public Health? Available at: http://www.whatispublichealth.org. Accessed April 24, 2009.

This site provides a short description of public health and lists public health activities. Watch the video until it shows the top 10 achievements of public health in the 20th century. Review them, and identify which ones involve medications.

Stolley PD, Lasky T. *Investigating Disease Patterns: The Science of Epidemiology*. New York, NY: Scientific American Library; 1995.

This text is a readable account of epidemiology and how it is applied to public health problems. Numerous examples are presented of epidemiological investigations and studies; some of them are related to medications and other products.

Allan J, Barwick TA, Cashman S, et al. Clinical prevention and population health: curriculum framework for health professions. *Am J Prev Med*. 2004; 27(5):417–22.

This article is the outcome of a collaboration among the educational organizations of health sciences colleges from a variety of health care professions. It identifies a suggested content for the public health curriculum of all health sciences colleges. Their work is based on the premise that all health professionals should have working knowledge of public health.

Schroeder SA. We can do better—improving the health of the American people. *N Engl J Med.* **2007; 357:1221–8.**

This is a recent article on improving the health of the American people. The article reviews the relatively poor rank of health status in the United States compared to other industrialized nations and then discusses the primary contributors to premature death. Only 10% of premature death is thought to be related to health care. The author then advocates for focusing on factors that can improve health and for assuring that the less fortunate benefit.

Chapter 1 Review Questions

1. Define public health.

Public health is the action taken by governments or groups to enable residents (populations) to be healthy.

The answer should include population; involvement of government or other groups; and a focus on health or disease prevention, not with the treatment of disease.

2. Define health.

Health is having the capacity to function physically, mentally, and socially.

The answer should identify health as something more than the absence of disease.

3. The phases of the natural history of disease are listed below. Identify the type of intervention, public health or clinical treatment, that you would use for each phase by writing the corresponding letter in the blank provided.

(a) Public health   (b) Clinical treatment

___ Health (a)

___ At risk for disease exposure (a)

___ Initiate disease process (b)

___ Illness (b)

4. Suppose that the city council of a small rural town wants to assure that its residents are healthy. What approach do you think the city council should take—an individual approach or a population approach? Justify your answer.

A population approach would be best because actions to improve health need to affect all residents, not just those residents who are already ill. All residents in the town need to live in conditions that promote health so any actions taken by the city council have to benefit the entire population.

5. Identify aspects of the environment that are of interest using an ecological approach to public health.

(a) The house in which the person lives _____Yes _____No

The answer is yes.

(b) The conditions under which lettuce or other leafy green vegetables are grown

_____Yes _____No

The answer is yes.

(c) Air quality _____Yes _____No

The answer is yes.

(d) Availability of medications to treat headaches _____Yes _____No

The answer is yes.

All of the items are of interest using an ecological approach to public health because anything in the environment that might affect health is of interest. All of the items listed could affect health either positively or negatively depending on the specific situation.

Applying Your Knowledge

1. **When asked to define health, a pharmacist responded that a healthy person is one who comes to the pharmacy to buy greeting cards and magazines. The implication is that the person does not have health problems or else would be coming to get medication (e.g., prescription, OTC product). Do you agree or disagree with this definition? Why?**

2. **Identify the laws that regulate the sale of tobacco products in your community where your parents live or where you attend school. Do pharmacies sell tobacco products? Should they? Are laws prohibiting the sale of tobacco products to minors enforced?**

3. **One of the responsibilities of the local health department usually is restaurant inspection. It assures that restaurant foods are prepared and served under hygienic conditions. Check with your local health department to identify how they conduct restaurant inspections, for example, how often a restaurant is inspected. What do they look for? What happens if the restaurant receives a low score? You also could interview the owner and/or manager of a restaurant and ask what is done to assure that the restaurant is clean.**

4. Identify what you could do if you were in a situation like Daniel's mother and had cockroaches in your apartment and couldn't get rid of them. Look at a web site or call your local health department. Determine if they offer information or services or can refer you to other services for addressing a cockroach problem. Ask a local pharmacist what he or she could recommend for addressing a cockroach problem. You also could ask if you could call the public health department.

History of Public Health

Learning Outcomes

1. Using a general definition of public health, trace the history of public health concerns and practices from ancient eras to the beginning of the 21st century.
2. Describe how public health practices have changed or not changed from ancient to modern times.
3. Describe how the scientific method has changed public health practice.
4. Describe how the role of government in public health has changed or not changed from ancient to modern eras.
5. Differentiate between the prevention and treatment of illness or disease.

Introduction

This chapter reviews the history of public health to describe the earliest known public health concerns and practices and how they have evolved through time. This review will describe whether public health is a modern or, at least, recent invention or whether it has historical antecedents. To describe the roots of public health and how it has evolved, examples of what might be considered public health practice are reviewed from ancient Greece to the end of the 20th century. A contemporary case study introduces public health issues and practices relevant to the 21st century to illustrate how contemporary issues and practice may be similar to or different from earlier examples.

Public Health: An Historical Context

A broad definition of public health will be used for the purposes of illustrating how its practice has evolved through history. **Public health** is defined as the implementation of activities concerned with collective action to improve the health of a population.[1,2] The history of public health should be differentiated from the history of medicine or the history of **disease**, although it was clearly influenced by both. Medicine is typically concerned with restoring health to individuals who are ill; for example, the administration of a medication, quinine, to cure malaria, a parasitic disease spread by mosquitoes. While public health may be concerned with policies or procedures that would provide quinine to anyone who contracted malaria, in this discussion, the concern is primarily with preventing disease; that is, changing the environment so the mosquitoes that carry the disease cannot breed and consequently are not available to transmit malaria to humans. Another public health solution might be to spray insecticide to reduce the number of mosquitoes or use mosquito nets impregnated with insecticide to keep mosquitoes away from people.

Disease is a concept from biomedicine and is based on the pathophysiology of biomedicine.[3] Disease is usually conceptualized as a specific entity; for example, a person could have heart disease, malaria or **smallpox**, or arthritis. The history of disease will not be discussed except incidentally because the concept of disease is of relatively recent origin and did not exist before the advent of biomedicine. A focus on disease would by default eliminate the consideration of public health practices through much of recorded history.

By necessity, the focus must be on recorded history. For example, archeological evidence indicates that the Inca in South America had constructed sewers and baths.[4] Without some type of record, however, the purpose of these activities cannot be determined. The focus of the activities described in this chapter will be concerned with improving health or with preventing illness.

To determine if public health practice was used in a specific historical era, three characteristics will be examined: 1) whether the purpose of the practice was to improve health or prevent illness; 2) whether the focus was on a population rather than on an individual; and, 3) whether the practice was implemented by a government or other group responsible for or accountable to a community or population.

Infectious Disease: America in the 18th Century

In the late 18th century, **infectious disease** was a serious public health concern. No scientific understanding of infectious disease existed, and few if any medications or treatments were available. One infectious disease of particular concern and prevalence was smallpox. Smallpox is a disease caused by a virus, Variola. In 1775, about 30% of persons who became ill with smallpox were expected to die after a prolonged illness. It was characterized by severe malaise and the development of pustules covering the body, including the soles of the feet and the palms of the hands (see Figure 2.1). If individuals did not die, they developed **life-long immunity** (i.e., the ability to make antibodies to the virus).[5] Smallpox is spread by person-to-person contact typically through inhalation of droplets or particles containing the virus. A person is **contagious** as soon as sores develop and continues to be contagious until all scabs have been lost, typically a month after the beginning of the illness. Particles that adhere to clothing, blankets, and so on remain contagious indefinitely.

Colonists at the time of the Revolution relied on **inoculation** to reduce the impact of the disease. Inoculation procedures involved introducing infectious matter into a small cut or scratch, which produced a much milder version of smallpox than did natural infection. Like the natural infection, however, individuals undergoing inoculation would be contagious and would develop immunity.

Figure 2.1—Person with smallpox. Smallpox is caused by a virus, *Variola*. Note how the pustules completely cover the hands and feet, including the palms of the hand and the soles of the feet. The virus is spread through respiratory droplets or by particles from the scabs that develop over the pustules. If victims survive, they have lifelong immunity to smallpox.

Reprinted from http://www.ihm.nlm.nih.gov/ihm/images/A/14/034.jpg. Courtesy of the National Library of Medicine.

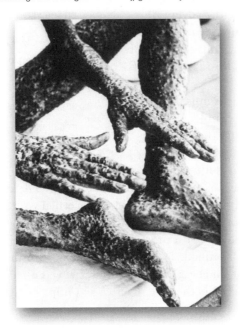

 CASE STUDY 1

How public health practice helped George Washington win the American Revolution

Washington assumes command of the American army

George Washington arrived outside of Boston on July 3, 1775, to assume command of the American army. The British army, consisting of professional soldiers well equipped with rifles, cannon, and ammunition, occupied Boston and controlled the harbor and shipping lanes into the city. The siege just after the Battle of Bunker Hill on June 17, 1775, is shown in Figure 2.2. The British had retreated into Boston so the Americans controlled the land access to the city. The American army outnumbered the British, 16,000 to 7000, but they lacked almost everything else. They lacked uniforms, ammunition (they had only 9 rounds per soldier), maps of the area, a

■ ■ ■

During the American Revolution, George Washington conducted the first successful public health campaign in America by:

- Using quarantine, then inoculation, to prevent smallpox among American troops;

- Requiring all new recruits not immune to smallpox to be inoculated; and

- Establishing inoculation hospitals for the care of the troops.

trained engineer, artillery, money, tents, and a flag. Additionally, the American troops lacked discipline and cleanliness; they preferred the fields to latrines and they had no way to wash their dishes, their clothing, or themselves. Consequently dysentery, typhus, and typhoid, infectious diseases spread by the fecal contamination of water or food or by lice, were present almost from the beginning of the siege.[6] The lack of materiel and training was daunting. It paled in comparison to their lack of immunity to smallpox because only a small portion of American soldiers were immune. Hence the American army could quickly become helpless and easily defeated if smallpox were to spread within the army, even though they outnumbered the British by more than 2 to 1. In contrast, the majority of the British troops were immune so the British army would be affected in only a minor way by smallpox.[5]

Quarantine

Smallpox was present in the civilian population of Boston when the siege began. Washington issued orders on his second day of command to prevent contact between civilians and soldiers. Smallpox hospitals were established, and any refugee from Boston suspected of having the disease was **quarantined** as was any soldier. The hospitals were closely guarded to prevent any contact between persons with smallpox and the susceptible American troops.

In November, the British ordered a few residents to evacuate Boston—some with smallpox—perhaps in an attempt to infect American troops.

When the British evacuated Boston on March 17, 1776, only soldiers with immunity to smallpox were allowed in the city. Most of the remaining troops quickly left the area en route to New York where General Washington anticipated the next big battle. The policy of quarantine, strictly enforced and possible because of the geographic location of Boston on a peninsula (see Figure 2.2), had prevented an **epidemic** of smallpox among susceptible American troops. In contrast, American troops sent to besiege Quebec were quickly defeated because at least a third of them were sick at any one time, most with smallpox, and reinforcements became sick shortly after arrival. The American forces sent to Quebec were almost destroyed, not by the British, but by smallpox.

Inoculation hospitals

In January 1777, General Washington established his winter camp near Morristown, New Jersey. To avoid further problems with smallpox, General Washington ordered the establishment of inoculation hospitals. All susceptible troops at Morristown were inoculated during the winter, and all suscep-

Figure 2.2—Map of the Siege of Boston, July 1775. Smallpox was present in the civilian population of Boston at the beginning of the siege. American troops controlled land access to Boston; any person leaving Boston suspected of having smallpox was quarantined. The location of Boston on a peninsula greatly facilitated General Washington's ability to keep smallpox away from susceptible American troops.

Source: Courtesy, American Antiquities Society.

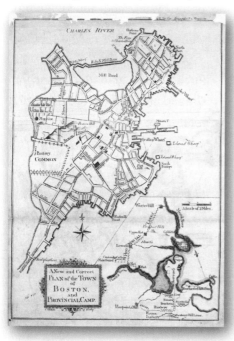

tible recruits were sent to an inoculation hospital before they joined the main body of the army. This policy continued throughout the Revolution. Subsequently most American soldiers were immune to smallpox, and susceptibility to smallpox ceased to be a factor in the war.[5]

General Washington clearly was engaging in public health practice according to the definition in the box. The quarantine of individuals with smallpox outside Boston and the establishment of the inoculation hospitals were intended to prevent the disease among the troops, a specific population. The activity was initiated by General Washington who was responsible for the health of a population, his troops. General Washington had successfully conducted the first public health campaign in American history.[5]

Public Health through Time

The timeline in Table 2.1 shows how practice evolved over several eras from a concern with the necessities of life (food, water, and sewage disposal) to the use of the **epidemiology**, a systematic approach to describing the causes, distribution, and risk factors associated with specific diseases. Public health concerns during the era of the ancient Greeks and Romans focused on supplying city residents with water, food, and the disposal of sewage. While these necessities continued to be an issue during the medieval era, widespread outbreaks of infectious disease known as epidemics resulted in actions to prevent or control the spread of disease. Antecedents of some public health practices to prevent the spread of smallpox, used during the Revolution by General Washington, are found in the medieval era.

Nineteenth-century public health practices marked the beginning of the use of the **scientific method**. The scientific method refers to the systematic collection and analysis of data that allowed public health researchers to identify how disease was transmitted and to identify strategies to prevent transmission. By the end of the 20th century, the focus had shifted from preventing infectious disease to preventing disease resulting from individual behaviors, for example, smoking. At the beginning of the 21st century, there is renewed concern with providing the necessities of life (water, food, and sanitation) and renewed concern with infectious disease.

Ancient times: water, sanitation, and food supply

Greece: 500 BC to 0 AD

In 500 BC, Greece consisted of many tiny city-states that were located on small areas of arable land between the rugged mountains and the sea.[7,8] The ancient city of Corinth[8] typically relied on locally produced foods as well as imported foods to feed the population. However, shipping was very primitive and unreliable so that too much reliance on imported foods could result in famine. Hence when the population became too large, a group of residents would band together and immigrate to another island or to another area and establish a new city.[7] Leaders in charge

Public health activities in ancient Greece and Rome were primarily related to:

- Selection of healthy environments for cities;

- Provision of clean water, removal of sewage, and adequate safe food; and

- Establishment of governance structures for administering and maintaining systems to perform public health activities.

Table 2.1

Historical Timeline for Public Health

500 BC–500 AD	Ancient era—Recorded evidence of public health activities
500 BC	Ancient Greece—Concern for living in healthy places based on drainage, winds, and soil; actual illness was usually treated by praying to gods
78 AD	Roman era—Continued Greek concern for a healthy environment but greatly expanded government role through engineering (e.g., constructing aqueducts) and regulations (e.g., regulation of food markets)
500 AD–1500	Medieval era—Multiple theories of illness including punishment for sin, astrological causes (position of planets and stars), and eventually miasma (poisoning from the foul odors emanating from garbage dumps, sewage, etc.)
1349	Bubonic plague swept through Europe; mortality rates are estimated to be 40–60%; city governments developed boards of health and quarantine strategies in an attempt to prevent and control the epidemic
1775	George Washington was faced with an epidemic of smallpox that could incapacitate his troops; quarantine and isolation procedures were reminiscent of medieval strategies to control plague
1800–1875	Sanitary era—Focus was on sanitation and collecting data on number and causes of death, which are the foundations of epidemiology
1848	Cholera epidemic in London during which John Snow used the scientific method to identify water contaminated with feces as the source of cholera infection
1875–1950	Infectious disease epidemiology; based on the germ theory where single agents related to a specific disease were identified; typical strategy for preventing disease was immunization or quarantine; concept of disease was developed
1950–2000	Chronic disease epidemiology; typical strategy for preventing disease was to modify individual behaviors, for example, smoking, diet, and exercise
After 2000	Shift to ecological framework for promoting health in which the influence of environment on health is examined; renewed concern with food, water, and sanitation as well as infectious disease

of establishing a new city were given instructions on how to locate the city so that the residents would be healthy. The treatise "Airs, Waters, and Places" advised leaders of new settlements to locate the city on higher ground where they would be warmed by the sun and catch salubrious winds. Marshy low lands and swamps were considered harmful to health. The soil also had to be examined carefully. Specific town officials were responsible for the water supply and drainage, presumably the drainage of sewage away from the city.[4]

The ancient Greeks thought that the preservation of health was important and seemed to have theories about how a person could retain his or her health. They believed that hygiene was important as well as nutrition, excretion, exercise, and rest. Further, the balance between the components and the balance with the surrounding environment was considered important. Unbalanced components would result in poor health and illness. One of the hallmarks of the Greek approach, compared to earlier approaches, was that it relied primarily on natural or rational explanations of health rather than on invoking gods. Individual Greeks did turn to the gods, especially Asklepios, but these actions seemed to be primarily aimed at cure of an illness, not prevention.[9–11]

Rome: 1 AD to 500 AD

The Romans adopted the principles of Greek medicine and, using their engineering skills, constructed aqueducts to supply their cities with water and sewers for drainage and sewage removal. Although not described in detail, the Romans seemed to associate clean water with health. Julius Frontinus, the water commissioner of Rome in 97 AD, supposedly stated that he had "…removed the causes of disease which previously had given the city a bad reputation."[4] (Note the use of the word 'disease'—a modern interpretation of a Latin word.) The Roman government assumed responsibility for providing water and maintaining sewers; they believed clean water was essential to civil life. Civic officials also oversaw the markets to assure that the food sold there was not spoiled.[12]

The State of Public Health Practice: 500 AD

Based on the broad definition of public health used in this chapter, both Greek and Roman governments were concerned about the health of populations, primarily the residents of specific cities. The ancient Greeks and Romans presumably provide the first written evidence of a concern with the health of a population. Actions were taken even though there seemed to be no strong theoretical foundations. The basis of their public health actions appeared to be experience; casual observation indicated that people tended to be healthier under some conditions than others. Neither the ancient Greeks nor the Romans appeared to rely primarily on gods, religious tenets, or the supernatural for justification of activities that characterize public health. As shown by the quote from Frontinus concerning the effectiveness of Roman aqueducts, they clearly believed that these actions promoted the health of residents. Notable also is the involvement of the government; for both the Greeks and the Romans, provision of services that promoted health was considered a role of the government and administrative structures were created to discharge these duties.

The medieval era, 500 AD to 1500, and its epidemics: the spread of infectious disease

Characteristics of the Medieval Environment

The development and governance of independent cities (formed by charter and governed by a council) throughout Europe[7,13] was one of the most influential factors affecting health during the Middle Ages (from the fall of the Roman Empire to the Enlightenment of the 16th century). Except for security, which was provided by armies maintained by the ruling nobility, the city council assumed responsibility for all governance of the city including issues related to the well-being of the population.

Despite repeated epidemics of bubonic plague, public health developments in the Middle Ages included:

- A change from religious- or superstition-based to observation-based policies;

- Establishment of city boards of health that included medical doctors; and

- Development of quarantine and related procedures for contagious disease.

Most cities were small, under 2000 people, and were built inside a wall[13] as shown in Figure 2.3. The city wall severely limited the area available for housing, resulting in houses that were crowded and dark because they were built with shared walls and few windows. Water was obtained from wells, which often were not protected from contamination by garbage and trash. Sewage was discharged into the street or into cesspits so wells were often contaminated. Most houses were constructed of wood and thatch—a perfect environment for rats and other vermin as well as for fire.

Medical care was extremely limited or not available. What was available, if not useless, was probably harmful or even fatal. Multiple theories existed to explain illness and poor health including retribution by God for sin, imbalanced humors, and astrological causes (i.e., confluences of stars and planets). Leprosy, the most common contagious disease, was treated according to precepts of the Christian Bible; sufferers were declared dead and were isolated in a separate compound outside the city walls. Another common problem was famine. City residents were dependent upon the surrounding farms for food; if the local crops failed, then famine ensued.[13] However, the rich did have access to spices from the Far East or to goods from other areas of Europe via trade routes.

Bubonic Plague Epidemic

The cities and their associated trade connections with the outside world set the stage for the bubonic (black) plague epidemic of 1347 to 1350. Bubonic plague is caused by Yersinia pestis, a bacterium in fleas that feed on rats. The disease is transmitted to humans when the host rat dies and the fleas seek an alternative host.[11] The plague epidemic began in 1346 in southern Russia between the Black and Caspian Seas and then spread to Constantinople, Greece, and Genoa, Italy, in 1347. By 1350, plague had spread through-

Figure 2.3—Medieval walled city. The small portion to the left is the original Roman city; the larger portion is the town and commercial district. Medieval walled cities were typically very crowded and dirty, a perfect environment for infectious disease.

Reprinted from Pounds N. *The Medieval City*. Westport, CT: Greenwood Press; 2005.

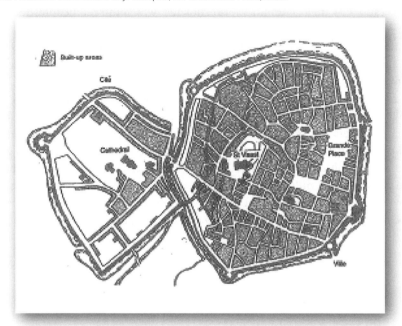

out Europe, through Scandinavia and to Moscow.[7] The mortality or death rate has been estimated at 25 to 60%. Thereafter the plague reoccurred periodically until about 1700.

Local Government Responds to the Plague

The contagious nature of the disease became evident, even though no theories of illness existed at that time to guide response. City governments began instituting quarantine and related procedures. Health boards were established by the city councils, and these boards established rules for responding to suspected plague cases. Ships were not allowed to dock and discharge passengers or goods if they had the plague aboard. Individuals suspected of having the plague would be quarantined in pest houses located outside the town, and travelers were not allowed into the city during epidemics. If city residents became ill with the plague, they would be isolated. In the medieval era, they were sent to the pest house until they recovered or died and their houses decontaminated. This often meant that most of their personal property was destroyed. Dogs and cats were slaughtered, a somewhat counterproductive move as they killed the rats that were hosts for the fleas.

The State of Public Health Practice: 1500

Despite the lack of documentation that medieval quarantine and isolation procedures were effective in treating the plague, the measures represent a positive development in the history of public health. Quarantine was promulgated by health boards at the local level, indicating that local governments had assumed responsibility for the health of their citizens. Additionally, the existence of local health boards meant that governmental structures had been created and could address other health-related problems. One outcome of increased governmental interest was the establishment of hospitals for the sick. The quarantine measures and the establishment of hospitals foreshadowed the use of similar measures by General Washington at the Siege of Boston in 1775.

The 19th century: birth of the scientific method

1848 London Cholera Epidemic

Cholera is caused by the bacterium Vibrio cholerae, which infects the intestine and results in diarrhea. If severe watery diarrhea, vomiting, and leg cramps develop, cholera can produce the rapid loss of body fluids resulting in dehydration and shock. Death can occur in a few hours. Typically the disease is spread through water contaminated with feces from a person who has the disease.[14]

In 1848, when cholera became epidemic in London, the mortality rate was 30% which, like other medieval cities, overwhelmed their capacity to bury the dead. Hence the bodies of cholera victims were left in the streets (see Figure 2.4). The generally accepted theory was that cholera was caused by **miasma**, the stench arising like a gas from garbage and other filth that was characteristic of a large city environment.[14] London with a population of about 2 million and rudimentary water and sewage systems was characterized by filth. Garbage rotted in the streets, and sewers contaminated the rivers from which local companies obtained water to pipe to city residents.

Figure 2.4—Evidence of the effect of cholera on a French town of the 1800s. The high mortality rate often overwhelmed the ability of the town to remove the dead so they were left lying in the streets while healthy residents fled the scene.

Reprinted from http://wwwihm.nlm.nih.gov/ihm/images/A/26/986.jpg. Courtesy of the National Library of Medicine.

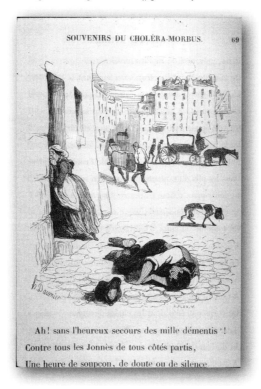

 CASE STUDY 2

John Snow, the father of anesthesiology and epidemiology

John Snow was a physician who moved to London to establish his medical practice in 1838; he had a general medical practice, which included obstetrical care. When ether anesthesia was introduced in late 1846, Snow began to administer ether and then chloroform as an anesthetic during childbirth and surgical procedures. Because chloroform was new and little was known about it, Snow began to conduct experiments with the drug in mice and birds. These experiments allowed him to relate the dose (i.e., the amount of anesthetic received) to the response and to describe the stages of anesthesia. Snow also invented a machine for the administration of ether and chloroform and became well known for his expertise in anesthesia. In fact, he was so well known that he administered chloroform to Queen Victoria for the births of two of her children.[14] Thus Snow's medical practice was focused on acute care. Nothing indicated in either Snow's practice or research that he was interested in public health.

The scientific method: gas anesthesia and cholera

Apparently Snow began to relate what he knew about gas anesthesia to the spread of cholera and soon realized that it did not behave like the diffusion of a gas. Snow proposed an alternative method of spread—through water contaminated with human feces from a person who had cholera. To test his hypothesis that cholera was primarily spread by contaminated water,

Snow began to systematically collect data. He retrieved all the information he could on cholera and then began to collect data on cholera cases to determine if it could be transmitted by water. Several water companies supplied piped water to London; consequently, adjacent houses could have different water sources. By identifying households that had a death from cholera and comparing them to households with no death, Snow was able to show that households using water from one company were four times more likely to have had a cholera death than houses using water from the second company. Example data are shown in Table 2.2.[14,15]

In 1854, Snow was able to use his knowledge of cholera transmission to end an outbreak of cholera in the Golden Street area of London. He discovered that the initial case of cholera had occurred in a house close to a water pump on Broad Street. With the help of the parish priest, Snow collected data on the cholera deaths for houses or businesses close to the Broad Street pump and compared them to houses that used other pumps. He used a map (see Figure 2.5) to identify where deaths from cholera occurred in the neighborhood. Most of the deaths occurred in households using the Broad Street pump. (The Broad street pump is in the center of the map; note additional pumps in the lower left, lower right, and upper right of the map. Few deaths occurred near these pumps.) Snow recommended to the parish priest that the handle be removed from the pump so residents could no longer access the contaminated water. After the pump handle was removed, the cholera outbreak ended.[13,14] Subsequently, laws and regulations were passed that prohibited London water companies from obtaining and selling water contaminated with sewage.

John Snow (1813–1858) is known as the father of anesthesiology and the father of epidemiology because:

- Experimentation enabled him to develop doses and methods to control the amount of anesthetic gas administered to a patient;

- A scientific understanding of the characteristics of gases enabled him to rule out miasma as a cause of cholera; and

- Systematic data collection on the incidence of deaths due to cholera for comparative population groups enabled him to establish that contaminated water was the source of cholera infection.

The state of public health practice: 1900

The response to the London cholera epidemics differs in several important ways from responses to other earlier epidemics. One significant difference was the use of the scientific method to first, refute the theory that cholera was caused by miasma, and second, to establish that contaminated water was the primary way the disease was transmitted from person to person. Snow had carefully studied gases and knew from his experiments that the pattern of gas diffusion did not fit the pattern of cholera diffusion. To test his hypothesis of transmission by water, Snow first reviewed all the information he could locate about cholera (known as literature review) and then he proceeded to collect data. Collecting data is a particularly powerful approach; no longer does one have to rely strictly on experience and impression but can rely on the data to determine if the cause is likely or not. Although Snow did not know exactly what caused the disease, he hypothesized that some kind of particle present in the

Table 2.2

Example Mortality for Cholera by Water Supply Company, London, 1854— as Compiled by John Snow[a]

Parish	Estimated Population Served by Each Water Company		Total Deaths from Cholera	Deaths per 10,000 Population
	Southwark & Vauxhall	Lambeth		
St. Olave	8745	0	161	201
St. John	9360	0	152	134
St. Peter	14,274	10,724	391	131
Wandsworth	0	1066	10	25
Streatham	0	3244	15	17
S Borough Rd	8937	6672	271	171

Estimated overall rate for the population that obtained water from Southwark & Vauxhall = 100/10,000

Estimated overall rate for the population that obtained water from Lambeth = 27/10,000

[a]Adapted from Vinten-Johansen P, Brody H, Paneth N, et al. *Cholera, Chloroform, and the Science of Medicine: A Life of John Snow*. New York, NY: Oxford University Press; 2003.

Figure 2.5—Broad Street Pump (circled in the center of the picture) identified by Snow as the source of contaminated water, which caused the cholera outbreak in London in 1854. Bars indicate the number of deaths due to cholera at each address. Snow had the parish priest remove the pump handle to end the outbreak. Note additional pumps around the perimeter with few bars indicating deaths near them.

Reprinted from Richardson BW. *Snow on Cholera*. New York, NY: Hafner Publishing; 1965.

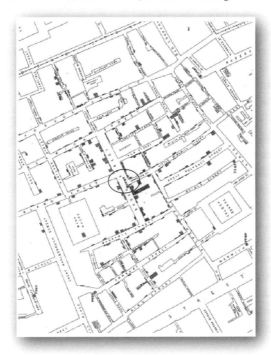

feces of cholera victims produced the disease when introduced into the gastrointestinal track of a healthy person.

A second difference was that Snow did not recommend quarantine and related procedures but recommended changing the source of water supplies to avoid water contaminated with feces. With removal of the pump handle from the Broad street pump, Snow showed that actions based on his understanding of cholera transmission could end an outbreak. The third significant difference was that Snow showed effective public health actions could be taken that did not involve curing the disease or even understanding exactly what and how the causative factor produced disease in an individual. Snow focused on the transmission of the disease, not on the cure of the disease. However the involvement of the government was inherited from the Middle Ages. The data on cause of death and number of deaths was obtained from the government. Then the government was involved in establishing the regulations, and enforcing them, related to water quality.

The 20th century: prevention as behavior change

Tobacco Use

Cigarettes were first marketed in the United States in the early 19th century, and development of the cigarette manufacturing industry after the Civil War made cigarettes a major tobacco product. By 1900, the average per capita consumption of cigarettes was 54 per year per person. Further development of the cigarette in the early 20th century by using milder tobacco blends decreased the discomfort of smoking and increased nicotine absorption into the bloodstream. At the time of World War I, doctors in the Army thought that cigarettes helped the wounded to relax. Cigarette smoking continued to increase; by 1945, the annual per capita consumption of cigarettes had reached 3449 and, by 1963, was 4345.[16,17]

Epidemiologic studies beginning in the 1950s established cigarette smoking as a cause of lung cancer. The classic epidemiologic study was conducted by Doll and Hill, with British physicians as subjects, and reported in 1956.[18] Doll and Hill sent a questionnaire to all physicians in the United Kingdom asking about smoking habits, and then they retrieved death data from the death registry for the United Kingdom. The findings for lung cancer are shown in Figure 2.6. The data showed that the deaths from lung cancer increased from 0.07 per 1000 non-smokers to 1.66 per 1000 heavy smokers, an increase of about 20 times with a difference that was statistically significant (probability of the difference being due to chance as less than 1 in a 100).

The 20th century public health approach to reducing tobacco use has become a model for changing individual behaviors that cause harm; it is characterized by:

- The use of epidemiologic studies to establish tobacco use as the cause of disease;

- Media campaigns to encourage individuals to stop or not to start smoking;

- Legislative action at the state and federal levels to regulate tobacco use (e.g., prohibition of smoking indoors);

- Availability of nicotine patches without a prescription; and

- Use of taxes on tobacco products to discourage use.

As shown in Figure 2.6, a dose–response relationship existed—non-smokers had the lowest rate, and the rates increased in response to the number of cigarettes smoked. Numerous epidemiologic studies were conducted with similar findings. They also showed that deaths from other diseases including respiratory disease other than cancer, other cancers, and coronary thrombosis increased with cigarette smoking.[19,20]

Multicomponent Approach to Changing Smoking Behavior

Figure 2.6—Death rates as percentage of rate for all men in the Doll and Hill study of smoking by British doctors.[18] Groups describe number of cigarettes smoked per day; 1 = non-smoker, 2 = 1–14 cigarettes per day, 3 = 15–24, and 4 = 25 or more. The rate is about 20 times greater for heavy smokers (Group 4); $p < 0.01$. Note the dose–response curve; the greater the number of cigarettes smoked, the greater the likelihood of having lung cancer.

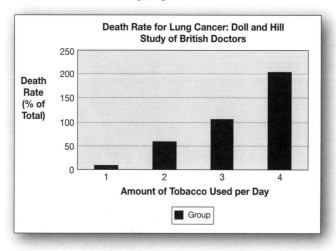

Fifty years after the Doll and Hill study,[18] smoking rates in the United States are about 20% for adults. The decrease in smoking has been attributed to a multicomponent approach to encourage individuals to stop smoking or to discourage them from beginning (see an example poster in Figure 2.7). Cigarette advertising on television and radio was banned in 1969, and laws were passed at the local level to restrict smoking in public places. The first law was passed in Arizona in 1973, to reduce non-smokers' exposure to second-hand smoke. In the 1970s, the federal government stopped providing cigarettes to service members as part of their rations. Federal legislation was passed in 1988 to prohibit smoking on all commercial U.S. flights. Taxes on tobacco products also have been levied at the state level. The increased cost of tobacco products has been instrumental in decreasing the number of teens who begin smoking.

Beginning in 1994, states began to sue the tobacco companies to recover the costs associated with providing medical care through **Medicaid** (the federal–state program for health insurance for low income individuals). By 1998, a **Master Settlement Agreement** had been reached with the major U.S. tobacco companies. Monies from this settlement were used by some states to develop media campaigns aimed at keeping teens from smoking. The effort to encourage individuals to stop smoking was enhanced by making smoking cessation patches available without a prescription. Additionally, several medications (e.g., bupropion) have been shown through **clinical trials** to help individuals stop smoking.

The State of Public Health: 2000

The tobacco cessation efforts of the 20th century have become a model for public health campaigns to change individual behavior. The campaign has relied on education through media efforts and intervention by health care professionals with support from legislative action. Messages encourage people to stop smoking, workplaces and other public venues prohibit smoking, and cigarettes are costly. At the end of the 20th century, similar strategies were applied to changing lifestyle to prevent obesity and diseases associated with it, for example, diabetes and heart disease.

Figure 2.7—Poster designed to encourage people to stop smoking. Posters and other types of media campaigns aimed at changing unhealthy behaviors were part of the multicomponent strategy used in the 20th century to reduce smoking. Behavior change was supported by regulations (i.e., no smoking indoors) and by increased taxes on tobacco products.

Reprinted from http://wwwihm.nlm.nih.gov/ihm/images/A/24/975.jpg. Courtesy of the National Library of Medicine.

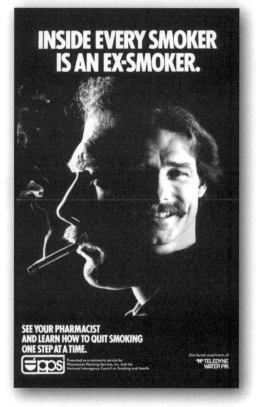

The 21st century: public health in daily life

CASE STUDY 3

Public health and a typical day in the life of a student

George reached out to turn off the alarm; it was only 6:30 AM, but he needed to get moving if he was going to get to his 8 AM class. There was supposed to be a quiz that day and then a lecture on the history of public health. George couldn't imagine what public health had to do with him; he was a pharmacy student who intended to practice in a community pharmacy after graduation. Regardless, he struggled out of bed and into the shower supplied with clean water in a structurally sound house without vermin (e.g., rats) or dangerous insects (e.g., mosquitoes carrying malaria). After his shower, George had clean clothes to wear and safe and effective medication to apply to the blister he had on his right foot from hiking last weekend. If George hurried, he would have time to drink some juice and eat a bowl of cereal with milk, all foods that had been fortified with vitamins and minerals, then stop on the way to class to grab a cup of cappuccino.

Because he didn't want to be late, George decided to drive so he got into his car and fastened his seat belt. He drove through streets where speed limits were posted, turn lanes clearly marked, and traffic lights operated to control the flow of traffic. As he paid for his cappuccino, George assumed that the beverage he purchased was safe to drink and would not result in any type of intestinal disease; he was unaware of the **county health inspector's** visit to the coffee shop last week. George did not notice that the sidewalk and curb were clear of trash and garbage as he ran to his car nor did he notice the garbage truck as it proceeded down the street picking up trash for local businesses. George parked in the lot a block away from the school of pharmacy and ran along the sidewalk as several cars passed him that apparently were driven by students, like him, who were almost late to class. George arrived in class just as the professor started handing out the quizzes.

Back to the Future: Public Health Issues in the 21st Century

George illustrates the perspective of many 21st century residents of countries with advanced economies such as the United States. Public health is a component of many of their daily activities, but the components are not recognized as protecting and maintaining their health. George can assume that there is no sewage running in the street, that the juice he drinks will not give him diarrhea because it is contaminated with a pathogenic organism, and that garbage and trash are collected and disposed of in a manner that does not endanger his health. George can assume that his car is safe to operate, that traffic is controlled to reduce the likelihood of an accident, and that there are sidewalks so that he does not need to walk in the street with the risk of being hit by a passing vehicle. Most of the laws and regulations related to safe food, household safety, the availability of safe water, and traffic safety were implemented in the last century before George was born. Thus, if George is typical of most Americans, he has not experienced life where the food may not be safe or where there is a high risk of being involved in a traffic accident.

Life in a representative government allows most citizens to pass the responsibility for public health onto other people, many of them professionals. Average citizens can enjoy the safety of their food and water supplies without understanding why their food and water are safe or knowing what person is responsible for assuring safety. Average citizens do not need to understand that individuals committed to having a healthy population advocated for the regulations and administrative structures required to make food and water safe. However George and other citizens who take public health for granted may experience real public health threats in their lifetime primarily through the rise of new infectious diseases, environmental threats, and the changing role of government.

Infectious diseases

Avian (Bird) Flu

One infectious disease causing a major concern in the 21st century is **avian or bird flu**. Avian or bird flu is a new type of influenza virus that has begun producing disease in humans. Influenza viruses occur naturally among wild birds; most strains do not produce significant disease and cause few problems. However, the H5N1 strain is deadly to domestic fowls and can be transmitted from birds to humans. Human mortality is very high with the H5N1 strain and has exceeded 50% in past outbreaks. Because influenza viruses readily mutate, the concern is that a human will become infected with the virus from a bird and then the virus will mutate so that it can be spread from human to human. Humans have no natural immunity, and there is currently no **vaccine** to prevent bird flu so the disease could spread quickly from person to person and become a **global pandemic**, that is, a worldwide outbreak of the disease.[21] (Imagine a person with bird flu traveling by air from Asia to Europe then the United States.)

Current efforts to address the threat of bird flu have included adding bird flu to the list of **communicable diseases** for which the CDC is authorized to apprehend persons suspected of having the disease, and isolating and detaining them as deemed necessary to prevent further spread of the disease.[21] If someone were thought to have bird flu, he or she would be isolated and kept in isolation until no longer contagious—reminiscent of the procedures used in the medieval and revolutionary eras to prevent the spread of plague and smallpox but now based on a scientific understanding of the disease, its cause, and method of transmission.

Extensively Drug-Resistant Tuberculosis

Another disease that could produce global pandemics in the 21st century is extensively **drug-resistant** tuberculosis. Extensively drug-resistant tuberculosis (**XDR-TB**) is caused by the bacterium, Mycobacterium tuberculosis, and means that the organisms are not sensitive to five different drugs used to treat TB infection.[22] XDR-TB is fatal in about 30% of individuals with the disease and is very expensive to treat, costing up to $500,000 to treat one patient. XDR-TB is already present in large parts of the world, especially the countries that made up the former Soviet Union and some countries in Africa. The CDC and local health departments also use isolation and detention procedures to limit the spread of XDR-TB.[22,23] XDR-TB has a unique history; it resulted from how antibiotics were used to treat TB, which in turn allowed the bacterium to develop resistance to antibiotics and produced a new form of TB that is difficult to treat.

Environment

Water, Sanitation, and Food Supply

Water and sanitation have re-emerged as public health problems in the 21st century. One billion people in the world do not have access to adequate amounts of clean water, particularly for drinking,[24] and are susceptible to the diseases transmitted through contaminated water supplies (e.g., cholera). Population growth will likely exacerbate the problem as the overall amount of clean water becomes inadequate for meeting the needs of humans. Related to the water issues are general living conditions such as housing, sewage disposal,[2] and garbage disposal. More people can be expected to live in conditions where untreated sewage flows outside their residence or where trash is scattered along streets and roads, which contaminates the environment and provides surroundings for vermin (e.g., rats).

Food supply also has re-emerged as a public health issue. The cost of staple foods such as rice, corn, and wheat has increased dramatically in the early 21st century. In some countries, the poor cannot afford to purchase an adequate amount of food. In other countries, including the United States, the poor are forced to purchase foods that have little nutritional value.

Global Climate Changes

Global climate changes also can affect health. Potential negative impacts on health include a change in environment that produces flooding or drought with attendant changes in the availability of food and clean water.[2] Additionally, disease patterns may be altered as some areas become warmer; for example, malaria and cholera could appear in areas of the world where it is currently too cold. Increased pollution and increased exposure to industrial and agricultural chemicals as well as other toxic waste will likely accompany climate change. Hence current public health problems may be exacerbated, and new problems develop in response to global changes in climate and environment.

Role of government

Restricted Role of Government

The government's role in public health has been a necessary component of the progress in public health, particularly to assure adequate water, sanitation systems, and adequate food supply as well as to minimize pollution from industry. However, contemporary governments, including the U.S. federal government, are restricting their role in public health. Fewer funds are available for public health activities, and there is less interest in passing new regulations or laws or in enforcing current laws related to public health.

Role of Citizens

Because governments are restricting their role in public health, citizen participation is important for two reasons—1) to assure that governments fulfill their role in protecting citizens and promoting their health and 2) to make informed decisions on public health interventions (e.g., fluoridation of water supplies to prevent dental caries). Only about half of the U.S. population lives in communities where the water is fluoridated, and these are primarily large cities. Fluoridation has not been possible in many small and medium-sized cities because of local citizens' opposition. To institute many public health measures, the population to whom the regulations apply must agree to the measures.

Pharmacists have a role in public health both as citizens and as highly educated health professionals. Pharmacists can take a more active role as citizens assuring that public health departments have adequate resources and engage in activities to promote the health of local residents. Pharmacists also have expertise in medications and the use of them so they can contribute to the solution of public health issues that involve medications.

Chapter 2 Summary

This review of the history of public health reveals that actions taken by governments to improve the health of a population are identifiable in ancient Greece and Roman eras; however, local government, specifically city government, assumed primary responsibility for public health during the Middle Ages. Policies related to quarantine of persons thought to have a contagious disease were developed in the Middle Ages and continue to be used in the 21st century as exemplified by the use of quarantine and isolation procedures to prevent pandemics of bird flu and extensively drug-resistant tuberculosis.

Throughout much of history, the primary concerns of public health have been with the supply of adequate nutritious and safe food, safe water, and safe housing as well as with controlling infectious disease. These concerns continue to be relevant in the 21st century because increased population levels threaten the availability of adequate safe water. Lack of water and climate change also threatens the world's food supply. Additionally, most countries also have chronic diseases resulting from lifestyles that include smoking, lack of exercise, and excessive consumption of calories.

References

1. Beaglehole R, Bonita R, Horton R, et al. Public health in the new era: improving health through collective action. *Lancet.* 2004; 363:2084–6.

2. Beaglehole R. *Public Health at the Crossroads: Achievements and Prospects*, 2nd ed. West Nyack, NY: Cambridge University Press; 2004.

3. Kagawa-Singer M, Kassim-Lakha S. A strategy to reduce cross-cultural miscommunication and increase the likelihood of improving health outcomes. *Academic Med.* 2003; 78:577–87.

4. Rosen G. *A History of Public Health*. Baltimore, MD: John Hopkins University Press; 1993.

5. Fenn EA. *Pox Americana: The Great Smallpox Epidemic of 1775–82*. New York, NY: Hill and Wang; 2001.

6. McCullough D. *1776*. New York, NY: Simon & Schuster; 2005.

7. Bellan RC. *The Evolving City*. Canada: Copp Clark Publishing Company; 1971.

8. Barefoot P. Buildings for health: then and now. In: King H, ed. *Health in Antiquity*. New York, NY: Routledge; 2005:205–15.

9. Porter D. *Health, Civilization and the State: A History of Public Health from Ancient to Modern Times*. New York, NY: Routledge; 1999.

10. King H. Introduction: what is health? In: King H, ed. *Health in Antiquity*. New York, NY: Routledge; 2005:1–11.

11. Hays JN. *Epidemics and Pandemics: Their Impacts on Human History*. Santa Barbara, CA: ABC-CLIO; 2005.

12. Morley N. The salubriousness of the roman city. In: King H, ed. *Health in Antiquity*. New York, NY: Routledge; 2005:192–204.

13. Pounds N. *The Medieval City*. Westport, CT: Greenwood Press; 2005.

14. Vinten-Johansen P, Brody H, Paneth N, et al. *Cholera, Chloroform, and the Science of Medicine: A Life of John Snow*. New York, NY: Oxford University Press; 2003.

15. Richardson BW. *Snow on Cholera*. New York, NY: Hafner Publishing; 1965.

16. Centers for Disease Control and Prevention. 2000 Surgeon General's Report: Tobacco Timeline: Highlights. Available at: http://www.cdc.gov/tobacco/data_statistics/sgr/sgr_2000/highlights/. Accessed July 6, 2007.

17. Centers for Disease Control and Prevention. Economics: Total and Per Capita Yearly Consumption of Manufactured Cigarettes. Available at: http://www.CDC.gov/tobacco/data_statistics/tables/economics/consumers. Accessed July 6, 2007.

18. Doll R, Hill AB. Lung cancer and other causes of death in relation to smoking. *BMJ*. 1956; 233(ii):1071–81.

19. Friedman GD. Cigarette smoking and geographic variation in coronary heart disease mortality in the United States. *J Chron Dis*. 1967; 20:769–79.

20. Doll R, Hill AB. Smoking and carcinoma of the lung. *BMJ*. 1950; 2:739–48.

21. Centers for Disease Control and Prevention. Avian Influenza (Bird Flu). Available at: http://www.phppo.cdc.gov/flu/avian/gen-info/. Accessed July 9, 2007.

22. Centers for Disease Control and Prevention. Extensively drug-resistant tuberculosis—United States, 1993–2006. *MMWR*. March 23, 2007; 56:250–3.

23. Stobbe M. Ga. Honeymooner with TB saw Europe, then hospital. Arizona Republic. May 30, 2007:A8.

24. Centers for Disease Control and Prevention. Healthy Drinking Water. Available at: http://www2a.cdc.gov/ncidod/ts/. Accessed July 5, 2007.

Suggested Readings

Diamond JM. *Guns, Germs, and Steel: the Fates of Human Societies*. New York, NY: WW Norton & Co.; 1998.

This text describes available technology and how the development and spread of infectious disease influenced societies. This account requires the reader to reassess his or her beliefs about the importance of disease in history.

Woodham Smith CBF. *Florence Nightingale, 1820–1910*. New York, NY: McGraw-Hill; 1951.

Florence Nightingale is known as the founder of the profession of nursing, but she was also a major contributor to the development of public health practices (e.g., development and use of statistics in public health).

Fenn EA. *Pox Americana: The Great Smallpox Epidemic of 1775–82*. New York, NY: Hill and Wang; 2001.

This book provides a fascinating account of the little known smallpox epidemic during and after the Revolutionary war and its impact on the patriot army as well as its impact on the native peoples of the Western Hemisphere.

Rosen G. *A History of Public Health*. Baltimore, MD: John Hopkins University Press; 1993.

This definitive history of public health offers a 471-page synopsis of almost any topic related to public health; the book was published in 1958.

Vinten-Johansen P, Brody H, Paneth N, et al. *Cholera, Chloroform, and the Science of Medicine: A Life of John Snow.* New York, NY: Oxford University Press; 2003. This book offers a readable account of Snow's early life and practice and how he generalized scientific skill from one area, anesthesiology, to another area, infectious disease.

Chapter 2 Review Questions

1. **Water, sanitation, and food supply were identified as the primary public health concerns in ancient Greece and Rome. Identify which of the three would be considered a public health concern at the beginning of the 21st century. Justify your answer.**
   All are concerns at the beginning of the 21st century. Population growth and pollution are threatening the availability of clean water. Sanitation is an issue because of possible water shortages, inability to dispose of garbage, and threats from natural disasters resulting from climate change. The food supply is threatened by the increasing population and climate change.

2. **A scientifically based cure of a disease is required before public health actions can be taken.** _____ **True** _____ **False**
   False. Because public health is primarily concerned with preventing disease, actions that will prevent the disease can be taken even if a cure is not known for the disease. Refer to the examples: John Snow was able to prevent the spread of cholera, even though there was no understanding of how to treat the disease once a person became sick. General Washington did not know how to cure smallpox, yet he was able to prevent it from affecting his troops.

3. **Match the government action to its corresponding public health era. There is one correct response for each government action.**
   (a) Ancient   (b) Medieval   (c) Revolutionary war
   (d) 19th century   (e) 20th century   (f) 21st century

   _____ Established inoculation hospitals to inoculate against smallpox (c)

   _____ Reduced funding for public health activities (f)

   _____ Recommended healthy locations for cities (a)

   _____ Established local boards of health to respond to epidemics (b)

   _____ Collected data on deaths (d)

   _____ Prohibited certain types of behavior (i.e., smoking) indoors (e)

4. **A response to an epidemic in the medieval era would consist of:**
(a)   Using quarantine to restrict the movement of persons who might have been exposed to the epidemic illness.

Quarantine as a practice to prevent exposure of a population to an epidemic disease originated in the medieval era with bubonic plague and continues to be practiced in the 21st century for certain diseases.

(b)   Collecting data to identify the cause (e.g., contaminated water) of the illness.

Data collection did not become part of a response to an epidemic until the middle of the 19th century when John Snow collected data to show that miasma could not because of the cholera epidemic.

(c)   Collecting data to determine if a specific action (e.g., boiling water) is related to prevention of a disease.

Data collection did not become part of a response to an epidemic until the middle of the 19th century when John Snow collected data to show that changing water supplies could prevent the spread of cholera.

(d)   Isolating anyone who appeared to be sick with the epidemic illness in a house outside the town.

The establishment of pest houses was a typical town response to an epidemic disease in the medieval era. Isolation continues to be used in the 21st century for certain diseases, for example, extremely drug-resistant tuberculosis.

(e)   (b) and (c)

An incorrect response; see comments with the two choices.

(f)   (a) and (d)

The correct response; see comments under other choices.

5. **Science has contributed to public health by enabling certain actions to be taken to prevent a specific disease.   _____ True   _____ False**
True. Until the middle of the 19th century when John Snow used scientific methods to identify contaminated water as the source of cholera and then recommended avoiding contaminated water as a way to prevent cholera, many different strategies (e.g., quarantine) would have seemed appropriate with no way to select among them.

Applying Your Knowledge

1. Numerous public health concerns were identified in this chapter including concerns with water, food, sanitation, infectious disease, and behavior (i.e., smoking). On the Internet, locate the web site for your county or state health department. How many of the public health concerns described in this chapter can you identify on the web site?

2. John Snow was a physician who had no formal training in public health; in fact, most physicians of the era would have thought that the prevention of disease was not the responsibility of a physician. (Physicians were supposed to treat people after they became ill.) Why do you think Snow would add public health concerns to his regular medical practice? Do you think that you might have a role in public health in the 21st century? Justify your answer.

3. As you attend class at your college, identify as many aspects as possible of your environment and human behavior that are related to public health. Identify both things that promote health and things that might expose you to adverse health effects.

4. John Snow established how cholera could be prevented 150 years ago. Why do you think cholera still produces disease?

Public Health at the Local, State, National, and Global Levels

Learning Outcomes

1. Explain why public health issues in one country often become a concern in other countries.
2. List the key functions of public health organizations or systems.
3. Explain the role of surveillance in mitigating the spread of disease.
4. Describe how the U.S. public health system is structured at the national, state, and local levels.
5. Describe the roles of the World Health Organization, Pan-American Health Organization, and non-governmental organizations such as the Red Cross, International in addressing public health issues.

Introduction

Public health activities are performed at many levels from local to national to global. The organizations and agencies devoted to public health at these different levels share many of the same functions including disease surveillance, policy development, and provision of access to health care. To better understand how all these agencies fit together to provide public health services, this chapter will look at public health organizations within the United States and organizations that exist for international public health needs. Agencies of particular interest to pharmacists, such as the Food and Drug Administration, will be emphasized. To illustrate how the various agencies work, a case study based loosely on the 2002–03 SARS pandemic will be used.

Public Health from Local to Global

The primary site of activity for most public health interventions is within individual communities or neighborhoods. This locale is where the members of the population and the public health practitioners interact. For issues that are unique to the community or do not spread beyond the community, the local approach is effective. However, many public health problems extend beyond local borders, for example toxic waste spills, infectious diseases, wars, and **natural disasters**. Any of these problems may require involvement of counties, states, the nation, or even other countries to fully understand the scope of the problem and respond to it. National and global organizations can often facilitate communication among the affected populations, provide access to expertise not available locally, and coordinate efforts to respond. The most effective responses to public health problems are those that involve local, state, national, and international partners.

Many international **outbreaks** of infectious disease often begin as a single episode of illness or injury that quickly spread if not contained. In the case of an outbreak of a new viral disease, public health organizations at all levels need to minimize the spread of the disease and reduce the **mortality** and **morbidity** rates because of interdependence and the global nature of our world today. More than at any other time in history, trade, travel, and communication span the globe and connect populations in ways never imagined 100 years ago. It has been said that an infectious disease outbreak in any part of the world can be in a person's backyard half a world away within 24 hours. Luckily, information about an approaching virus can be transmitted even faster via web and telecommunications, so a population can prepare if it is warned. That is where the **SARS**-inspired case begins—a single patient who has an unknown respiratory illness. The case is designed to show how this disease impacts patients and practitioners in other continents. What starts as a local outbreak quickly becomes a global health issue.

CASE STUDY 1

How a local outbreak can become a global public health issue

Yi Chen gets a mysterious viral illness

Yi Chen is a 52-year-old male who was born and raised in the Guangdong province of southern China. His work as a shrimp salesman requires travel to many communities within his sales region. He averages six trips a month via the local train system. During those trips, he often stays at nice hotels where businessmen from countries also lodge. He chats with other travelers as he enjoys his after dinner cigarette and cup of beer.

After his most recent trip, Yi Chen began to feel feverish and achy. Ming, his loving wife of 34 years, made a broth soup called qing fei jiy du tang (a soup for clearing the lungs) to help him fight the illness. Her herbal remedies for fever did not seem to work for this illness. By the next morning, Yi had developed a cough that was dry (no sputum or congested sound), which compounded the diarrhea that began during the night. Ming Chen loaded Yi into a taxi and took him to the local hospital just 8 miles away where he was admitted for treatment. Yi was placed in a room where he could be separated from other patients, health care workers, and visitors.

The mystery illness begins to spread

When Ming returned in the morning, she found her husband quite ill. Pneumonia had developed, and his breathing was labored and painful. The physicians had called an infectious disease specialist and asked medical students to examine Yi. By noon, they decided he should be treated at the larger regional hospital in Guangzhou and transported him via ambulance to the large medical center. Several physicians, including Dr. Zhang, seven nurses, and four medical students worked closely with Yi during the course of his illness that lasted almost 2 weeks. Yi Chen was their eighth case that week.

By the time Yi left the hospital, his local hospital had received another six cases, three of which were health care workers from the hospital. The regional medical center in Guangzhou had admitted around 45 people that week—many were transferred from smaller hospitals in the province. In spite of the growing number of cases of this mystery illness, Dr. Zhang and his colleagues did not have much information about the outbreak or disease. They were not aware that the illness had begun to appear in other provinces and major cities such as Beijing where hundreds of residents were now diagnosed with a mysterious disease (Figure 3.1).

Figure 3.1—November 2002: A cluster of mysterious atypical pneumonia cases appear in southeastern China. Total cases: unknown.

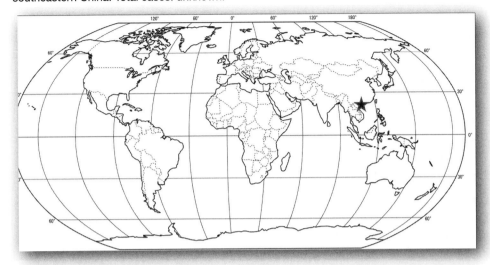

Key Functions of Public Health Organizations and Agencies

Regardless of whether an organization is a local **health department** or an international entity, several key functions are typically performed. As Table 3.1 shows, the activities include monitoring the population's health as well as the presence of disease, developing policies to promote health or reduce preventable disease or death, advocating for vulnerable members of the community, and supporting programs that improve community

Table 3.1

The Ten Essential Public Health Services

General Area	Specifics
Monitor	Health status to identify and solve community health problems
Diagnose and investigate	Health problems and health hazards in the community
Inform, educate, and empower	People about health issues
Mobilize	Community partnerships and action to identify and solve health problems
Develop	Policies and plans that support individual and community health efforts
Enforce	Laws and requirements that protect health and ensure safety
Link	People to needed personal health services and assure the provision of health care when otherwise unavailable
Assure	Competent public and personal health care workforce
Evaluate	Effectiveness, accessibility, and quality of personal and population-based health services
Research	For new insights and innovative solutions to health problems

Source: Centers for Disease Control and Prevention (CDC). National Public Health Performance Standards Program. Available at: http://www.cdc.gov/od/ocphp/nphpsp/EssentialPHServices.htm. Accessed September 28, 2008.

infrastructure and quality of life. Some interventions may be directly related to health (e.g., access to medical care and pharmaceuticals through public insurance and clean drinking water), while others may be indirectly related to health (e.g., improved educational system and higher wages known to positively influence health). Because the case scenario in this chapter is focused on an outbreak of an infectious disease, additional information about **disease surveillance** is included.

> Surveillance refers to actively monitoring a population for the appearance of a new disease or the sudden increase in an existing disease. The disease under surveillance may be an infectious disease, chronic disease, or preventable injuries or exposures. International travel has made surveillance a global activity because of its ability to spread disease quickly and widely.

Disease surveillance

Disease surveillance is the process of monitoring the number of new and existing cases, **incidence** and **prevalence rates**, respectively, of a disease in a population. The information can indicate whether there is a higher-than-usual number of cases of a particular illness. Although originally used for infectious diseases, surveillance could include any disease of interest to decision-makers in the community. Examples include monitoring the level of substance abuse, chronic diseases like diabetes or heart disease, and the number of medication error cases that caused death. This chapter will focus on the use of surveillance to monitor an infectious disease outbreak.

Not all infectious diseases are monitored and reported through surveillance programs. For infectious diseases, the surveillance focuses on a limited list of diseases that spread easily through intimate or close contact. They are called **reportable diseases**, which indicate they are being monitored by public health agencies and must be reported when they are suspected or confirmed. Historically, physicians and medical laboratories were most likely to identify reportable diseases so they were usually the people who reported them to a local health department; however, any health care professional including pharmacists could submit the report.

Figure 3.2 shows an example of a state reporting form used to pass information about a disease under surveillance to state and federal agencies. There is a national list of **notifiable diseases** for which each state is required to report cases, but states may have additional diseases of interest that they are tracking so their list may include more reportable diseases. The diseases on the national and state lists will fall into several general categories: sexually transmitted infections, childhood infectious diseases, and bioterrorism-related infections. Most lists will include a catch-all category such as the "unusual cluster of disease" category to ensure that new diseases like SARS as well as any unusual behavior of existing diseases are also reported.

The individual reports of a reportable disease are forwarded to state and then national health departments where they are compiled, analyzed, and disseminated via the web and publications (e.g., Weekly Morbidity & Mortality Report) to keep all health officers informed about possible outbreak in their area and surrounding communities.

Figure 3.2—Example of Infectious Disease Reporting Form

Source: Texas Department of Public Health Services.

TEXAS
Department of State Health Services

Infectious Disease Report

Form is published at
http://www.dshs.state.tx.us/idcu/investigation/conditions/

General Instructions

This form may be used to ***report suspected cases and cases of notifiable conditions*** in Texas, listed with their reporting timeframes on the reverse side of this form or available at www.dshs.state.tx.us/idcu/investigation/forms/101A.pdf. In addition to specified reportable conditions, ***any outbreak, exotic disease, or unusual group expression of disease that may be of public health concern should be reported*** *by the most expeditious means available.* A health department epidemiologist may contact you to further investigate this Infectious Disease Report. Information needed to classify cases of infectious disease is outlined in the Epi Case Criteria Guide found at www.dshs.state.tx.us/idcu/investigation/forms/EpiCaseGuide.pdf.

Suspected cases and cases should be reported to your local or regional health department at the following address, phone or fax number.

Information for your local or regional health department can be found at:
http://www.dshs.state.tx.us/regions/default.shtm

As needed, cases may be reported to the Department of State Health Services at 1-800-252-8239, 512-458-7676, or after-hours at 512-458-7111

Disease or Condition			Date: ______ *(Check type)* *(Please fill in onset or closest known date)*		☐ Onset ☐ Absence	☐ Specimen collection ☐ Office visit
Physician Name	Physician Address ☐ See Facility address below				Physician Phone ☐ See Facility phone below ( ) -	
Diagnostic Criteria (Diagnostic Lab Result and Specimen Source or Clinical Indicators)						
Patient Name (Last)		(First)		(MI)	Telephone ( ) -	
Address (Street)		City		State	Zip Code	County
Date of Birth (mm/dd/yyyy)	Age	Sex ☐ Male ☐ Female	Ethnicity ☐ Hispanic ☐ Not Hispanic		Race ☐ White ☐ Black ☐ Asian ☐ Other ☐ Unknown	
Notes, comments, or additional information such as other lab results/clinical info, pregnancy status, occupation (food handler), school name/grade, travel history						

Disease or Condition			Date: ______ *(Check type)* *(Please fill in onset or closest known date)*		☐ Onset ☐ Absence	☐ Specimen collection ☐ Office visit
Physician Name	Physician Address ☐ See Facility address below				Physician Phone ☐ See Facility phone below ( ) -	
Diagnostic Criteria (Diagnostic Lab Result and Specimen Source or Clinical Indicators)						
Patient Name (Last)		(First)		(MI)	Telephone ( ) -	
Address (Street)		City		State	Zip Code	County
Date of Birth (mm/dd/yyyy)	Age	Sex ☐ Male ☐ Female	Ethnicity ☐ Hispanic ☐ Not Hispanic		Race ☐ White ☐ Black ☐ Asian ☐ Other ☐ Unknown	
Notes, comments, or additional information such as other lab results/clinical info, pregnancy status, occupation (food handler), school name/grade, travel history						

Disease or Condition			Date: ______ (Check type) *((Please fill in onset or closest known date)*		☐ Onset ☐ Absence	☐ Specimen collection ☐ Office visit
Physician Name	Physician Address ☐ See Facility address below				Physician Phone ☐ See Facility phone below ( ) -	
Diagnostic Criteria (Diagnostic Lab Result and Specimen Source or Clinical Indicators)						
Patient Name (Last)		(First)		(MI)	Telephone ( ) -	
Address (Street)		City		State	Zip Code	County
Date of Birth (mm/dd/yyyy)	Age	Sex ☐ Male ☐ Female	Ethnicity ☐ Hispanic ☐ Not Hispanic		Race ☐ White ☐ Black ☐ Asian ☐ Other ☐ Unknown	
Notes, comments, or additional information such as other lab results/clinical info, pregnancy status, occupation (food handler), school name/grade, travel history						

Name of Reporting Facility	Address	
Name of Person Reporting	Title	Phone Number ( ) - extension
Date of Report (mm/dd/yyyy)	E-mail	

Above Information is CONFIDENTIAL. Please notify sender if received in error, and return or destroy. **EEPI-1(Rev. 2/09)**

Once a **sentinel case** (i.e., initial case) of an infectious disease is detected in a community, the reporting system is used to alert local health care providers who will watch for additional cases. The general public may receive instructions about how to limit exposure or which symptoms require medical care, and adjoining communities and the state may be alerted about the existence of an outbreak in the area. The state health department receives information from the local agency and forwards it to the **Centers for Disease Control and Prevention (CDC)** where it becomes part of the ongoing statistics of disease outbreak. The CDC also provides support back to the local health department via the state. In cases of outbreak where the organism is unknown or the spread of disease is rapid, the CDC will provide additional expertise to identify cause and technical assistance for limiting spread of disease. The CDC will also alert its international partners about outbreaks since global travel makes the spread of many diseases quick and easy.

International travel has added a new dimension to disease surveillance and quarantine efforts. As Figure 3.3 shows, travel aids in the spread of disease in several ways. First, a person traveling to an area where a disease outbreak exists may become infected and bring the disease with him or her upon return home. Second, a person with a contagious disease who is not yet experiencing illness may travel to another area and infect local residents. Third, a traveler may infect or be infected by fellow travelers who then go to their destination or return home and inadvertently expose others. If the infecting organism can exist outside the human body, the luggage may also be a source of infection when handled by others. As a result of these pathways for spreading disease, many surveillance programs include plans for screening international travelers and using quarantine for people, pets, or luggage as needed.

Figure 3.3—How Trade and Travel Can Spread Disease and Exposures

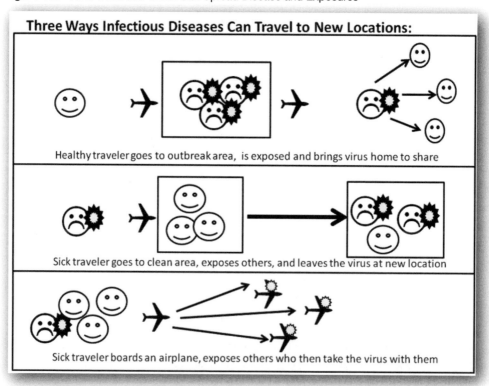

Failure of local surveillance delays response efforts

Local surveillance and communication fails

Within the Guangdong province there was a lack of communication about a new mystery illness that was spreading among residents. The local health care providers, including Dr. Zhang who cared for Yi Chen, did not know that they were a high-risk group for contracting the illness due to their prolonged close contact with infected and ill patients. Although some efforts to isolate the sick patients were made, stringent precautions to avoid exposure were not immediately taken since the scope of the outbreak was not known.

When Dr. Zhang first noticed the fever, he had been in close contact with at least 60 patients, his colleagues at the clinics, numerous nurses, and other hospital and clinic-based health care workers. His greatest concern was a recent flight he took to Hong Kong to attend a medical convention—he knew enough about infectious disease to be concerned about the other attendees, other hotel guests, and fellow travelers on the airplane. When several of his colleagues began complaining of similar symptoms, they quickly polled their closest co-workers to see if anyone else was potentially infected. They found four other physicians, six nurses, and three medical students with fevers and early symptoms, so they voluntarily put themselves in quarantine in one wing of the hospital where they planned to stay until they were sure that they were not sick or the illness ran its course. They took these measures to protect their families and others from exposure to the mystery illness. The loss of these health care workers from their usual routine put a great strain on the hospital, but the severity of the illness and the sheer mystery of it kept the accountants and CEO from complaining about the lost revenue.

The health care worker quarantine wing soon became an **isolation** medical wing as each one developed the mystery illness. Of the 16 workers in the isolation wing, seven died from the disease or its complications. The remaining nine recovered, but were not fully returned to health for another 4 weeks. The experience of being confined to a single wing in the hospital had been incredibly difficult, and most of the survivors found themselves facing depression and anxiety. Access to reports of other outbreaks were limited so Dr. Zhang and his colleagues did not know that the disease had taken a toll in their province or that it was beginning to appear in other countries in southeast Asia. Provincial and national officials in China did not notify other provinces or other countries about an outbreak of a viral pneumonia of unknown cause for another 3 months.

Mystery illness spreads to other countries

By February 2004, Dr. Zhang had recovered sufficiently to be released from the isolation wing. He resumed his practice and cared for more patients with the mystery illness. His own illness had conferred active immunity, and he was one of a few medical providers who could work with patients without fear of contracting their mystery illness. He had recently heard from his old medical school friend, Dr. Trang, who was now practicing in Hanoi; he was treating a patient with a pneumonia that appeared to be viral but was not a known illness. It was an interesting case, and he wondered if Dr. Zhang had ever seen anything like it.

Dr. Trang had time to email Dr. Zhang because he had taken the day off due to a slight fever. Before leaving work the day before, he had contacted the local health officials to report this unusual and potentially contagious illness. This time, the health report made its way from local officials to national agencies that contacted the **World Health Organization (WHO)** where similar reports had recently arrived from Hong Kong and Singapore (Figure 3.4).

Figure 3.4—March 31, 2003: Outbreaks of mysterious atypical pneumonia cases first appear in other southeastern Asia countries then other continents as travelers return home. Total cases: 1,622.

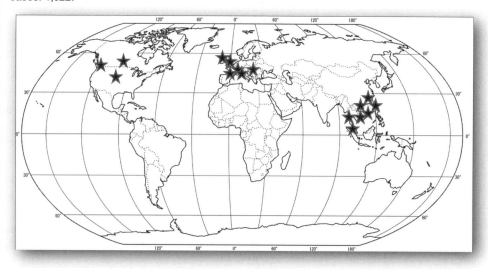

International Public Health Network

Because so many public health issues occur across borders, an international system or network is needed to coordinate efforts and transfer information. As the SARS case will show, the spread of a contagious, infectious disease can be worldwide. Only a global effort to mitigate the spread of the disease will stop the outbreak before it becomes a full-blown **pandemic** (a global outbreak of disease). This section will look at the various international organizations that share information and coordinate actions across borders as well as some of their key functions.

International organizations devoted to public health issues depend upon the voluntary reporting and cooperation of nations around the globe to identify, communicate, and respond to public health emergencies and issues.

Participation in international organizations is voluntary; not all countries participate.

Voluntary collaboration instead of mandates

A key difference between international and national public health systems is whether the organization has the ability to mandate and enforce behaviors. Because international public health organizations are not associated with a particular government, they do not have the inherent powers to pass or enforce laws that will protect health. All efforts to intervene are voluntary and succeed only if each country involved in the issue takes steps internally to follow the recommendations of the international organization.

Voluntary participation instead of required membership

Another key difference between international and national public health systems is the voluntary nature of participation in the international public health system. Not all countries are members of the international organizations, which creates gaps in the global system. Because participation cannot be enforced, the international public health organizations attract countries by providing information and expertise that they need to keep their populations healthy.

The World Health Organization (WHO, International)

The World Health Organization (WHO) is the primary international public health organization. The role of WHO in public health can be defined by its core functions of providing leadership and engaging partners in issues of critical importance to health; promoting areas of research and ensuring findings are disseminated widely; developing standards and promoting their use; promoting the use of ethical and evidence-based options; monitoring and assessing health and trends; and developing its own capacity to ensure that its efforts can be sustained.[1] In essence, WHO exists to promote communication and collaboration among nations on important matters of health. Its key functions are summarized in Table 3.2.

WHO was created in 1948 by the **United Nations** as the global health authority that would coordinate and guide health policy, practice, research, and disease surveillance in participating countries. It has become a respected partner in many public health endeavors. Any nation that participates in the United Nations can

The World Health Organization (WHO) is the primary international, intergovernmental public health entity. Countries considered members of the United Nations are WHO member countries. WHO cannot mandate action but it can provide expertise, support, and guidance to each country while it promotes communications and collaborations. WHO's efforts are supported by regional offices and non-governmental entities.

Table 3.2

Functions of the World Health Organization (WHO)

- Provide leadership on important health matters
- Partner with other public or private organizations as needed
- Shape the research agenda and ensure new knowledge is disseminated
- Develop standards and set norms and monitor implementation
- Promote policy options that are ethical and evidence based
- Provide technical support and expertise
- Monitor and assess the trends in health
- Promote change and support the development of its own sustainable institutional capacity

Source: World Health Organization, International. The Role of WHO in Public Health. Available at: http://www.who.int/about/role/en/index.html. Accessed September 23, 2008.

also be a member of WHO. The international headquarters for WHO is located in Geneva, Switzerland, a historically neutral country. The organization is headed by the Director General who is appointed by the World Health Assembly, which is the decision-making body of WHO and consists of representatives from the member nations.[2]

The member countries are divided into six regions that span the globe. Each region represents countries within a distinct geographic area, such as the "**Region of the Americas**," which consists of North, Central, and South American countries including the United States.

Table 3.3 lists the eight regions. WHO conducts its work and communication primarily through these regional groups. Each region is able to concentrate on public health issues that may be unique to its geography and populations. Like its parent organization, each region is an international entity.[3]

As an international entity, WHO can serve as a focal point for reporting disease outbreaks and sharing information across many countries. Because membership and participation in WHO and its programs are voluntary and limited to nations that are participants in the United Nations, some gaps exist in membership and participation. Not all countries are represented, and recommendations for practice or policy within countries cannot be enforced.

Pan-American Health Organization (PAHO)

Another international health organization to which the United States belongs is the **Pan-American Health Organization (PAHO)**, which includes North, Central, and South American countries. This regional organization was actually created about 50 years before WHO. It came into existence as a result of coordinating regional efforts to control the spread of infectious disease through increased sea travel.[4] At the time, global air travel did not exist, so disease outbreaks were generally contained within a continent or region.

When WHO was created in the 1940s, the PAHO assumed the role of the "Regional Office of the Americas." The headquarters for PAHO are in Washington, DC, where staff members focus their efforts on getting member nations to collaborate on international health issues that are found in the Americas.[4] As a regional office for WHO, PAHO has the same issues associated with voluntary membership and compliance with policies and standards as its parent organization. Although PAHO is primarily linked with WHO, it also serves other agencies of the United Nations (e.g., World Bank).

The mission of PAHO is to improve the health of the people in the Americas and to strengthen health systems from local to national levels. It does this by promoting health care programs that increase access and add efficiency to systems, promoting education and social communications, reducing the spread of transmissible diseases and chronic diseases, and fighting outbreaks of disease in countries in the Americas.[4] **Vulnerable populations** such as mothers, young children, poor, elderly, and refugees or displaced individuals are the target groups for health improvement. Focus areas for interventions

Table 3.3

Six Regional Offices of the World Health Organization (WHO)

African Region
Region of the Americas (PAHO)
South-East Asia Region
European Region
Eastern Mediterranean Region
Western Pacific Region

Source: WHO—its people and offices. Regional offices. Available at: http://www.who.int/about/structure/en/index. html. Accessed September 23, 2008.

are the safety of the blood supply, safe drinking water, sanitation, and tobacco use. To accomplish its mission, PAHO partners with other UN and WHO agencies, national public health agencies, and private, non-governmental organizations.

Non-Governmental Organizations (NGOs)

In addition to international agencies whose membership is comprised of countries, some private organizations are not representative of a particular country or government. These **non-governmental organizations (NGOs)** frequently partner with governmental and intergovernmental organizations to achieve a health goal. Members of NGOs may be private citizens or businesses; the organizations may be supported by private, public, or both types of funds. Even NGOs receiving public funds (i.e., funds from governments) are considered non-governmental as long as their governing boards do not include representatives from the government providing the financial support. The NGOs often supplement services or provide programs within countries when the local public health system lacks sufficient funds or resources, which further differentiates them from WHO and PAHO.

Many NGOs begin as an effort to fill a specific niche that the governmental and intergovernmental organizations are unable fill. Like their public counterparts, the NGOs grow and expand over time often making the scope of their missions broad and overlapping their work with other NGOs and government organizations. For example, CARE, International began as a nongovernmental food relief agency after World War II when its sole purpose was to provide packages (CARE packages) to starving families in war-ravaged Europe. Today, CARE's humanitarian aid now includes fighting global poverty and its related health issues. The organization focuses on women since they can impact the entire family. Projects supported through CARE include efforts to improve basic education, reduce spread of HIV, increase clean water and sanitation, grow economic opportunities, protect natural resources, and provide emergency aid.[5] Other examples of international NGOs that focus on health and vulnerable populations are the International Federation of Red Cross and Red Crescent Societies (IFRC), which provides emergency services in areas struck by disaster as well as basic health care services.[6] Oxfam, International is a famine-relief NGO, and Doctors without Borders (*Médecins Sans Frontières*) provides international teams of health care providers to countries and areas where services are not available or other NGOs will not go.[7]

Global network of public and private public health partners

As Figure 3.5 shows, the public and private elements of the global public health system form a network that is designed to improve communication and coordinate responses to issues that extend beyond the borders of individual countries. Over time, the intergovernmental agencies such as WHO and nongovernmental agencies

The global network of public health organizations consists of a complex web of governmental, intergovernmental, and non-governmental organizations that have formed many partnerships to address public health issues. The NGOs are often able to implement local services based on national or international policies and standards set by intergovernmental groups such as WHO.

such as the IFRC have expanded the scope of their missions so that they now often have overlapping missions. This forms a complex network of partnerships and activities for many public health concerns.

Figure 3.5—Relationships among Public and Private Participants in the Global Public Health System

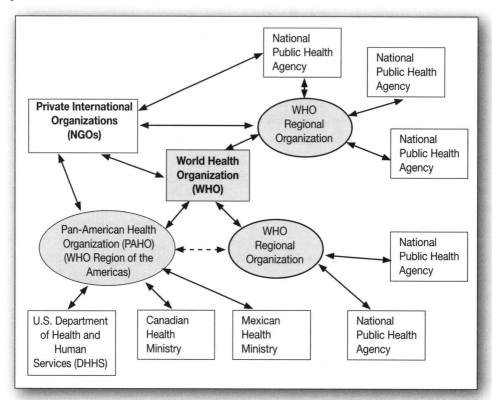

 CASE STUDY 1 (*continued*)

WHO gets the world involved in the mystery illness

WHO epidemiologist Urbani names the mystery illness SARS

Although Yi Chen had recovered from his illness, the virus that caused the disease was spreading to other countries. During a recent trip to Hong Kong, Yi Chen had noticed people wearing face masks. He tried to buy some masks for himself and his family, but the local pharmacies and hospitals had already sold their supplies. Like many of his neighbors, Yi asked a distant relative living in Kansas City to send him a supply of face masks. He had just begun to hear about the mystery illness, and it sounded like it was spreading to other towns, provinces, and countries.

During March, the mystery illness had been named SARS for Severe Acute Respiratory Syndrome by a physician who was investigating the outbreak for WHO. Yi was sorry to hear that the physician, Dr. Urbani, had contracted SARS and died several weeks later. During those early spring months, Yi had to rethink his travel plans because travel advisories and alerts were appearing for many southeastern Asian countries. Many alerts were for other provinces in China and the city of Beijing, which had reported over 400 cases of SARS. Yi also found that his business contacts in other provinces and countries were not eager to have him conduct business in person since he was from an outbreak area and may have had SARS.

Global collaboration to fight the spread of SARS

Yi was not aware of a concurrent international effort to isolate and identify the virus that caused SARS. News reports about the disease and international efforts were still limited in his hometown and did not describe the international team of 11 leading research labs that were working on the genetic sequence of the virus. During a business trip to Singapore, he learned that the virus was a coronavirus from the same group of viruses that also causes the common cold. The newly identified virus had been named SARS co-V. Apparently, it was a small germ; those face masks he had shipped from the United States could not block it. From his conversations with other businessmen, Yi learned that the disease was now appearing all around the world. It was interesting to hear stories about how various countries were taking different approaches to detecting and controlling the SARS outbreaks (Figure 3.6).

Figure 3.6—May 1, 2003: Clusters of SARS cases appear on six continents and spread within China. Total cases: 5,663.

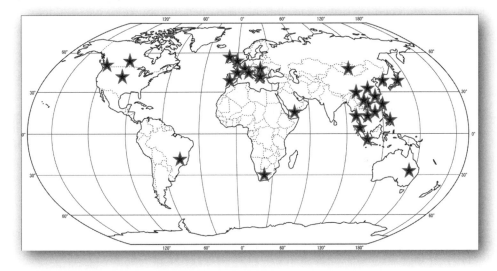

Public Health Systems within Countries

While efforts to address public health problems at the international level are based on the voluntary cooperation of countries, efforts within a country may actually be enforceable depending on how the nation has established its public health system. Although the structure of these public health systems within different countries varies and their issues are not the same, the key functions of the public health systems remain similar. Unlike their international counterparts, public health

Public health systems within a country often have the authority to mandate and enforce behaviors that are deemed to be in the interest of the public's safety and welfare. This authority may be delegated to local governments or agencies.

organizations or agencies with a country often have the ability to mandate behavior and require participation. This section of the chapter will look at the U.S. public health system beginning with the federal level. After looking at the federal agencies, the state and local levels of public health will be examined.

The U.S. Public Health System

Federal authority

The establishment of health or public health services in the United States was not specifically addressed by our founding fathers in the U.S. Constitution. In other countries, such as Mexico, constitutional provisions establish public health services. In the United States, public health services were established indirectly through several mechanisms. First, the commerce clause of the Constitution gives the federal government the power to regulate trade with other nations, including tribal nations, and between states. An example of this type of power is seen with the regulation of the pharmaceutical industry and the advertisement of pharmaceuticals. Second, the power to tax citizens and spend tax dollars allows the federal government to raise funds that support national public health programs and initiatives and allocate the monetary resource to state and local governments that will conduct the programs.[8]

State and local authority

Powers not specifically given to the federal government via the U.S. Constitution were retained by the states. This state-level authority, which is called police power, allows a state to set laws and enforce them for the welfare of its citizens; however, these powers are subject to limitation by the U.S. Constitution, state constitution, and a balance of individual rights and public welfare. The 10th Amendment, which granted authority for each state to act on behalf of its citizens for matters not specified by the Constitution, made this implicit authority more explicit.[8]

In general, federal laws related to public health take precedence over state laws, which in turn take precedence over local laws. When federal laws do not exist, the state sets its own. As a result of the delegation of most public health authority to the states, great variation exists in the structure and function of local and state health agencies across the country. Tribal health authority results from negotiated treaties with the federal government, and the extent to which that authority is granted to local governing bodies is determined by each tribe.

U.S. public health system functions include:

- Interacting with international organizations;

- Interacting with state and tribal public health systems;

- Delegating authority to states to care for the health of their citizens;

- Regulating activities that cross state lines or are specifically named in the Constitution; and

- Determining how public funds are distributed and used.

Structure of the U.S. Public Health System

As Figure 3.7 shows, three levels or tiers exist in the U.S. public health system: local, state, and federal. The local agencies may be established at the county, city, or neighborhood level depending on the state system and the size of the population served. Public health agencies may be as simple as a single health officer or as complex as a multi-state, multi-center, complex of services provided by thousands of individuals. Tribal agencies operate at a level that is most similar to the state level public health agencies; they are shown at the same level in the figure.

The flow of information, funding, and policy-making between local, state, and national health departments helps to delineate the relationships among the different entities. For example, health care, which is a component of public health, is practiced at the local level but may be affected by state licensing laws and national policies on access. In return, health care providers and their professional organizations may help to shape policies at the local, state, and federal levels. Many other organizations and agencies contribute to the public's health, including law enforcement, environmental quality, agriculture, and schools. Although this chapter will not focus on their contributions, remember that most public health issues affect and can be affected by virtually every aspect of the community.

Figure 3.7—Public and Private Elements of the U.S. Public Health System

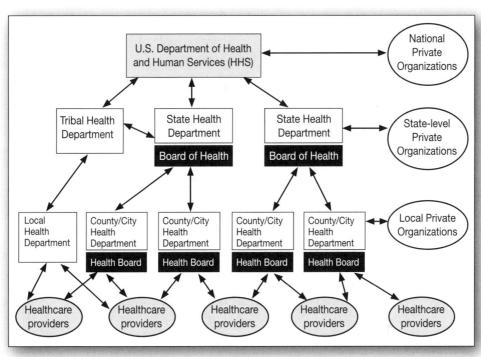

Department of Health and Human Services (HHS)

Mission

The U.S. Department of Health and Human Services (HHS) is the principal national organization charged with both protecting health and providing essential human services for Americans. As a federal program, the HHS serves more as a source of policy, guidance, and funding but does not directly administer the programs. Administration is delegated to state health departments or their designees. Therefore, HHS works with state and local (i.e., county or city) governments to ensure information and services reach the public. The support often comes in the form of financial resources, technical assistance, education, and goals for the program. It has been estimated that almost one-fourth of the federal budget is spent on HHS programs, which indicates the size of the department and the focus on keeping residents healthy and productive.[9]

Background

The HHS was officially established in 1980 from two groups of pre-existing agencies: those that were in the **U.S. Public Health Service** and those that were devoted to the welfare of citizens. As Table 3.4 shows, HHS now consists of 11 operating divisions or agencies that can still be roughly divided into those that focus on health and those that focus on the welfare of vulnerable populations such as children and the elderly.[9] Many divisions and departments are within each agency. For example, within the **Food and Drug Administration (FDA)**, six centers and three offices are devoted to various regulatory and review functions related to food and product safety. These 11 agencies and their departments are responsible for over 300 programs that address health and human service needs including research in health and social sciences, food and drug safety, educational programs for children, disaster preparedness, and substance abuse prevention or treatment.

U.S. Public Health Service (USPHS)

The U.S. Public Health Service (USPHS) is perhaps the oldest of the federal services or departments focused on public health. USPHS began as the Marine Hospital Service, which was dedicated to the care of sick or disabled seamen. Over time, the service expanded to include more public health duties and agencies that were eventually incorporated into the HHS.[10] Table 3.4 indicates the HHS agencies that are considered part of the USPHS. To fulfill its mission, the USPHS established its own health care staff called the commissioned corps.

The commissioned corps of the USPHS has around 6000 health care providers and researchers in its ranks. Pharmacists are one of a number of health professions included in the corps. Most USPHS pharmacists work with one these four agencies: the Indian Health Service (47%), the Food and Drug Administration (26%), Bureau of Prisons (14%), and the National Institutes of Health (13%).[10] In addition to their usual clinical duties, PHS pharmacists are also expected to assist with responses for disasters such as hurricanes. These positions may be located in Washington, DC, or spread throughout the country. Most are clinical pharmacy positions, but some have additional advisory or consultative aspects. For example, a PHS pharmacist working with the Health Resources and Services Administration (HRSA) is required to provide medications for HIV/AIDS to patients in an underserved population and study national pharmacy manpower requirements.[11]

As a federal employee, pharmacists are not required to be licensed in the state where they are stationed as long as they have a current license in at least one of the states in the union. With regard to the SARS outbreak, PHS pharmacists in clinical positions were affected in the same manner as health care providers in other settings.

Table 3.4

Major Agencies of Health and Human Services (HHS) and Their Primary Roles

Agency		Primary Roles
HHS agencies for health (public health) services		
AHRQ	Agency for Healthcare Research and Quality	Supports research on the health system, including quality and cost issues
ATSDR	Agency for Toxic Substances and Disease Registry	Works to prevent exposure to hazardous substances created by wastes
CDC	Centers for Disease Control and Prevention	Provides a system of disease surveillance and reporting
FDA	Food and Drug Administration (FDA)	Assures safety and efficacy of medications; safety of food and cosmetics
HRSA	Health Resources and Services Administration	Provides access to basic health care services in underserved populations
IHS	Indian Health Service	Works with tribes to provide health services to American Indians and Alaska Natives
NIH	National Institutes of Health	Promotes and funds biomedical research
SAMHSA	Substance Abuse and Mental Health Services Administration	Works to improve availability and quality of prevention and treatment programs
HHS agencies for human (welfare) services		
CMS	Centers for Medicare & Medicaid Services	Administers the Medicare and Medicaid programs
ACF	Administration for Children and Families	Promotes the economic and social well-being of children, families, and their communities
AoA	Administration on Aging	Provides services to the elderly to help them remain independent

Source: U.S. Department of Health and Human Services. Available at: http://www.hhs.gov/about/whatwedo.html. Accessed September 14, 2007.

Centers for Disease Control and Prevention (CDC)

The Centers for Disease Control and Prevention (CDC), which supports surveillance of health status and disease, maintains the related statistics and promotes disease prevention. This division of the DHHS is tasked with monitoring and preventing international transmission of disease. The director of the CDC also leads the Agency for Toxic Substances and Disease Registry (ATSDR), which is dedicated to reducing exposure to toxics in the environment, particularly those found in waste sites designated as priorities by the Environmental Protection Agency (EPA).[12]

In the 2002–03 SARS outbreak, the CDC served as a source of information and the group to which state health departments reported both suspected and confirmed cases of SARS. The CDC web site has numerous resources for a variety of diseases that can be used by practitioners as well as the general public. For pharmacists, this site can provide just-in-time information about topics of concern for patients such as travel vaccination recommendations, epidemiology of diseases, and in the present case, information about how SARS is spread, early symptoms, best treatment options, and areas where travel restrictions or cautions exist. Information about SARS can still be found on the web site because of concerns that it will reappear.

Food and Drug Administration (FDA)

One of the divisions in the HHS that is most familiar to pharmacists is the Food and Drug Administration (FDA), which is deeply involved in the drug development and production process. FDA works with the manufacturers rather than researchers to ensure products are both safe and effective. As one might expect, pharmacists are included among the employees of this division.[13] The mission of the FDA is to protect the health of the public by assuring medications, food, cosmetics, and products that emit radiation are safe, effective, and secure (i.e., not tampered with or contaminated). Its goal is to do this in a speedy and efficient manner that does not compromise safety.[13] Virtually all efforts to ensure drug product safety come from the FDA with one notable exception being child safety caps, which are regulated by the **U.S. Consumer Product Safety Commission (CPSC)**.

The FDA is best known for its work to promote legislation that regulates pharmaceutical manufacturers and the drug approval process. The FDA has many other roles that promote safety. It has several voluntary reporting systems for issues related to medication including its safety reports for adverse events (**MedWatch**), vaccines adverse events (**VAERS**), **counterfeit medications**, and problems with online pharmacies. Through its **Center for Drug Evaluation and Research (CDER)**, FDA provides oversight of marketing of new medications, generics, new indications for existing products, and post-marketing surveillance. Personnel in this center are primarily MDs and PhDs, but some pharmacists are in key positions and on the staffs. In addition to drug approval duties, the CDER also provides counterterrorism and emergency response support related to medication supplies and access.[14]

■ ■ ■

At the national level, public health activities focus on issues that are interstate and international. In the United States, the primary federal agency for public health is the Department of Health and Human Services (HHS). Through its 11 agencies, HHS provides a broad array of services, support, and policy for states. Among those divisions are several with strong ties to pharmacy, including the FDA and USPHS.

The FDA has created a Counterfeit Drug Task Force to combat counterfeit medications in the United States and abroad. Its efforts complement those of the **International Medication Products Anti-Counterfeiting Taskforce (IMPACT)**, which was created by WHO. In addition, it provides travelers with advice about the dangers of purchasing medications while traveling since counterfeit medications in some areas are more common than genuine products and problems can arise with buying medications via the Internet.[14] Pharmacists are among the personnel and consultants that work with the FDA. As an employee, pharmacists are technically hired as USPHS pharmacists who are assigned to the FDA. In addition to being an employee of the FDA where duties reflect standard clinical practice as well as proposal review duties, pharmacists can also be found on the rosters of the various FDA advisory committees.[15]

With regard to the 2002–03 SARS outbreak, the FDA could potentially become involved in expedited approval of a vaccine found to be effective against the virus if such a vaccine were discovered. FDA could also be involved with approval of off-label use of existing medications if they showed efficacy against the SARS virus. In the case as presented in this chapter, the role of the FDA is minimal.

State public health structures and functions

Basis of Authority and Ability to Delegate

The 10th Amendment to the U.S. Constitution made state governments the primary protectors of the health of people living within their borders. A state may undertake a myriad of activities to meet this responsibility, including the creation of an administrative agency called the health department (or public health agency). Activities conducted by the state health department in one state may be quite different that those in another due to differences in state priorities, politics, and ability to delegate to local governments.

State Health Departments and Boards of Health

Like their local counterparts, state health agencies are under the direction of the **Health Officer** (or Medical Officer) whose work is guided by the state's **Board of Health**. The structure of the state health departments and boards vary by state. In general, the state health departments may be organized in several different ways. The traditional public health agency limits its oversight to just public health and primary care services. If a health department is organized as a "super public health agency," it also oversees mental health and substance abuse services in the state; one that is a "super health agency" may include supervision of Medicaid instead of mental health and substance abuse services. The largest of all organizations, the "umbrella agency," oversees all of the above mentioned services plus other human services programs.[16]

At both the state and local levels, two separate but related entities are the Board of Health and the health department. The Board of Health is comprised of a group of volunteers from the community or state that represent various points of view including health care. The board provides oversight and guidance for public health agencies. These volunteers are usually appointed by the local government and selected to represent a variety of interests and expertise. The duties of the health board focus on oversight of the health agency's progress towards meeting its mission and its fiduciary responsibilities.

Most of the authority to act on public health issues on behalf of the population resides within the state health boards and departments. This authority, which was conferred upon the states by the federal government, can be and is often delegated to the local public health organizations. Tribal public health organizations are similar to state health departments in their authority to act on behalf of their citizens.

Health boards generally hire and evaluate the Health Officer who serves as the director of the local health agency. The Health Officer is responsible for ensuring that programs and services are implemented and carried out. This usually means delegating duties to divisions within the organization where the staff members actually conduct the work. Historically, Health Officers were physicians, but some now have other graduate credentials such as a Master of Public Health (MPH) degree.

Some local health agencies are so small that the Health Officer is technically the agency; most others are true health departments with several divisions, numerous programs, and more than one person on staff. When the health agency is large enough to employ more than one person, it is generally referred to as a health department. The health department is the organization that does the work deemed necessary to protect the health of the citizens.

Both health departments and Boards of Health are created by the local government and have their authority bestowed upon them by those governments as an extension of the same authority that was given to the state. Some municipal and county departments are combined into a single city-county organization through agreements between the municipal and county governments.

Local public health structures and functions

Boards and departments of health also exist at the city or county level. Larger metropolitan areas may have a city health department in addition to a county department. In rural or frontier areas where the populations are sparse, the department may consist of a single person. In other areas, the city and county departments may be combined into a single entity. The local government decides how it will delegate the authority and the scope of that authority.

The local level is where public health really meets the population it serves. Most programs are administered at this level, local citizens are involved on the Boards to provide the community perspective, and disease reports are collected case-by-case and fed to the state's epidemiologist for analysis before being forwarded to the CDC for national statistics to be monitored and reported.

At the local level, the policies and funds dedicated to public health work are put into practice. This is the level where the governmental entity interacts directly with the populations for which it exists to serve. The local level is also where much of the disease monitoring data is collected and sent back to state, federal, and international public health entities.

CASE STUDY 1 (*continued*)

The United States prepares for the arrival of SARS

Kansas prepares for its first case

In Kansas City, Lai Chen, a fourth-year pharmacy student, arrived at her community retail pharmacy for a 6-week experience in clinical pharmacy activities in a retail setting. She had a vested interest in the SARS outbreak because one of her great aunts, Ming Chen, had apparently died from the disease just last winter. Her great uncle, Yi, had been corresponding with Lai's mother who naturally asked Lai for information. Her first task had been to find face masks to mail to her extended family in Guangdong province. She had been surprised to learn that she was not the only one looking for this scarce commodity.

As Lai settled into her rotation, she became one of many health care workers preparing for the inevitable arrival of SARS in the U.S. heartland. Recent cases in Toronto had piqued interest in early detection of SARS cases and implementation of safety precautions for health care providers working with SARS patients. Lai was asked to find information on the disease, guidelines for clinicians, and treatment options. Lai began with a search of the CDC and WHO web sites where the latest information was being posted. Her preceptor suggested that she also look at the Canadian national health service site (**Health Canada**) for additional updates and information.

Based on her search of the literature, Lai prepared a brief list of potential issues that the retail store could face if a SARS outbreak occurred in Kansas City. Her list is shown in Table 3.5 along with possible methods for addressing them. Key components included providing information to patrons of the store without scaring them, clarifying or correcting misunderstandings of reported literature or news reports, providing patients with tangible things they can do to reduce their risk, discouraging purchases of devices or medicines that are not effective, and keeping the pharmacy personnel safe while working with exposed or sick patients or handling or discarding their unused medications.[17,18]

Case post-mortem

By the time the SARS outbreak ended in late 2003, over 8000 probable SARS cases and 774 deaths were reported across 29 countries.[19] In the United States, eight cases out of 29 were confirmed and no deaths were reported. All the confirmed U.S. cases were tied to travel to areas where SARS outbreaks were known to exist and were not caused by human-to-human transmission while in the states.[20] Figure 3.8 shows all countries with one or more cases of SARS.

Fears that the following 2002–03 winter season would produce another outbreak were largely unfounded with only few cases reported in China and no evidence of another global SARS event. The experience from the SARS outbreak did provide valuable information for individuals who are preparing plans for responding to an **avian flu pandemic**, which has been predicted to occur at any time.

Table 3.5

Lai's List of Potential SARS-Related Issues for a Retail Pharmacy

Prepare for:	Cause	Issues
Patient surge (increased number of patients)	If local hospitals are closed or put under quarantine, patients will seek other sources of care and information	Increase staffing to handle increased traffic Prepare information for patients
Sicker patients	These patients may be sicker than usual but barred from hospital	Review info and help triage patients
Worried well	Patrons who have respiratory symptoms but no history of exposure	Provide information and reassurance
Poor communication or information	Health officials may change information frequently to adjust to evolving situation	Seek reliable information sources Seek local info for current quarantine/treatment info
Protecting workforce from exposure	Health care workers are highly likely to become infected if they work closely with a SARS patient Need to limit exposure time and closeness	Use standard and respiratory precautions Handle items for potentially exposed SARS patients while wearing gloves Frequent hand washing Use face masks if counseling coughing or feverish patients Use telephone for counseling Drop off prescriptions at homes Bill via credit card numbers to avoid handling checks or money
Monitoring pharmacy staff	Fever is an early sign of SARS; if a family member is sick, put employee on sick leave	Take temperature of workers once a shift; if fever is present, send worker to designated SARS clinic site
Requests to dispose of potentially contaminated medications	Family members of potential SARS cases may have unused medications they want to throw away	Determine local health department recommendations for disposing of unused medication products that had been dispensed to a SARS patient
Requests for ineffective prevention and treatment options	Remedies for self-treating SARS may be requested by patients even though they are not effective	Provide patients with most current treatment and prevention information

Sources: 1. Revised U.S. Surveillance Case Definition for Severe Acute Respiratory Syndrome (SARS) and Update on SARS Cases—United States and Worldwide, December 2003. *MMWR*. 2003; 52(49):1202–6. Available at: http://www.cdc.gov/mmwr/preview/mmwrhtml/mm5249a2.htm. Accessed September 23, 2008. 2. Centers for Disease Control and Prevention. Severe Acute Respiratory Syndrome (SARS). Fact Sheet: Basic Information about SARS. Available at: http://www.cdc.gov/ncidod/sars/factsheet.htm. Accessed September 23, 2008.

Figure 3.8—August 7, 2003: SARS cases appeared in 26 countries around the world. Total cases: 8,422. Total cases in health care workers: 1,725 (20%).

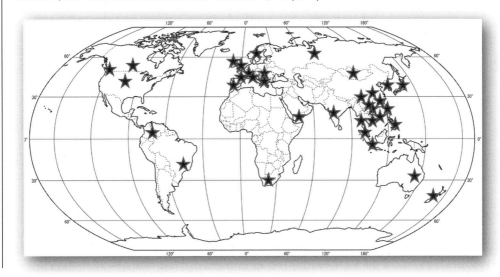

Local to Global Roles for Pharmacy in Public Health

As the SARS case showed, many facets and levels exist in public health. Almost all are places where pharmacists can become involved. Table 3.6 shows, local, state, national, and international organizations offer numerous opportunities for pharmacists to participate. It may be easiest to start close to home at the local level when the Health Board requests nominees to fill open positions.

Table 3.6
Pharmacy Roles in Local to Global Public Health

At the local or state level

- Contact Health Boards and task forces
- Use education and awareness programs
- Report unusual sales volumes for medications or patient complaints
- Be an advocate for local citizens and keep eyes open for issues

At the federal level

- Contact task forces with professional organizations
- Serve on review panels or government committees
- Use national voluntary reporting systems

At the international level

- Participate in voluntary medical and humanitarian aid
- Raise awareness for international travelers of risks and prevention
- Donate money or supplies

Pharmacists will be affected by and can provide interventions for global public health issues, which include identifying and reporting new or emerging cases of resistance to antibiotics and antivirals, the quality of products purchased via the web, and counterfeit medications obtained from supposedly reliable wholesalers and secondary wholesalers. Pharmacists can also ensure access to medications during emergencies and for vulnerable populations who lack sufficient resources or insurance to purchase them.

Chapter 3 Summary

To learn about the various levels of the U.S. and international public health systems, this chapter looked at the flow of information during the 2002–03 SARS pandemic. Local health departments are the point of contact with the individual residents, and care and data collection occur primarily at that level. State departments of health provide support to local department as well as a conduit for information to federal agencies. At the national level, policy, guidance, funding, and interaction with international partners become the primary activities. Globally, the public health system is a voluntary network of countries and private organizations that work to facilitate the flow of information and expertise to parts of the world where it is most needed. These systems are interdependent, and pharmacists have the potential to be involved at any level of the public health system.

References

1. World Health Organization, International. The Role of WHO in Public Health. Available at: http://www.who.int/about/role/en/index.html. Accessed September 23, 2008.

2. World Health Organization Basic Documents, 46th ed. Geneva, Switzerland: WHO Press; 2007. Available at: http://www.who.int/gb/bd/PDF/bd46/e-bd46.pdf. Accessed September 23, 2008.

3. WHO—its people and offices. Regional offices. Available at: http://www.who.int/about/structure/en/index.html. Accessed September 23, 2008.

4. Basic Documents of the Pan American Health Organization, 17th ed. Official Document No.325. Washington, DC: PAHO/WHO Regional Office; 2007. Available at: http://www.paho.org/English/D/OD_325.pdf. Accessed September 23, 2008.

5. CARE, International. About CARE. Available at: http://www.care.org/about/index.asp. Accessed September 23, 2008.

6. International Federation of Red Cross and Red Crescent Societies. Available at: http://www.ifrc.org/index.asp. Accessed September 23, 2008.

7. The Role of Nongovernmental Organizations. International Information Programs U.S. Department of State. Available at: http://usinfo.state.gov/products/pubs/principles/ngos.htm. Accessed September 23, 2008.

8. Gostin LO. Public health law in a new century: Part II: Public health powers and limits. *JAMA*. 2000; 283(22):2979–86.

9. U.S. Department of Health and Human Services. Available at: http://www.hhs.gov/about/whatwedo.html. Accessed September 14, 2007.

10. U.S. Public Health Service Commissioned Corps. Available at: http://www.usphs.gov/default.aspx. Accessed September 23, 2008.

11. Department of Health and Human Services. Agencies with Pharmacists. Available at: http://www.hhs.gov/pharmacy/agencies.html. Accessed September 28, 2008.

12. CDC Organization webpage on the Centers for Disease Control and Prevention. Available at: http://www.cdc.gov/about/organization/cio.htm. Accessed September 23, 2008.

13. Food and Drug Administration (FDA). Available at: http://www.fda.gov/default.htm. Accessed September 23, 2008.

14. Center for Drug Evaluation and Research (CDER). Available at: http://www.fda.gov/cder/index.html. Accessed September 28, 2008.

15. Food and Drug Administration. FDA Advisory Committees: Human Drugs. Available at: http://www.fda.gov/oc/advisory/drugscommlist.html. Accessed September 28, 2008.

16. Association of State and Territorial Health Officials (ASTHO). Innovations in Public Health: Understanding State Public Health. PUB-0703004. April 2007. Washington, DC: ASTHO. Available at: http://www.astho.org/pubs/UnderstandingPHASTHO.pdf. Accessed October 3, 2008.

17. Austin Z, Martin JC, Gregory P. Pharmacy practice in times of civil crisis: The experience of SARS and "the blackout" in Ontario, Canada. *Res Soc Admin Pharm.* 2007; 3:320–35.

18. Chin TW. Severe Acute Respiratory Syndrome (SARS): the pharmacist's role. *Pharmacotherapy.* 2004; 24(6):705–12.

19. Revised U.S. Surveillance Case Definition for Severe Acute Respiratory Syndrome (SARS) and Update on SARS Cases—United States and Worldwide, December 2003. *MMWR.* 2003; 52(49):1202–6. Available at: http://www.cdc.gov/mmwr/preview/mmwrhtml/mm5249a2.htm. Accessed September 23, 2008.

20. Centers for Disease Control and Prevention. Severe Acute Respiratory Syndrome (SARS). Fact Sheet: Basic Information about SARS. Available at: http://www.cdc.gov/ncidod/sars/factsheet.htm. Accessed September 23, 2008.

Chapter 3 Review Questions

1. **Explain why an outbreak of poliomyelitis in Mexico may be a concern to the citizens of Canada.**
   Polio is caused by a virus that may be transmitted to others who have not been vaccinated or have had acquired immunity from a prior infection. An outbreak of polio in Mexico could easily travel to any part of the globe via international air travel, so all countries, not just Canada, should be concerned about a large outbreak of the disease.

2. **Which of the following best describes a key function of WHO?**
   (a) Monitor health and disease trends   (b) Provide technical support

   (c) Set standards   (d) All of these

   The answer is (d).

3. **Explain the role of surveillance in mitigating the spread of disease.**
   Surveillance should allow for early detection of an outbreak so that steps can be taken to slow or stop its spread before it becomes an epidemic. Surveillance also provides information about the level of disease in the community; therefore, it can be monitored to determine when an outbreak is over.

4. **Describe how the U.S. public health system is structured at the national, state, and local levels.**
   The national or federal level of the U.S. public health system is anchored by the large HHS department that includes key agencies such as the FDA, CDC, and PHS. The Public Health Service is the medical or health care corporation of the HHS, which employs pharmacists for clinical pharmacy and dispensing roles. The FDA ensures products are safe and effective, while the CDC serves as the surveillance and reporting sector of HHS.

At the state level, Boards of Health and departments of health are given authority to act on behalf of their residents by the federal government. The health departments are usually large and complex, while the health boards are relatively simple in composition and small in size. Boards of Health provide oversight of the department.

At the local level, the city or county health department is headed by a Health Officer who is hired by the local health board. Local health departments may be small (one person) or larger multi-divisions departments that administer programs to the local populace.

Tribal health departments work at a level similar to the state health departments in regard to their relationship with the federal government.

5. **Describe the roles of the World Health Organization (WHO), Pan-American Health Organization (PAHO), and non-governmental organizations such as the Red Cross, International in addressing public health issues.**
   The WHO is the primary organization for the international public health network. It does much of its work through its regional offices, which includes PAHO. Non-governmental organizations such as the Red Cross, International often provide supplementary support at the local level when local systems cannot.

Applying Your Knowledge

1. **Describe how pharmacists can become involved in disease surveillance.**

2. **Using the CDC web site, determine the prevalence of malaria, polio, and pertussis (whooping cough) in the United States and in your home state. Using the WHO web site, determine the prevalence of these diseases in Somalia. Find the country with the highest prevalence of HIV/AIDS.**

3. **Look for information about West Nile virus on the CDC web site. When did it arrive in the United States and how did it get here?**

4. **Think about a recent food recall or warning. How was the FDA involved? Why was it so difficult to determine the source?**

5. **What are WHO, CDC, and FDA doing to reduce the problem of counterfeit medications? Where is this problem especially bad and what types of medications are being counterfeited?**

Role of Law in Public Health

Learning Outcomes

1. Describe the source of state police power and federal authority to pass laws that support public health goals for people and communities.
2. Explain how public health laws are used to modify behavior, regulate goods or services, and protect the environment.
3. Describe the public health events or issues that led to pharmacy laws to regulate the manufacturing and use of medications.
4. Discuss the role of law in addressing international public health issues related to pharmaceuticals and pharmacy practice.
5. Identify ongoing and emerging public health issues related to medication use or pharmacy practice that may require future legislation or regulation.

Introduction

The ability to enforce policies and mandates that will benefit the populace through the use of police power is a tool used by public health officials. This chapter will look at the role of law in public health as it is applied to efforts for controlling disease and making communities healthy. A particular emphasis is placed on public health laws that impact how pharmacy is practiced. To illustrate some current public health concerns related to safety and effectiveness, a medication-oriented case will be used. The chapter will end with examples of public health issues that led to key federal pharmacy laws. This approach was used to emphasize the reasons all those laws and regulations that restrict and guide pharmacy practice exist today.

Public Health Law in the Context of Medication Use

Virtually all aspects of life in the United States are touched by public health policies and laws; medications and the practice of pharmacy are no exception. Like many other products and food items, the production of medications is heavily regulated to ensure safety and effectiveness. Advertising claims are subject to review and revocation if they exceed results of research. Practitioners and pharmacies are controlled and competence assured through licensure, inspection, and continual professional education requirements. Ensuring access to needed medications is the role of public health insurance and community health centers, both of which are supported by public funds and supervised by public agencies. In spite of all these laws and regulations, medication use still involves risk.

Recent medication issues that are now public health concerns include the human errors associated with their use (i.e., medication errors); uncontrolled access to prescription medications via web sites based outside of the United States; tainted products; and counterfeit medications designed to fool unwary consumers and make money for the criminals who produce them. Efforts to contain and control these sources of potential risk will require new laws, better enforcement, and international cooperation.

CASE STUDY 1

Counterfeit medication purchased via the web

Bill looks for more affordable medications on the web

Bill is a healthy young man in his late 20s who is planning to travel to Southeast Asia to see the sights and enjoy the local cuisine and culture. As part of his preparations, he checked the CDC web site for travel vaccination requirements and got vaccinated at the local health department. He saw that prophylaxis with oral anti-malarial medications prior to departure and upon return to the states was also recommended. The cost of the medication from the health department and local pharmacies was too high for Bill, so he decided to find a cheaper alternative. One of his travel-wise friends said he bought the same stuff on the web for a fraction of the cost. Another friend told him he would be able to buy anti-malarial medications as well as medications for travelers' diarrhea once they were in the foreign country.

Before the trip, Bill purchased preventive medication for malaria. His friends told him online pharmacies would sell him what he needed without a prescription and for a fraction of the price. This sounded like a good idea, so Bill went online and purchased a supply of a potent anti-malarial, mefloquine 250-mg tablets. He chose the mefloquine because it was effective against organisms causing malaria that were resistant to older medications like chloroquine or doxycycline. The site was identified as Canadian and offered free Viagra® with an order of 30 mefloquine tablets at $14.24 per tablet. Bill didn't need the second medication, but it was hard to resist getting something for free!

Bill receives a counterfeit medication

Unbeknownst to Bill, the web-based company he decided to do business with was able to offer great deals on medications because it sought sources that were low cost and not necessarily trustworthy. The product he purchased had been produced and designed to deceive—it was counterfeit mefloquine. Because Bill had never used the product before, he did not notice that the tablets looked larger than the real product. According to the instructions, Bill began taking his preventive medication 1 week prior to the start of his dream vacation. He would be taking it once a week throughout his stay, then 4 weeks after returning home. He took the first dose, which he tolerated very well, and had no unpleasant side effects. He didn't think about the lack of usual side effects as a possible indication that the medication lacked 250 mg of active ingredient.

Law as a Tool for Public Health

One of the biggest differences between health care interventions and public health interventions is the ability of public health officials to enforce mandates designed to reduce risks and improve health. This ability to use law to change behavior is an important tool for public health. Unlike public health, effort made by pharmacists to change the behavior of patients requires their voluntary cooperation.

Sources of authority

The source of authority for local, state, and federal governments to enforce public health laws comes from different sources. In the United States, each state is a sovereign entity entitled to make its own laws and control the behavior of its residents as long as it does not counteract or undermine federal law or contradict its own constitution. This authority is often referred to as **police power**. Most federal laws are written in a manner that allows each state to interpret and apply them in a manner that is most appropriate to that state. This usually means state laws are stricter than federal laws, but with some exceptions. In addition, **case law**, which is the judicial review of legally challenged laws and legal decisions (i.e., appeals), is used to further refine understanding of federal and state public health laws and the extent of their power.

Federal laws can address interstate issues (e.g., commerce) and taxation (e.g., federal tax codes). Because states are sovereign entities responsible for their own citizens, most of the laws affecting public health and pharmacy exist at the state level. Laws, even within states, often require additional work by agencies in the state to become operational. Agencies are tasked with preparing rules and regulations that contain very specific details based on an interpretation of the law.

When interpretations of federal, state, and local laws differ, the court system is used to hear arguments and provide interpretations via case law. Populations that are not guided by state laws such as the U.S. military and entities such as American Indian tribes have their own governments.[1] In addition to creating laws, federal and state legislators often create agencies or departments to enforce new laws. For example, the **Food and Drug Administration (FDA)** was created as part of a federal law to ensure safe medications, cosmetics, and food.

When discussing law related to pharmacy or public health, one does not generally think of international laws. It is worth noting, however, that **International Health Regulations (IHRs)** are developed and voluntarily enforced by countries under the leadership of the **World Health Organization (WHO)**. A recent revision of the IHRs designed to provide a worldwide approach to all potential hazards, not just a few specific infectious diseases, has been released.[2]

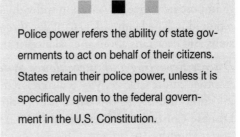

Police power refers the ability of state governments to act on behalf of their citizens. States retain their police power, unless it is specifically given to the federal government in the U.S. Constitution.

Laws to mandate and enforce behaviors

Public health laws at all levels are used to make unsafe behaviors illegal and to promote behaviors that improve health or reduce the risk of disease or injury. Laws that require seatbelts, restrict the sale of tobacco and alcohol to minors, allow speed limits to be established, and regulate where and how garbage may be disposed of are all designed to improve the health of a community. Virtually every local ordinance, state law, or federal act requiring or forbidding a behavior has its roots in either a public health or economic issue. Some have particular relevance to health care and pharmacy, so they are explored in more depth in this chapter.

Restricting Personal Movements to Contain a Disease

Laws that allow the government to restrict movement have their origins in efforts to control the spread of contagious diseases. To control the spread of infectious disease in a community, health departments may restrict the movement of individuals or transportation vehicles into and out of areas. Such measures may also be used to prevent the spread of chemical or radioactive contaminants. Interfering with the freedom of individuals to go where they wish when they wish is an especially sensitive action in the United States because individual rights are highly regarded. The decision to impose restrictions is made only when failure to do so may result in great harm to the community or population.

Movements are restricted for several reasons. One reason involves removing a person who is sick with an infectious disease from the population; this is called **isolation**. Because contagious diseases are often transmitted before any apparent signs of illness are evident, isolation measures alone may not be enough to halt the spread of disease. For individuals who have been exposed and are most likely to become ill, they are separated from others through **quarantine**. Families of an ill person also may be placed in quarantine during a severe outbreak of disease. Isolation and quarantine practice may also involve closing borders or transportation and trade routes. Because some infectious organisms can survive on objects or spread through animal-to-human transmission, quarantine may also apply to inanimate objects, animals, birds, and fish.

The concepts of compulsory vaccination and enforceable quarantine clash with the concept of personal freedom. An outbreak of smallpox in Boston around the turn of the 20th century led to the implementation of required vaccination. Many residents were opposed to this action because of a prevailing opinion that the vaccines were unsafe. The statutory penalty for refusing to be vaccinated was $5 (today's value would be over $100). In one particular case, Mr. Henning Jacobson refused to be vaccinated because he had had a bad reaction to an earlier vaccination, so he was fined. His case was eventually appealed to the U.S. Supreme Court where the Court upheld the right of the state to impose its police power upon individuals when the welfare of the whole population required it. The landmark case of *Jacobson v. Massachusetts* continues to shape discussions and decisions about the balance of state police power and individual rights.[3,4]

Disease Reporting and Surveillance Systems

Another enforceable activity is also related to historical efforts to control the spread of infectious disease. To this day, a list of notifiable diseases is posted on the **Centers for Disease Control and Prevention (CDC)** web site; a similar list resides on the web sites of state health departments. The list contains vaccine-preventable diseases, sexually transmitted diseases, and other communicable diseases. When a physician diagnoses a case or a medical lab identifies a microorganism that causes one of the diseases, that information must be reported to the local health department. The reporting chain then goes to the state health department and ultimately to the CDC where it is added to reports from other states. The information is used to track trends in the level of disease activity in the community. The authority to require reporting originates in the state legislatures where the power may appear as a statute or delegated to the state's board of health or department of health. Federal involvement to compile the state information was established in 1933 in the **U.S. Public Health Service**. This activity is currently performed by the CDC.[5]

Another legally supported action for public health officials is access to **personal health information (PHI)** for the purposes of disease surveillance and monitoring. Most pharmacists are familiar with the **Health Insurance Portability and Accountability Act (HIPAA)** and its guidance for patient information confidentiality. This act includes a privacy rule that limits access to protected health information. Because the need to protect the public is of greater concern than the need to maintain privacy of the individual patient at times, the rule grants an exception to public health personnel who are authorized by law to gather and use such information for preventing or controlling disease.[6] This exception removes the requirement to obtain permission from each individual patient prior to accessing the information. While this exception provides easier access, it is important to remember that access to and use of protected health information is regulated by other state and federal laws.

Public health laws that are used to modify behaviors keep the population healthy in two ways:
(1) reduce behaviors that are risky and tend to lead to injury or death and
(2) promote behaviors that keep people healthy.

Laws to regulate goods and services

In addition to regulation of human behavior, public health laws are also used to regulate the products used or consumed by the public and the businesses and individuals who provide services to ensure the health of the population is not put at risk by faulty products or inept providers. Federal laws are used when goods or services are sold across state or international borders. Within a state, regulation may occur at the state level or within a county or community, depending on the scope of the distribution of goods and services.

Licensure for professionals such as pharmacists occurs at the state level. This means a pharmacist who wishes to practice in another state must also be licensed in that state. Because pharmacy practice laws can vary among states, this requirement is necessary to ensure the pharmacist is knowledgeable about the local laws and requirements. An exception to this rule involves pharmacists who are employees of the federal government; as long as they have a license in good standing in one of the states, they are allowed to practice at the federal care site.

Regulation of Professionals and Care Sites

State governments are responsible for licensing businesses and individual providers for many businesses, including pharmacy. This is done to ensure that the individuals who provide care are competent and the sites where care is provided are safe. At the state level, health care practitioners are controlled through two primary mechanisms: licensure and practice acts. The licensure process is designed to ensure practitioners entering the field have minimal required knowledge and, through re-licensing requirements at regular intervals, that practitioners remain competent. **Pharmacy Boards** protect the public's health by ensuring all the pharmacists and technicians practicing in the state meet some minimum standard of training and practice. These boards also monitor practice through complaints from patients and others in the community and on-site inspection of pharmacies.

To help define which activities can be performed by a health care professional, the state will have practice acts. **Pharmacy practice acts** are used to define the scope of practice for pharmacists and pharmacy technicians. The acts affect practice through the development and implementation of rules and regulations by the state's pharmacy board. In addition, federal laws for controlled substances also impact pharmacists' professional actions; these laws are enforced by the Drug Enforcement Agency (DEA). Like pharmacists, pharmacies are also subject to licensure and regulation.

Regulation of Manufacturers and Distributors

Because most manufacturers seek a large market, their sales will cross state and national borders. This means their activities and products are subject to federal regulations and agency inspections. Likewise, the interstate transportation of products from one wholesaler to another will involve federal agencies and regulations. If sales and distribution are limited to an area within a state or county, local laws and agencies will provide most of the control.

Issues related to the regulation of manufacturers and distributors involved in international trade—where products are produced in one country and sold in another—can raise public health issues. Problems may emerge because there are differences in the manufacturing standards, inspection of the manufacturing process, product quality assurance measures, and accountability for faulty products. Because there is no international police power, problems created by these differences require cooperative measures between the countries and possibly internal steps to reduce use of faulty products. Voluntary product recalls of already marketed products are used to warn U.S. wholesalers, retailers, and consumers about an unsafe product. A more proactive approach is to require the foreign manufacturer to enter into a contractual agreement that specifies the level of manufacturing standards and product quality required to sell the product in the receiving country. This is described in the 1995 Compliance Policy Guide on International Memoranda of Understanding (MOU) for the FDA.[7] For example, the U.S. and European Union have a **Mutual Recognition Agreement (MRA)**, which assures that products produced in Europe but marketed in the U.S. will meet U.S. manufacturing and labeling standards.[7] These products enter the U.S. market through wholesalers and retailers. It is generally illegal for a person to directly purchase medications from a foreign manufacturer in another country.

> Public health laws may be used to ensure products are safe and effective and professionals are competent providers.

Laws to Protect Vulnerable People and Environments

A community has a vested interest in having healthy and productive residents as well as a healthy environment in which to live and work; therefore, laws have been passed to protect those who are most vulnerable to disease, injury, and contamination. Such laws may be used to increase access to services and products and decrease negative treatment created by discriminatory practices.

Ensuring access to health care services and products

While most laws apply to the general population, some groups in the population are especially vulnerable to health risks or are unable to care for themselves. One such group is the very young (infants and children); other groups that may be vulnerable are the elderly, individuals with reduced cognitive abilities, homeless people, and some mentally ill individuals. Legislation creating new agencies or approving funding to support health care, housing, and food for these populations as well as laws to reduce discrimination against those needing care have been used in public health. These laws may be federal or state level actions. For example, older and disabled citizens have access to medical services through Medicare, a public health insurance program created in the 1960s; likewise, children and disadvantaged families have increased access to care through other public health insurance programs such as state-run Medicaid and children's health insurance programs (CHIPs).

Regulating impact on the environment

Clean air and water are essential to human existence, so it is no surprise that efforts to minimize impact on the environment are needed. Laws are needed because many individuals do not see how their actions will affect others or how their actions may have a cumulative effect over time. As a result, public funds are used to monitor air and water quality, restrictions are made regarding how household garbage is disposed, and discharge of materials from factories is regulated. An example of a federal law created to control disposal of wastes and products includes the 1976 Resource Conservation and Recovery Act (RCRA), which required the U.S. Environmental Protection Agency (EPA) to develop regulations for controlling how solid and hazardous wastes are disposed.[8] Like many laws, it has been amended since it was originally passed to further refine it and make it relevant for current problems.

Based on the local environment and risks, local ordinances may require the use of catalytic converters in automobiles to reduce emissions or outlaw burning garbage or fireplaces when the air is stagnant. Controlling where community members build or requiring dog owners to pick up pet wastes are other examples of local zoning and pet ordinances designed to protect the environment in the long and short term. Because air and water can easily cross borders, national and international laws or agreements may be used to ensure protection of the resources for all populations. In these cases, the source of potential contamination is controlled through regulations and mutual agreements.

> Public health laws may be used to protect those individuals who are particularly susceptible to harm or frequently lack access to services. The environment may also be protected through the use of public health laws.

Table 4.1

Examples of Historically Important Public Health Laws and Court Decisions

Year	Act	Purpose
1905	Jacobson v. Massachusetts	Upheld mandatory vaccinations as an acceptable use of state police power at U.S. Supreme Court
1935	Social Security Act	Addressed social welfare through retirement benefits and health insurance and was the first federal law to do so
1938	Federal Food, Drug, and Cosmetic Act	Required proof of safety prior to marketing medicines
1946	Hill-Burton Act	Promoted improvements and expansions of health care infrastructure
1964	New York Mental Hygiene Law	Abolished mandatory hospitalization by judicial decision and replaced it with medical decision
1964	Civil Rights Act (Title VI)	Designed to address issues created by discrimination
1969	National Environmental Policy Act	Required environmental impact studies prior to initiating new programs

Source: Adapted from Landmark Public Health Laws and Court Decisions, Encyclopedia of Public Health. Breslow L, ed. New York, NY: Macmillan Reference USA; 2002.

CASE STUDY 1 *(continued)*

Bill's assumptions about the safety of his medication

Bill has never personally experienced injury from a faulty product or tainted food, so the idea that something he can buy is possibly fake or dangerous never crosses his mind. This is not an unusual state of mind. Because so many aspects of U.S. life are regulated, many people just assume that someone is watching out for them and items wouldn't be sold if they are unsafe. While Bill's risks may be minimal with a medication product produced within the United States by a licensed manufacturer, those same guarantees do not exist for products produced and sold by companies not based in the United States that do not have contractual requirements to meet the same standards. Because the product Bill purchased contains only 25 mg of active ingredient (10% of the 250 mg amount on the label), he is at risk of contracting malaria as well as promoting the development of resistant strains of *Plasmodium falciparum,* the main causative organism for malaria. The good news is that his particular fraudulent product does not contain any toxic ingredients.

Public Health Issues that Inspired Landmark Pharmacy Laws

Many reasons exist for the creation and amendment of laws designed to reduce risks and promote health in a population. Often, a new law is enacted in response to an emerging problem or new issue not previously encountered. Pharmacy laws have often been created and amended in response to patient and public safety problems. Because laws have changed the nature of practice, it is often difficult to recall exactly why they were needed. As the precipitating event fades in memories, the laws and regulations that guide practice can seem more like hoops through which pharmacists have to jump rather than responses to critical public health issues. A study of the prevailing attitudes and practices prior to the passage of key federal pharmacy laws can expose the underlying public health issues encountered and addressed through legislation.

Faulty or dangerous medications

In the late 1800s and into the 20th century, concern had been growing about the number of patent medicines being sold to an unsuspecting public. There were no enforceable regulations requiring labels to list active and inactive ingredients, no requirement to show proof of safety or efficacy, and no restrictions on how the items were sold or the promises made in the advertisements. As a result, a series of laws were enacted and agencies created to ensure that products made or sold in the United States are both safe and effective. The laws address faulty products and false claims, and hold the person or company selling the products liable regardless of intent.

Unsafe Medication

Perhaps one of the most well-known public health issues related to an unsafe medication is the 1937 Elixir of Sulfanilamide tragedy. This occurred at a time when antibiotics were just beginning to be accepted as treatment for infectious diseases, and effectiveness and safety were regarded with suspicion. Sulfanilamide, a sulfa antibiotic, was marketed as a tablet for adults. Because of its dosage form and taste, it was difficult to administer to children. As a result, the manufacturers of medicinal products worked to create a liquid form of the medication for use in children. Solubility and taste were obstacles to creating a useful product. One chemist determined that diethylene glycol (DEG) would both dissolve and sweeten the sulfanilamide and prepared a batch of Elixir of Sulfanilamide that was sold to pharmacies in several states (Figure 4.1). Because the label did not indicate the diluent, other pharmacists were not aware of the deadly diluent. Within a short period of time, the product caused the death of over 100 people, mostly children, and led Congress to finally heed the FDA's advice to pass the new Federal FD&C Act in 1938.[9]

Figure 4.1—Elixir of Sulfanilamide Bottle and Label

Source: U.S. Food and Drug Administration, Center for Drug Evaluation and Research. Portion of photo on Food and Drug Administration website; URL: http://www.fda.gov/AboutFDA/WhatWeDo:History/ThisWeek/ucm117880.htm. Accessed July 24, 2009.

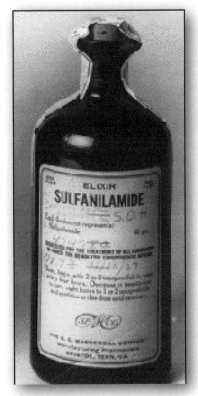

Ineffective Medications and False Claims

Another public health issue created by medication products was the marketing of products that were not necessarily unsafe, but were not effective. A well-known example of these **patent medicines** is *Lydia E. Pinkham's Vegetable Compound*®. While ineffective medicines may not directly harm the patient, they can cause harm if

Figure 4.2—Article Cover Page for Adam's Series "The Great American Fraud" in 1905–1906 in Collier's Weekly

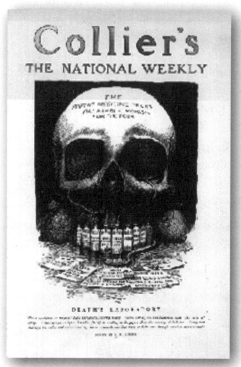

their use delays the patient from seeking legitimate care. Sales of these products raise two public health concerns: spending limited funds on ineffective treatment and delaying effective treatment if available. The predominance of **quack medicines** had reached its heyday in the late 1800s and early 1900s when a series of exposés, *The Great American Fraud*, by Samuel H. Adams in *Collier's Weekly* magazine described the practice in such detail that public furor resulted in legislation to reduce fraud by listing ingredients on the labels[10] (Figure 4.2).

Although a series of legislation designed to improve labeling (Figure 4.3) and control advertising claims was enacted, requirements to actually prove effectiveness were not fully realized until after mid-century when a potential public health disaster was narrowly averted through the delayed approval of thalidomide, a mild sedative/hypnotic and anti-emetic. It had been used in European countries for several years, and the manufacturer was now seeking approval for its release in the United States as a treatment for morning sickness. Approval was delayed by the chief medical officer of the FDA because results of neurological studies raised concerns. During that delay, reports from Europe that the drug was causing a specific type of birth defect called phocomelia began to surface. As a result, the drug was never approved for use in the United States for treating morning sickness.[11]

This incident caused great public outcry and inspired the passage of the 1962 Kefauver-Harris Drug Amendment that increased requirements for bringing a new product to market. The requirements now included proof of efficacy as well as safety. Today, new drug products undergo four phases of human subject research to determine their safety, effectiveness for a given condition, appropriate doses and duration of therapy, side effects, and pharmacokinetic properties. The fourth phase of study is called the **post-marketing surveillance or phase IV** study; these studies are conducted to detect serious but rare adverse events that may be caused by a recently released medication.

Figure 4.3—Evolution of the Medicine Bottle and Label through the 20th Century

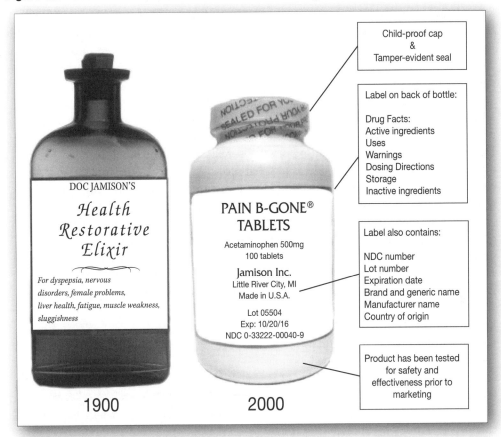

Counterfeit, Adulterated, and Tampered Medications

A third area of concern with medication products focuses on the integrity of genuine products after they are shipped from a legitimate manufacturer as well as of false products intended to deceive. As before, the public health issues are related to the use of products that contain toxic ingredients or fail to fully treat due to a lack of labeled ingredients. One example of a public health issue that resulted in a revision of the dosage form and packaging is the series of poisonings that occurred in the 1980s with Extra-Strength Tylenol® capsules laced with cyanide. At least six people died as a result of taking the tampered product. Sadly, one couple who was attending the funeral of a victim had experienced headaches, saw the bottle of extra-strength capsules on the kitchen counter, each took a couple, and also succumbed to the poison and died. As a direct result, the product, which had been a standard capsule that could be twisted open, was discontinued and replaced by a capsule-shaped (caplet) dosage form. In addition, all over-the-counter medications were required to have tamper-resistant packaging that is still seen today (Figure 4.3).[12]

Issues with **counterfeit medications** have existed for many years, but recent advances in technology have made it easier for criminals to reproduce labels and create tablets, unit-dose packages, and cartons. These counterfeit medications can enter the U.S. medication supply through secondary wholesale distribution systems and via sales on the Internet. Many of the web-based sources are physically located outside of the United States to avoid regulatory agencies and prosecution. Control of the problem is difficult because a counterfeit operation can set up, sell, and dismantle quickly. The World Health Organization (WHO) has estimated that one out of four medicines used in developing countries are either counterfeit or substandard. This estimate doubles in Southeast Asia and Africa to around 50%.[13]

Weaknesses in the U.S. drug distribution system, which employs primary and secondary wholesalers to move products from manufacturers to retailers, have been used as a point of entry for counterfeit and substandard medications into the health care system. **Diversion,** the inappropriate routing or sale of medications, is another problem created by these weaknesses. A 1987 study found that secondary wholesalers were the source of counterfeit and substandard medicines.[14] The Prescription Drug Marketing Act (PDMA) was designed to strengthen the drug distribution system in the United States.[15]

Two solutions for these problems are licensing the wholesalers and requiring **pedigrees** (i.e., paper trail that documents the chain of custody from manufacturer to pharmacy). Wholesalers are licensed in the state where they are physically located as well as any state where they do business, and they are licensed through the drug Enforcement Agency (DEA) if they handle controlled substances. The PDMA requires pedigrees for any wholesaler who is not an **Authorized Distributor of Record (ADR),** which most **secondary wholesalers** are not. State laws can also be used to close the loophole in the PDMA that also requires ADRs to file pedigrees for any product that leaves and re-enters the normal distribution channels as defined by the state. Although the pedigree requirement may not stop the practice, it will help identify offenders and serve as useful evidence in prosecuting them.

Medication safety and effectiveness is an ongoing public health issue that is addressed by a series of pharmacy laws. These assurances do not necessarily extend to products made or sold by foreign sources.

Table 4.2

Selected Pharmacy Laws Inspired in Part by Faulty or Dangerous Medications

Year	Act	Purpose
1906 (1912)	Food and Drug Act (Sherley Amendment)	Eliminates the sale of adulterated products and false claims of therapeutic effectiveness. Intent to defraud must be proven
1938	Federal Food, Drug, and Cosmetic (FDC) Act of 1938	Has many purposes, including a requirement for new drugs to be proven safe prior to marketing and eliminates the need to prove intent to defraud consumers
1962	Kefauver-Harris Drug Amendment	Ensures new drug products are proven both safe and efficacious prior to marketing
1972	Over-the-Counter Drug Review	Ensures non-prescription medications are safe, effective, and appropriately labeled
1982	Tamper-Resistant Packaging Regulations	Makes it a crime to tamper with packaged products and requires tamper-proof packaging

Adapted from U.S. Food and Drug Administration. Center for Drug Evaluation and Research. FDA Centennial at CDER: the History of Drug Regulation in the United States. Web page available at: http://www.fda.gov/Cder/centennial/history.htm. Accessed May 13, 2009.

 CASE STUDY 1 *(continued)*

Caveat emptor and medications of dubious quality

Although some risk of a manufacturing error may make a medicine unsafe, the manufacturing and packaging standards for medications in the United States have greatly improved product safety and effectiveness. As a result, consumers like Bill are confident about the products being sold. Because the web site he used to buy mefloquine looked official and was available to him, he subconsciously assumed it had been inspected and approved by some government agency. Regulating web-based sales of medications is a tricky business. If the server is located within the United States, the site can be held to U.S. standards if the site owners can be located. There is a voluntary program used to identify online pharmacy sites that are reliable—it is called **Verified Internet Pharmacy Practice Sites (VIPPS)** and is run through the **National Association of Boards of Pharmacy (NABP)**. Unfortunately, the site that Bill visited did not display the VIPPS logo and was not a verified site.

Because the web-based business that sold the medication to Bill is not based in the United States, he is dealing with a lot of unknowns and should exercise caution. Not all foreign-based sources of medications sell inferior quality products; rather, the opportunity for criminal mischief or poor manufacturing standards is greatly increased. The old maxim of *caveat emptor* (let the buyer beware) should guide Bill's actions and decision-making.

Luckily, Bill also visited the CDC and WHO web sites for additional information about traveling in a malaria-endemic country. There he found sound recommendations to use DEET (a potent mosquito repellent), avoid the outdoors at dusk and dawn, and sleep with a mosquito net covering the bed. Since certain mosquitos carry the disease-causing organisms, he should avoid mosquito bites to prevent infection.

Unsafe use of otherwise safe medicines

Once product manufacturing and testing regulations were in place, the focus of concern shifted towards a lack of patient safety. Problems with inappropriate or unsafe use of otherwise safe medications led to additional legislation and amendments of key pharmacy acts. In addition, regulation of the practitioners through licensure was needed to ensure competent care. Some of the main issues related to patient safety are presented here.

Unsupervised Use of Potent Medications

Until 1951, manufacturers of medications were allowed to determine whether their product required a prescription. Because a clause in the FDC Act of 1938 allowed any product designated as a prescription medication to be exempt from the patient labeling requirements for over-the-counter products, manufacturers often designated products as prescription only. This led to prescription requirements for products that could be safely used without that level of supervision. In 1951, the Durham-Humphrey Amendment (also called the Prescription Drug Amendment) was passed; it created two classes of medications: prescription and over-the-counter. In addition, all prescription medications were required to include the phrase "*Caution: Federal law prohibits dispensing without a prescription.*" Products would be deemed legend (prescription) medications if they had abuse potential or were potentially harmful if not used correctly.[16]

Medication Errors

Once safe and effective medication products were generally available, it became apparent that they could still injure and kill people if they were not used appropriately. Early efforts to require increased supervision of patients using medicines with a high potential for harm, if misused, resulted in several federal laws that created prescription and non-prescription classes of drugs. For medications with the potential to be addictive, federal laws created five categories or schedules with even more stringent requirements on their use and distribution. While the classifications help to restrict the distribution of medications, patients were still at risk of injury and death due to human errors related to prescription writing, dispensing, and administration of medications.

The scope of medical and **medication errors** was not fully appreciated until a 2000 report (*To Err is Human*) by the **Institute of Medicine (IOM)** propelled the problem into the public spotlight and subsequently made medical errors a national public health concern.[17] Since then, additional reports in the Quality Chasm series have been published. Later estimates of medication errors are thought to be low because many errors go unreported if they do not result in injury or death. With that in mind, the rate for medication error-related injuries and deaths in hospitals, long-term care facilities, and elderly outpatients have been estimated at 400,000, 800,000, and 530,000 each year, respectively.[18] To date, reporting medication errors is a voluntary activity and no federal laws have yet been enacted to require reporting errors. One of the primary issues is the lack of an agreed-upon definition of what the term "medication error" actually includes.

Abuse of Clinically Used Medications

Abuse of alcohol and psychoactive drugs has occurred through the ages. Concerns with the addictive characteristics of alcohol and then opiates and cocaine grew to critical levels as the 20th century began. Initially, some viewed cocaine as a legitimate treatment for depression and opium or one of its derivatives like heroin as a treatment for alcohol addiction. Sales of these substances were not regulated, and patent medicines often included one or more of them. In the later years of the 1800s, prohibition movements began to emerge and a groundswell of reform started to build. Although some manufacturers changed their products to avoid the negative associations, others continued to manufacture their patent medicines and tonics with ingredients that would one day be deemed narcotics and subjected to taxation and regulation. Even Coca-cola®, a tonic that had been reformulated to replace wine with sugar to avoid the alcohol prohibitionists, probably contained miniscule amounts of cocaine from the fresh coca leaves used to flavor it. To remove the possibility of including cocaine in the product while still retaining its flavor, subsequent formulations used processed coca leaves.[19]

Public outcry focused primarily on alcohol, but international opium conferences in 1909 and 1911 led to an international opium agreement that would require countries to control the sales of the narcotics within their borders. The 1914 Harrison Narcotic Act was passed as a result. Although it appeared to be a law to organize and regulate sales, it contained wording that was interpreted by law enforcement as a means for restricting the sales of narcotics to known addicts. Even though it was amended numerous times, and then repealed in 1970, the attitude of addiction as an illegal behavior rather than a disease persists to this day.[20]

Today, narcotics are classified into five classes or schedules based on their medical usefulness and potential for physical dependence and addiction. The risk of addiction or abuse relative to medical benefit is greater at a lower number. For example, drugs that are Schedule I do not have any apparent medical benefit and have a high risk for physical dependence and addiction.

Table 4.3

Laws Inspired in Part by Unsafe Use and Access Issues

Year	Act	Purpose
1914	Harrison Narcotic Act	Requires prescriptions for products with higher levels of narcotics and increases recordkeeping requirements
1951	Durham-Humphrey Amendment	Restricts the sale of medications that require medical supervision to prescription status (VERIFY)
1970	Comprehensive Drug Abuse Prevention and Control Act	Categorizes drugs on basis of abuse and addiction risk compared to therapeutic benefit
1988	Prescription Drug Marketing Act	Designed to eliminate diversion of products from legitimate channels of distribution and requires wholesalers to be licensed
1997	Food and Drug Administration Modernization Act	Expands scope of agency activities and moves agency to the DHHS
2003	Medicare Prescription Drug Improvement and Modernization Act of 2003	Includes Medicare Part D, which increases access to medications through private insurers

Adapted from U.S. Food and Drug Administration. Center for Drug Evaluation and Research. FDA Centennial at CDER: the History of Drug Regulation in the United States. Web page available at: http://www.fda.gov/Cder/centennial/history.htm. Accessed May 13, 2009.

CASE STUDY 1 *(continued)*

Who can Bill turn to if something goes wrong?

One of the most important aspects of pharmacy practice is ensuring that patients understand their medications and use them appropriately. Counseling and monitoring patient progress is a key activity that promotes better health outcomes. One of the greatest concerns with online pharmacies is whether patients are still receiving the full pharmacy service. Sites that are VIPPS eligible will have methods for interacting with patients, although it may be via the computer or telephone rather than in person. In Bill's case, the site did not list a pharmacist. Instead, Bill was asked to complete a form that would be reviewed by a physician who would then write the prescription so it could be filled and sent.

When Bill returned from his trip and began to show signs of an influenza-like illness (ILI) — fever, shaking chills, and night sweats — he called the support phone number to find out if he was reacting to the medicine or if he was sick. He called the contact phone number listed on the web site, but it was out of order. He began to get suspicious about the site; when he noticed that the web site was no longer posted, he became convinced that he had been tricked. He then did two things: contacted his family physician to seek treatment for what he suspected was malaria and called the state's fraud prevention hotline to report the web-based company.

Inappropriate disposal of medications

Pharmaceuticals enter the waste system and eventually the environment in several ways. Raw materials may come directly from compounding and manufacturing; medications may be discarded by pharmacies or patients; medications may be sent to disposal facilities or returned to manufacturers via a reverse distribution process; and medications used in animals and humans may be excreted into sewage systems. While households may contribute to pharmaceuticals entering the environment, the primary sources are hospitals and other health care institutions.[21]

Barnes et al. found measurable levels of several prescription medications, including female hormones and antidepressants, in the ground water.[22] Handling and disposal of chemicals are controlled by the Environmental Protection Agency (EPA) through the 1976 Resource Conservation Recovery Act (RCRA).[8] The Act regulates medication disposals and requires specific steps in disposing products that contain human blood products or items contaminated by human blood or tissue (biological wastes) as well as medications that are chemical entities with high risks of toxicity or hazard (hazardous wastes). But these regulations are designed for hospitals, long-term facilities, manufacturers, and pharmacies but not individual households. Institutions or pharmacies may also get rid of expired medications through reverse distributors that, in turn, will return the pharmaceuticals to the manufacturers or dispose of the products. Ultimately, the disposal of waste from pharmaceutical products by businesses is regulated by the RCRA. Patients or households, however, receive little or no guidance on proper disposal of unused medications. As a result, many are discarded via garbage (landfills) and toilets (sewer system).

Wastes are created in the manufacturing and use of medicines. Although full impact on the environment is not fully understood, laws are being enacted to ensure unused products and manufacturing wastes are disposed of in a proper manner.

CASE STUDY 1 *(continued)*

How should Bill dispose of the leftover medications?

Fortunately for Bill, his malarial infection was caught early and successfully treated so he recovered fully. During the final followup visit with the physician, he was advised to get rid of the unused medications that he purchased online since he was not sure they were actually mefloquine and he didn't need the free Viagra.

Getting rid of the unneeded medications was difficult. Bill paid a lot of money for them and wanted to hang on to them "just in case." However, when he considered that the products may in fact be fakes, he decided to throw them away. That was when Bill discovered that he was not sure how to dispose of them safely. His friend told him to flush them down the toilet; he is the same guy who told him to buy the cheap mefloquine online. As he hovered over the toilet with a handful of tablets, he recalled recent news reports of pharmaceutical contamination in the ground water and the poor advice he received from his pal last time. This time he decided to look into the issue himself.

Bill called the medical clinic to see if they had any information about safe disposal, but they were not able to help him. He then called a local retail pharmacy to see what they would recommend. Luckily, they had information about a local program conducted through the health department's water quality department and provided him with a copy of the household pharmaceutical wastes disposal guidelines. His instructions told him to remove the labels to ensure his private information was protected, but to keep the tablets in their vials and bubble packaging. He then had to put them in a sealable plastic bag that he should pack inside a small cardboard box to disguise the contents. Bill then waited until close to garbage pickup time as possible to actually place them in the trash. Bill could now enjoy his photos and recall the details of his vacation.

Chapter 4 Summary

Laws are an important tool for public health. As the need for prevention and intervention increase and change with the emerging public health issues, laws are written, revised, and refined through case law to ensure that they are appropriate and sufficient. Maintaining a balance between individual rights and public needs requires ongoing assessment too. Pharmacy is heavily regulated through laws that impact the manufacturing processes, practitioner licensure, sales of medications, and disposal of products. In the daily grind of pharmacy, it is easy to forget that the many regulations and laws that shape practice have their roots in public health issues. As new problems emerge, pharmacists will need to be actively involved in promoting new laws or amending existing ones. The widespread use of the Internet is adding a whole new dimension to efforts to ensure that products sold to patients are safe and effective and used with sufficient supervision to ensure that they do not create new health problems. Not all public health issues can be addressed through laws as the case illustrates of the unsuspecting young man who purchased a low-cost, counterfeit product from a web-based source.

References

1. Gostin LO. Public health law in a new century. Part II: Public health powers and limits. *JAMA.* 2000; 283(22):2979–86.

2. Gostin L. The international health regulations and beyond. Reflection & reaction. *Lancet Infect Dis.* 2004; 4:606–7.

3. *Jacobson v. Massachusetts, 197 U.S. 11 (1905).* Available at: http://www.supreme.justia.com/us/197/11/case.html. Accessed May 10, 2009.

4. Colgrove J, Bayer R. Manifold restraints: liberty, public health, and the legacy of *Jacobson v. Massachusetts. Am J Public Health.* 2005; 95:571–6.

5. Department of Health and Human Services, Centers for Disease Control and Prevention. Mandatory reporting of infectious diseases by clinicians. Reports and reconmmendations. *MMWR.* June 22, 1990; 39(RR-9):1–11, 16–17.

6. Department of Health and Human Services, Centers for Disease Control and Prevention. HIPAA privacy rule and public health: guidance from CDC and the U.S. Department of Health and Human Services. Early release. *MMWR.* April 11, 2003; 52:1–12.

7. Food and Drug Administration. A Plan that Establishes a Framework for Achieving Mutual Recognition of Good Manufacturing Practices Inspection. Available at: http://www.fda.gov/oc/fdama/fdamagmp.html. Accessed May 15, 2009.

8. U.S. Environmental Protection Agency. Wastes—Laws & Regulations: Hazardous Waste Regulations. Available at: http://www.epa.gov/wastes/laws-regs/regs-haz.htm. Accessed May 13, 2009.

9. Wax PM. Elixirs, diluents, and the passage of the 1938 Federal Food, Drug and Cosmetic Act. *Ann Intern Med.* 1995; 122(6):456–61.

10. Adams SH. The great American fraud, *Collier's,* October 7, 1905. Reprint of original article text posted at URL: http://www.museumofquackery.com/ephemera/oct7-01.htm. Accessed May 1, 2009.

11. World Health Organization. Use of thalidomide in leprosy. Available at: http://www.who.int/lep/research/thalidomide/en/print.html. Accessed July 29, 2008.

12. Beck M, Monroe S, Prout LR, et al. The Tylenol scare. *Newsweek* (U.S. edition). 1982; Oct 11:32.

13. World Health Organization. WHO calls for an immediate halt to provision of single-drug artemisinin malaria pills. News Release 2006. Available at: http://www.who.int/mediacentre/news/releases/2006/pr02/en/. Accessed May 15, 2009.

14. Gaul GM, Flaherty MP. U.S. prescription drug system under attack: multibillion dollar shadow market is growing stronger. *The Washington Post.* 2003; Sunday, October 19. Available at: http://www.washingtonpost.com/wp-dyn/content/article/2007/06/28/AR2007062801011_pf.html. Accessed May 15, 2009.

15. U.S. Food and Drug Administration. Combating Counterfeit Drugs: A Report of the Food and Drug Administration. February 2000. Available at: http://www.fda.gov/oc/initiatives/counterfeit/report02_04.pdf. Accessed May 15, 2009.

16. U.S. Food and Drug Administration. Center for Drug Evaluation and Research. FDA Centennial at CDER: the History of Drug Regulation in the United States. Web page available at: http://www.fda.gov/Cder/centennial/history.htm. Accessed May 13, 2009.

17. Institute of Medicine of the National Academies; Committee on Quality of Health Care in America. *To Err Is Human: Building a Safer Health System.* Kohn LT, Corrigan JM, Donaldson MS, eds. Washington, DC: National Academy Press; 2000.

18. Institute of Medicine of the National Academies; Committee on Identifying and Preventing Medication Errors. *Preventing Medication Errors: Quality Chasm Series.* Aspden P, Wolcott JA, Bootman JL, et al., eds. Washington, DC: National Academy Press; 2006.

19. May CD. How Coca-Cola obtains its coca. Business Section; *The New York Times.* Friday, July 1, 1988. Available online at: http://www.nytimes.com/1988/07/01/business/how-coca-cola-obtains-its-coca.html. Accessed May 15, 2009.

20. Brecher EM and Editors of Consumers Reports. Licit and Illicit Drugs: The Consumers Union Report on Narcotics, Stimulants, Depressants, Inhalants, Hallucinogens, and Marijuana – including Caffeine, Nicotine, and Alcohol. Boston, MA: Little Brown & Co.; 1972.

21. World Health Organization. Wastes from health care activities. Fact Sheet no. 253. Reviewed November 2007. Available at: http://www.who.int/mediacentre/factsheets/fs253/en/. Accessed May 15, 2009.

22. Barnes KK, Kolpin DW, Furlong ET, et al. A national reconnaissance of pharmaceuticals and other organic wastewater contaminants in the United States—I. Groundwater. Science of the Total Environment; 2008.

Suggested Readings

Institute of Medicine of the National Academies. Quality Chasm Series, which includes *To Err Is Human: Building a Safer Health System* (2000) and *Preventing Medication Errors* (2006).

This series provides insight into the current issues related to safe medication use.

Sinclair U. *The Jungle.* Doubleday: Page & Co.; 1906.

This novel is available from numerous publishers; it is about the meat packing industry in Chicago around the turn of the 20th century. It has been identified as the primary cause of the public outcry that pushed Congress to pass the 1906 Food and Drug Act to protect the food supply.

Adams SH. The great American fraud, *Collier's*, October 7, 1905. Reprints of several original articles in the series are available at: http://www.museumofquackery.com/ephemera/oct7-01.htm/.

These articles were another important catalyst for the passage of the 1906 Food and Drug Act. They provide great descriptions of patent medicines and practices of the time.

Chapter 4 Review Questions

1. The U.S. Constitution specifies that states are the primary authority for ensuring the health of their citizens. _____ True _____ False

False. The source of authority for state governments to act on behalf of their citizens in health matters comes from inherent police powers retained by the states because the U.S. Constitution did not specifically give that power to the federal government.

2. List situations where the federal government has authority to act on behalf of citizens of all states.

The federal government has authority to regulate any activity or good that involves multiple states or other countries through its regulation of interstate and international trade. In addition, the federal government has the authority to determine how tax dollars are spent, which may include expenditures for public health activities.

3. Give four examples of local or state laws that are used to prevent a potentially dangerous behavior, promote a healthy behavior, or protect a community.

Prevent potentially dangerous behaviors: enforcing speed limits for automobiles, age limits for purchasing tobacco or alcohol, age limits for driving, and requirements for seat belts or helmets.

Promote healthy behaviors: Making vaccination of school children mandatory, using tax dollars to support public health insurance programs, and creating parks and safe walking or bicycling paths.

Protect a community: litter laws and waste disposal regulations and housing ordinances.

4. Describe the public health tragedy that led to the passage of the 1938 Food, Drug, and Cosmetic Act.

The tragedy known as the "Elixir of Sulfanilamide" tragedy of 1937 occurred when a chemist used a kidney-toxic diluent, DEG, to prepare the liquid form of the antibiotic for children. Because the labeling requirements did not include inactive ingredients or diluents, the pharmacists who dispensed the product did know it contained DEG. As a result of its use, about 100 people died of kidney failure. The next year, the federal Food, Drug, and Cosmetic Act of 1938 was passed.

5. Describe emerging issues related to pharmacy services and pharmaceuticals that may lead to future legislation and regulation.

There are several areas of concern, which include ongoing occurrence of medication errors; unregulated business of online, web-based "pharmacies"; increasing number of counterfeit medications created and sold at the international level; decreasing access to quality health care; and a renewed concern with the impact of manufacturing and patient pharmaceutical wastes on the environment.

Applying Your Knowledge

1. Think about laws or local ordinances that you do not like. Discuss how you feel about "criminalizing" a behavior that others consider risky. Finish the discussion by exploring underlying public health issues—how would your behavior impact others?

2. Pick a federal pharmacy law, which was not described in the chapter, and research the public health issues that led to its passage or repeal.

3. Discuss possible methods for addressing the emerging public health issues related to medications and pharmacy practice such as counterfeit medications, online pharmacies, medication errors, and pharmaceutical wastes.

Ethics and Economics in Public Health

Learning Outcomes

1. Describe how the values or principles underlying public health ethics differ from those that form the basis for bioethics.
2. Explain what a professional code of ethics is and how it is used by someone in that profession.
3. List the steps to take for working through an ethical dilemma.
4. Explain why an economic decision should consider immediate and downstream costs and results.
5. List the steps to take for comparing two or more options on an economic basis.

Introduction

Understanding how ethics and economics can guide and impact decision-making and policy formulation in public health can be critical to an understanding of public health priorities, laws, and programs. Because decisions are made at a population (often called societal) level, some of the guiding principles are essentially different from those used in health care to guide decisions made about individual patients. This chapter will begin with an introduction to two different ways of viewing problems and potential solutions: ethics and economics. Using a case that highlights the ethical and economic issues related to injectable drug abuse (IDA) programs, these two important aspects of public health decision-making and policy formulation will be explored. Concepts in ethics and an approach to solving ethical dilemmas will be addressed first, then economic concepts used to guide the use of public funds and resources will be considered. By the end of the chapter, you should be aware of the various implicit ethical and economic arguments or concerns that a public health problem raises and how they should be explicitly considered in a decision or proposed solution.

Role of Ethics and Economics in Public Health Decision-Making

The goal of public health is to ensure "conditions in which people can be healthy."[1] To achieve this goal, public funds are used to create programs, policies, and laws that promote conditions conducive to healthy living. As good stewards of these public funds, national, state, and local health departments often face tough decisions about which programs to fund, where to place efforts to develop new policies or laws, and when to eliminate or remove programs, policies, or laws that

Public health agencies should consider ethical and economic aspects of issues and proposed programs to ensure that they are serving the best interest of the community and its residents as well as being good stewards of public funds.

no longer serve their purpose. The decision process used to reach conclusions should be informed by ethical and economic considerations as well as scientific data (i.e., population or epidemiological data). The best way to apply ethical or economic reasoning to a public health issue is to make the assumptions and concepts as transparent and explicit as possible so others can clearly see how that reasoning affected the final decision. This requires an increased personal awareness of the ethical and economic concepts that guide decision-making.

Figure 5.1—Intravenous methamphetamine abusers are at an increased risk of infection with HIV, in part, from sharing dirty needles.

Source: Corbis Corporation.

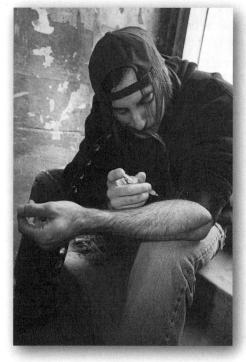

Substance abuse as a public health problem

In 2007, almost one in two (46%) people said they had used an illicit drug at least once in their lifetime, and one in 12 (8%) had used an illicit drug at least once within the past month.[2]

It has been estimated that 12 million (4.9%) Americans age 12 years or older tried **methamphetamine** at least once in their lives, and 600,000 (0.2%) had used it during the past month.[3] Rates of methamphetamine abuse are tracked in various ways through **self-report surveys**, emergency room admissions data, arrests and law enforcement data, and reported causes of death. All methamphetamine abusers are at an increased risk of infection with HIV in part from sharing dirty needles, but primarily from dangerous sexual behavior like not using condoms or having multiple partners (Figure 5.1). Studies have shown a two-fold or greater increase in risk from dangerous sexual behavior.[4] Outbreaks of hepatitis A and B have occurred in methamphetamine users, resulting in several hundred cases and some deaths; long-term injectors of methamphetamine also have a higher risk of exposure to the hepatitis C virus. Other health risks that appear to be greater in the methamphetamine-abusing populations include violent behavior and abuse of other illicit drugs.[4]

The burden of methamphetamine abuse in the United States was estimated at around 900 deaths and the loss of over 44,000 **quality-adjusted life years (QALYs)** in 2005.[5] Cost of the consequences created by methamphetamine abuse was estimated to be between $16 to $48 billion dollars. This estimate includes **costs** to society that are associated with drug treatment, health care, premature death, intangible costs of being addicted, **lost productivity**, crime, child endangerment and, in the case of meth labs, damage to the environment.[5]

 CASE STUDY 1

Ethical and economic issues associated with injected methamphetamine

Although the characters and community are fictitious, the issues are real and continue to be a source of conflict and confusion for pharmacists and public health officers alike. This case includes many details that are not pleasant, but do reflect behaviors frequently employed by those who have an addiction disease. Because ethical issues are explored, it is important to be both aware of your own beliefs and be open-minded to those of others.

Ethan abuses methamphetamine

Ethan is a young man in his 20s who currently has a methamphetamine habit that requires using the drug twice a day to avoid withdrawal symptoms. Although he may appear relatively normal to the casual observer because he is still employed at a local grocery store, has his own apartment, and dresses relatively well, Ethan has tell-tale signs that his addiction is beginning to wear down his body and mind.

Ethan was not always an addict. In fact, he used to be quite athletic and an excellent student. Those who knew him in high school predicted he would become a successful businessman after being a star of the state college's track and field team. He was a good-looking young man with a serious girlfriend and a no-nonsense approach to schoolwork. He was well known for his risky behaviors, and he always enjoyed pushing his physical limits through hang gliding and motorcycle racing. His family, very religious and hardworking, was one of the "good families" in town. Because he was bright, no one noticed signs of stress and then addiction during his junior year of high school. Ethan had not intended to become an addict—he would later say, "It just sort of happened."

Ethan had experimented with beer and marijuana several times in his sophomore year of high school. The experiences had been fun, and he did not suffer any long-term effects. He could party at night and go out and win a race or hang glide without any problem. He even avoided temptations to take supplements to increase his athletic prowess in track. The problem for Ethan began one Friday night when he had just broken up with his longtime girlfriend, and his buddies took him to a party where he could meet other girls and forget his troubles. While drinking his beer, a nice-looking girl who was a senior at the school offered Ethan her meth pipe and asked him if he wanted to try it. He did, and the drug-induced mania made him feel invincible. He was awake for almost 24 hours talking and getting physically close to his new friend. By Saturday night, the euphoric effects finally ended and he crashed so badly that he could not function.

The experience led him to seek more of the drug. Ethan was one of those individuals whose physiology was altered with the first dose. As his **dopamine** stores depleted, his cravings grew and grew until all he could think about was how to get that next dose. As much as he tried, he could not replicate that first high. After a while, he sought the drug merely to avoid withdrawal because in addition to his addictive behavior, he was physically dependent. He quickly learned that injecting meth would ease his symptoms much faster than smoking, so he became quite adept at using syringes and needles.

Ethan exposes himself and others to hepatitis and HIV

In pursuing the next dose of meth, Ethan would often share syringe and needle setups with others. Sometimes, he would dig through garbage cans at homes of people he knew had diabetes to find used syringes or needles. Since the needles remained sharp with several uses, he could re-use them several times. Through his job as a clerk at a pharmacy, he had once stolen a packet of 1-cc insulin syringes but discovered that the short needles were not long enough for intravenous injections. He was fired from the job shortly thereafter because his work performance had slipped and he was constantly not showing up for his shifts. So, he was content to use the same syringe and needle repeatedly and share it with others since it was difficult to get new ones.

Ethan also found that he could trade sexual favors for meth. Since he was a good-looking young man, he was quite successful in finding "dates." Ethan was not homosexual, but he tolerated the advances of other men because his sole purpose in life was to obtain more meth. Most of his male partners did not use condoms, but Ethan was not too concerned about it. He was focused solely on getting his meth; once he had it, he quickly forgot what he had to do to get it. Ethan supplemented his meth funds with stolen property that he took from unlocked cars and purses he found unattended in shopping carts at local stores.

Ethical Issues in Health Care and Public Health

This case shows there are risks to Ethan's personal health and well-being as well as risks to others in the community. In determining the best course of action to take in addressing the various issues, decision-makers will be guided by their underlying personal and professional values. Because the underlying value systems in health care and public health do not align completely, most situations can be viewed in different ways. This can lead to different approaches in addressing the same situation. One of the most apparent differences between the health care and public health value systems is how individuals, their community, and the relationship among them are viewed. These different values can be seen in a review of the underlying principles of **bioethics** (the **ethics** of medicine and health care) and public health ethics.

First, a definition of ethics is in order. Ethics is the branch of philosophy concerned with human values of right and wrong (i.e., morals) and how those values manifest in decisions and behaviors by individuals or entire groups of people. Ethics may also refer to a set of rules or principles intended to guide behaviors or decisions; for example, professions have **Codes of Ethics** that their practitioners are expected to uphold.[6] The underlying values or ethics that guide the development of programs or policy are often not explicitly stated and must be inferred from the manner in which the program or policy will affect the individual, the environment, and the community. For example, a bicycle safety program that allows patients to voluntarily choose to wear helmets to reduce their risk of a serious head wound would seem to favor autonomy of the individual over a reduction in avoidable head trauma. For both public health and health care, several major ethical principles can be identified and they tend to come from bioethics and human rights traditions.

Guiding principles for health care work and research

Bioethical principles lay the foundation for the medical and health professions. Over the years, these guiding principles have increasingly emphasized the individual's free will and control of his or her own body and personal information. Bioethics consists of four main ideas or principles that frame the codes of ethics for professional behavior and responsible human subjects' research: non-maleficence, beneficence, respect for autonomy, and justice.

Non-Maleficence

This value can be loosely translated as "do no harm." This may be one of the oldest principles of bioethics. It emphasizes taking appropriate steps to avoid negative results when working with others. As a guiding ethical principle, it makes clear that actions in health services and research should not create new illness or injury. In a clinical practice or a public health program, this principle means using interventions that have been tested and shown to be safe and effective (i.e., evidence-based practice). In research in medicine and public health, this would mean minimizing risks from dangers posed by the unknown.

Beneficence

This principle focuses on the positive aspect of providing treatments or intervention that will be beneficial to others. Unlike the first principle that advises avoiding injury, this principle tells practitioners to act in a manner that will leave their patients in a better state than the one they were in prior to the intervention or treatment.

Respect for Autonomy

This bioethical principle focuses on the rights of the individual to retain control of his or her own body and personal information. Within this principle, one finds the right of a patient to refuse treatment; the need to tell patients the truth about a treatment, including potentially bad outcomes (i.e., informed consent); the right of privacy and confidentiality of medical information; honesty; and the right to noninterference (i.e., others cannot impose their will upon the patient or make the patient do something he or she does not want to do). This principle usually refers to the patient or research subject, and not to the practitioner or researcher.

Justice

The fourth bioethics principle focuses on the equity of access to resources in care and participation in research. In biomedical research, this principle refers to how subjects may be included or excluded from participating in the study while in clinical care and public health. This principle refers to how resources are distributed and who has access to them. For resources that are abundant, equity can be achieved rather easily. But, such abundance is not usually found. Situations are typically encountered where funding is not sufficient to support all programs for all people, so some method for equitably dividing the limited funds or resources is needed.

Bioethics principles

Ethan's situation, when viewed as a medical or health care ethical issue, will focus on whether he has control over his person (autonomy) when he is addicted to methamphetamine. The bioethics principles will want any intervention that is implemented to respect that autonomy, so it will probably be voluntary, not mandatory, and will promote the beneficial effects of abstaining from further methamphetamine use. An intervention such as a **needle exchange program** where **injectable drug abusers** can exchange used "dirty" needles for clean ones may be considered unethical from a bioethics point of view since it potentially enables the addict to continue using a drug that is known to be harmful, thus violating the non-maleficence (do no harm) principle. This underlying value system can be inferred from comments about how a needle exchange program will "promote more injected drug use" and "fails to help the patient overcome his or her addiction."

Guiding principles for public health work and research

Because the principles of bioethics focus on the individual, they are usually not comprehensive enough to serve as ethical guides for public health decisions that need to consider the community as well as the individual. For this reason, the concepts within human rights, which look at the many factors that can affect dignity and freedom, have become part of the public health ethics perspective. The connection between health and human rights has its modern origins in the **1948 Universal Declaration of Human Rights**.[7] Unlike bioethics, which emphasizes the individual, a human rights approach takes a broad view of the treatment of individuals in a larger society. This approach recognizes that many factors including social and economic ones can impact health and that the government has a responsibility to ensure those rights are protected.[5] The human rights approach recognizes the interdependence of people with their environment and community as well as the need for governments to exercise appropriate use of their powers to promote conditions in which health is possible. Three general categories of values have been identified as the foundation of public health ethics: health, community, and bases for action.[8]

Health

The belief that all humans have the right to the resources necessary for health is one cornerstone of the values underlying the public health ethics. It coincides directly with the Universal Declaration of Human Rights. This value emphasizes the outcome of health for everyone, not the equal distribution of resources.[8]

Community

Six key values comprise this category. First, people are inherently social and interdependent. A sign of a health community is the presence of positive relationships between people and institutions. There is also a need to balance the right of the individuals against the fact that a person's action can affect others.

Second, the effectiveness of institutions is heavily dependent on the public's trust. Actions that promote that trust include two-way communication (listening to the needs of the people as well as providing information), honesty, sharing of information, accountability for actions and words, and reliability.

Third, collaboration is a key function of public health. To be effective, public health endeavors will require many different agencies and professions. As new issues and challenges arise in public health, new partners will be needed.

Fourth, people and their environment are interdependent. This is a reciprocal relationship because people benefit from an environment rich with resources needed to sustain healthy life, and the environment benefits from good stewardship by the people who use it.

Fifth, each person in a community should have the opportunity to contribute to discussions about public matters. Although a final policy, law, or program may not address all concerns voiced by community members, all concerns should be given a chance to be aired during the planning process.

Sixth, a primary concern for public health should be identifying and promoting the basic requirements for health in the community. Because the manner in which a society is structured is reflected in the health of the community, public health must be concerned with the structural influences that cause disease and poor health. So, in addition to providing care for those who are sick, public health should seek out and prevent those underlying causes.

Bases for Action

Within this category, four beliefs describing the need for fact-based action are found. The first belief addresses the power and importance of knowledge in terms of our need to discover new knowledge (research) and share it with others. There is also a moral obligation to protect information that is confidential, such as patient information.

Another basis for action in public health is the use of the scientific method to gather objective data about the factors affecting health. This does not conflict with the community value of giving everyone an opportunity to voice concerns. Rather, this belief will complement that information and, together, form a more complete picture of community health and needs.

Action must be taken once people have knowledge of a need or cause of disease. Knowledge of a public health problem creates a moral obligation to take action to correct it, and this should be done in a timely manner. Sometimes the required action is additional research to better understand the situation and inform the response.

Finally, other reasons cause us to act and they should not be delayed because of a lack of information. Two situations illustrate where this can occur: 1) when the value and dignity of individuals is deemed to be a greater obligation than achieving optimal efficiency or **cost-effectiveness**, and 2) when action cannot be delayed because of imminent risk or danger.[8]

A comparison of health care (bioethics) and public health reveals that both prize the dignity of the individual, but public health values also consider the interaction of individuals with one another, their environment, and community.

Professional Codes of Ethics

To communicate their core values and beliefs, professions will often use public statements such as mission statements, codes of ethics, or guidelines to explicitly communicate how they will view and consider issues. These public statements serve as guidance for the practitioners as well as information for those who will be affected by the decisions. While rigid adherence to guidelines or codes of ethics is not always possible, these formal declarations can provide a starting point for discussions of an issue.[6]

Code of ethics for pharmacists

The first **code of ethics** for pharmacists was created in the late 1800s. Since then, it has been revised numerous times with the most current version approved in 1994.[9] Like many health care professions, the code of ethics for pharmacy incorporates the four bioethics principles along with being truthful and honest (i.e., veracity), meeting commitments and maintaining competence (i.e., fidelity), and respecting confidentiality and privacy.[9] Confidentiality refers to information, while privacy refers to a person; both terms describe limiting access and keeping personal information private. Figure 5.2 shows the 1994 Code of Ethics for Pharmacists.

The professional code of ethics for public health practice indicates an underlying value in finding a balance among the rights of the individual, the needs of the community, the protection of the environment, and the interdependence of these things.

Principles of the ethical practice of public health

In 2002, the first code of ethics for public health practice was approved. It formalized the values that had been used for years by public health practitioners. It went beyond the bioethical principles to include human rights principles and recognize the interdependence of humans, the environment, and the community. Table 5.1 shows public health's first code of ethics.[8]

Figure 5.2—Code of Ethics for Pharmacists (1994)

Source: APhA web site at http://www.pharmacist.com.

A *pharmacist* respects the covenantal relationship between the patient and pharmacist.

A *pharmacist* promotes the good of every patient in a caring, compassionate, and confidential manner.

A *pharmacist* respects the autonomy and dignity of each patient.

A *pharmacist* acts with honesty and integrity in professional relationships.

A *pharmacist* maintains professional competence.

A *pharmacist* respects the values and abilities of colleagues and other health professionals.

A *pharmacist* serves individual, community, and societal needs.

A *pharmacist* seeks justice in the distribution of health resources.

Table 5.1

Principles of the Ethical Practice of Public Health, v.2.2 (2002)

1. Public health should address principally the fundamental causes of disease and requirements for health, aiming to prevent adverse health outcomes.

2. Public health should achieve community health in a way that respects the rights of individuals in the community.

3. Public health policies, programs, and priorities should be developed and evaluated through processes that ensure an opportunity for input from community members.

4. Public health should advocate and work for the empowerment of disenfranchised community members, aiming to ensure that the basic resources and conditions necessary for health are accessible to all.

5. Public health should seek the information needed to implement effective policies and programs that protect and promote health.

6. Public health institutions should provide communities with the information they have that is needed for decisions on policies or programs and should obtain the community's consent for their implementation.

7. Public health institutions should act in a timely manner on the information they have within the resources and the mandate given to them by the public.

8. Public health programs and policies should incorporate a variety of approaches that anticipate and respect diverse values, beliefs, and cultures in the community.

9. Public health programs and policies should be implemented in a manner that most enhances the physical and social environment.

10. Public health institutions should protect the confidentiality of information that can bring harm to an individual or community if made public. Exceptions must be justified on the basis of the high likelihood of significant harm to the individual or others.

11. Public health institutions should ensure the professional competence of their employees.

12. Public health institutions and their employees should engage in collaborations and affiliations in ways that build the public's trust and the institution's effectiveness.

Source: http://www.phls.org.

CASE STUDY 1 (*continued*)

Economic principles

In Ethan's community, a task force has been assembled to collect information about the "meth problem" and determine a course of action that will reduce its impact on the town. Although Ethan will not be able to voice his opinions directly, he will be represented on the task force by two recovering meth abusers and by the information gathered from a sample of current meth users. The task force membership represents a diverse group of agencies and disciplines including law enforcement, health department personnel, local health care providers, mental health and substance abuse specialists, clergy, and recovering addicts. After gathering information about the scope of the problem, they are convinced that action is necessary to address the most pressing issue—a sudden increase in the number of new cases of HIV and hepatitis C in young adults using meth.

Their initial cordiality and goodwill is running thin as they discover they have some fundamental differences of opinion about what is an appropriate action. These differences became apparent as they discussed the possibility of creating a needle exchange program. Some task force members supported this approach because research showed it was a cost-effective method for reducing the spread of blood-borne disease. The health care representatives were opposed to it because it would facilitate future abuse of the meth, which would have its own deleterious effects on the health of the young adults. They wanted to consider a mandatory **abstinence program** to help end the use of meth because addiction is a disease. The substance abuse specialist argued that a mandatory program would backfire because, although addiction is a disease, changing behavior will require having a person who is at least willing to try to end the addiction. Needless to say, the meeting ended without a plan and much acrimony. The task force chair decided to seek help with mediating all these different opinions at the next meeting.

Steps for Working through an Ethical Dilemma

A group of individuals from a diverse array of disciplines will often discover that they do not share the same fundamental values. In the case study, their differences indicated the presence of an ethical dilemma that had to be resolved in order to move forward as a group towards a course of action. When more than one value system is involved in a decision-making process, an ethical dilemma is bound to arise. A series of steps for resolving **ethical dilemmas** can be used to identify the various value systems. The steps described by Slomka and colleagues is presented here.[6]

Identify the ethical issue

First, it is important to identify the ethical issue and who is affected by it. This requires an awareness of your own values and an ability to listen to others who may hold different values. Since people do not usually speak in terms of their underlying values, this information has to be inferred from their opinions or suggestions about how to resolve a problem.

Collect data and information

After the issue has been identified, you should gather information about the issue under consideration. For a public health issue, this may include ensuring that all affected populations are found, the scope of the problem is determined, impacts on health and risks to health are known, and options for action are uncovered. This step may also involve seeking information about costs, sources of power, and the various value systems of the different groups. So, data collection and analysis is the second step.

Frame the issue

The third step will be to frame the issue in a manner that makes potentially conflicting values more explicit. This is where the various approaches to ethics such as philosophical or social justice can be used to see where values lie. An example of this third step would be a public health program of mandatory HPV vaccination of all teenage girls to reduce risk of cervical cancer, which values long-term community benefit over individual choice. This approach may be opposed by their parents who believe they should make all medical choices for their children or by the teenaged girls themselves because they are not sexually active. Both of these approaches appear to value individual autonomy regardless of long-term consequences. Other community members may push for a sexual education program that promotes abstinence, which is another approach that values individual autonomy over community need; still others believe teens will experiment with sex, so the best approach is education about barrier methods and free condoms because they value the reduction in spread of disease and long-term risks to health in the community.

Consider various options

Once the issue has been framed in a manner that makes the values clear, the next step is to consider the various options and consider their potential impact. When framed as a public health issue, options to consider are often a balancing act between respecting individual rights and promoting the community's welfare. In the example involving HPV vaccine, the public health goals of reducing incidence of HPV infection and subsequent incidence of cervical cancer are paramount. Considerations about whether teens are having premarital sex are not part of this particular decision. An additional part of this step is to clearly describe the values underlying the decision so when it is presented to the community, the reasoning is as transparent as possible.

Implement the chosen option

After identifying a solution that appears to be justified by public health ethics, it may be implemented. Implementation is the fifth step. At this point, it would be advisable to consider the economic ramifications of the approach selected and to consider whether other approaches would achieve similar or better results with less cost.

Evaluate process and new program

Once implemented, a new policy or program should be evaluated to see whether it is achieving the intended goal and whether any unanticipated ethical issues have

emerged. The new program or policy is not the only thing that should be evaluated. In public health, where public funds are used on behalf of the community, the decision-making process itself should be evaluated. Evaluation of the process and new program or policy is the sixth and final step.[6]

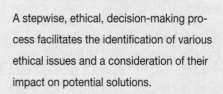

A stepwise, ethical, decision-making process facilitates the identification of various ethical issues and a consideration of their impact on potential solutions.

 CASE STUDY 1 (*continued*)

Steps for resolving an ethical dilemma associated with injected methamphetamine

At the next meeting of the task force, the team members met another community member who had agreed to walk them through the steps used to resolve ethical dilemmas. He had some training in medical ethics (bioethics) and lots of experience on the local hospital ethics board. He began by explaining the steps they would use to help each other see their respective points of view or values and then use that information to seek common ground and move them towards an action plan.

Task force members learned that they each valued the individuals' rights to be treated with dignity, but differed on the extent to which they thought someone with an addiction could make an appropriate decision about his or her health. Almost everyone agreed that stopping the spread of infectious disease was important in this population and that the issue could be considered separately from the question of addiction. One person sheepishly admitted that he had come to the task force thinking that addicts were bad people who deserved to die from infection or overdose. He told the other member that he had changed his mind after talking to Bill and Joan, the two recovering addicts who had shared their stories with the group. Now that he saw meth-addicted members of the community as people, he was more aware of their rights and need for respect.

After finding some shared values and articulating others that were not, the group agreed to move forward with the needle exchange program as long as one of its roles would be to provide information about how to access voluntary substance abuse rehabilitation services in the community. The scope of the program would depend on where it was conducted and the availability of funds and personnel.

Importance of Economic Issues in Public Health

The need for economic decision-making in public health exists because there are not enough resources (i.e., money, time, materials) available to do everything that is needed. As a result, decisions about where and when to expend funds or time must be made. As stewards of public funds, public health agencies seek ways to optimize results they get for the resources expended. This process is often described as looking for the most cost-effective approach or weighing the costs and benefits of various options. Full descriptions of the methods used to conduct the various economic analyses that compare alternatives can be found in other textbooks, so the following information will focus only on several key concepts related to those methods.

As discussed earlier in this chapter, some actions may need to be taken regardless of the economic consequence because they are simply the right thing to do. However, most of the time, finding the optimal and most cost-effective approach will be the preferred one.

Key economic principles

Actions and Subsequent Consequences

First, remember that any action or intervention will create consequences; second, some consequences are likely to require additional resources (i.e., costs). When comparing programs or considering total costs of a single program, it is important to consider all the costs that occur as a result of the program and not just the initial costs. For example, a public health influenza vaccination program may have high initial costs because of all of the vaccine used and personnel time to administer it, but later costs associated with treating those who get sick will be avoided. If this vaccination program is compared to a "no vaccination program," those later costs associated with people who get the flu, require treatment, and miss work will help to show that the initial costs of a vaccination program can reduce or even prevent later costs associated with getting the flu. Cost is a term that refers to any resource consumed as part of the initial intervention or any subsequent event that requires more resources. Those resources may be raw materials, products, and someone's time as measured in monetary terms.

Limited Resources

Economic decision-making, another key concept, means that decisions have to be made about how to use the resources when those resources are scarce. Naturally, decision-makers will want to use those scarce resources on programs or interventions that will produce optimal results for the resources expended. Obtaining optimal results will mean finding that point where using additional resources does not produce enough of an additional result to make it worthwhile using those resources.

Perspective of the Analysis

Another concept to consider is the effect that the perspective (i.e., point of view) has on any economic decision-making process. For public health, the decision will usually be very broad, encompassing a societal point of view. This means the economic analysis will include costs (i.e., resources consumed) that are directly related to either treating a condition or caused by a condition as well as costs related indirectly to the condition that reduce a person's productivity. Intangible costs may also be considered if fear or emotions are key parts of the problem being addressed.

Types of Economic Analyses

Several types of economic analyses may be seen in public health decision-making. **Cost benefit analysis (CBA)** has been used extensively in decisions about where to use public funds since it allows comparison of very different and diverse programs. Because the final results of each program are measured in dollars, they can be compared. For example, a CBA could be used to compare an adult influenza vaccination program with a children's nutrition program. By converting the outcomes produced by each program into dollars, decision-makers can decide which one produces the most benefit (i.e., cost savings) for the resources used.

A second type of analysis is a **cost-effectiveness analysis (CEA)**. This method differs from a CBA in that the results or outcomes are measured in natural units like number of cures or lives saved rather than monetary terms. This means a CEA can only compare interventions that produce the same type of outcome.

Another type of analysis that can be used when the outcome is focused on preferences or other quality-oriented result is called a **cost utility analysis (CUA)**. One of its most frequently used outcomes is the **quality-adjusted life year (QALY)**, which combines length of life with level of quality of life into a single number. Also, **cost-of-illness (COI) studies** are conducted when the costs of a disease or condition are needed in order to determine the magnitude of the problem and set policy or research funding priorities.

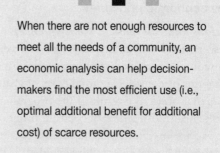

When there are not enough resources to meet all the needs of a community, an economic analysis can help decision-makers find the most efficient use (i.e., optimal additional benefit for additional cost) of scarce resources.

A framework for considering the economic impact of a program

Like ethical decision-making, economic decision-making can be made easier by following a stepwise framework. The following steps are adapted from a more detailed 10-step checklist used to review pharmacoeconomics literature or conduct an analysis.[10]

Frame the Question

The first step involves framing the question and setting the approach that will be used. This step will include deciding which type of analysis should be used, length of time over which the programs will be compared, and perspective of the analysis (usually societal for a public health question).

Identify Relevant Alternatives

In the second step, the alternative interventions that will be compared are identified, and the important cost and downstream event variables are determined. Deciding what will be measured as the outcome is determined at this step.

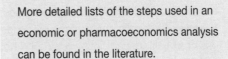

More detailed lists of the steps used in an economic or pharmacoeconomics analysis can be found in the literature.

Determine the Monetary Values

Step three involves placing values on the costs (resources), downstream events, and outcome. For the downstream events, their likelihood of occurring with either a weight or probability is also considered.

Perform an Initial Analysis

In the fourth step, an initial comparison will be performed. If more than two options are available, an incremental analysis can be conducted to review the additional costs for additional results.

Test the Robustness of the Initial Results

The fifth step will test the robustness of the initial results by varying the value of cost or event variables to determine whether uncertainty in estimating their value will affect the initial results. This is accomplished either through the use of variance, if the analysis is statistical in nature, or through one or more sensitivity analyses if the analysis uses probabilities instead.

Interpret Results and Select Alternative

The final step is interpreting the results of the analysis to make a determination about which program best optimizes the use of resources. This is often the program that produces the most overall benefit without the additional costs exceeding the additional benefits achieved.

CASE STUDY 1 (continued)

Resolution of ethical and economic issues associated with injected methamphetamine

Ethan heard clean needles were available through two local pharmacies and the health department. Apparently he could turn in used needles and receive new clean ones. He hesitated at first because he wondered if it was just another rumor or a way for the police to identify meth users. When Carl, an outreach worker from the health department, confirmed that it was a new program and that its purpose was to reduce the spread of infectious disease and not catch users, Ethan decided to check it out.

Ethan went to a small pharmacy near his apartment after discovering that his old employer's store was not one of the pharmacies participating in the program. He was pleasantly surprised by how kind and respectful the technician and pharmacist were when he requested a pack of clean needles. They did not preach to him about the virtues of quitting—always a turn off. They did let him know they had information about rehab programs that he could use when he was ready to quit. Ethan knew he would want to quit someday, but he just couldn't face doing so now.

From the community perspective, the needle exchange program appeared to be most effective in reducing the number of new hepatitis C cases and moderately effective in reducing the incidence of HIV. So far, only one person voluntarily sought rehab services, and it was too early to know if the rehab would be successful. Because the two local pharmacies volunteered to participate, the costs of the program were purchase of needles and syringes and use of a health department worker for 8 hours of outreach each week. Based on these initial results, the city planned to continue the program for at least 2 more years.

Chapter 5 Summary

Decision-making in public health should involve consideration of ethical and economic issues. For ethical decision-making, you can use the public health code of ethics as a guide for framing the issues and working through potential ethical dilemmas created by proposed programs or policies. Because public health agencies are tasked with using public funds wisely and efficiently, decisions to implement new programs or policies should also consider the immediate and future economic impacts. These two separate processes can be used to help decision-makers gain a more complete understanding of the issues and the impact that a new program will have in the community. As our case of the methamphetamine abusers illustrated, finding a solution is often a balancing act between what is best for an individual and what is best for the community.

References

1. Committee for the Study of the Future of Public Health, Division of Health Care Services, Institute of Medicine, The Future of Public Health. Washington, DC: National Academy Press; 1988:7.

2. SAMHSA Table 1.11B—Illicit Drug Use in Lifetime, Past Year, and Past Month, by Detailed Age Category: Percentages, 2006 and 2007. Available at: http://www.oas.samhsa.gov/nsduh.htm. Accessed February 5, 2009.

3. Centers for Disease Control and Prevention, CDC HIV/AIDS Fact Sheet: Methamphetamine Use and Risk for HIV/AIDS. Updated January 2007. Available at: http://www.cdc.gov/hiv. Accessed February 5, 2009.

4. Vogt TM, Perz JF, Van Houten Jr CK, et al. An outbreak of hepatitis B virus infection among methamphetamine injectors: the role of sharing injection drug equipment. *Addict.* 2006; 101(5):726–30.

5. Nicosia N, Pacula RL, Kilmer B, et al. The economic cost of methamphetamine use in the United States, 2005. RAND Drug Policy Research Center. Santa Monica, CA: RAND Corporation; 2008.

6. Slomka J, Quill B, DesVignes-Kendrick M, et al. Professionalism and ethics in the public health curriculum. *Public Health Reports.* 2008; 123:27–35.

7. United Nations 1948 Universal Declaration of Human Rights. Available at: http://www.un.org/Overview/rights.html. Accessed February 9, 2009.

8. Public Health Leadership Society, Principles of the Ethical Practice of Public Health, version 2.2 (2002). Available at: http://www.phls.org/products.htm. Accessed December 10, 2008.

9. American Pharmacists Association. Code of Ethics for Pharmacists (1994). Available at: http://www.pharmacist.com/AM/Template.cfm?Section=Code_of_Ethics_for_Pharmacists&Template=/CM/HTMLDisplay.cfm&ContentID=5420. Accessed February 9, 2009.

10. Drummond MF, Obrien BJ, Stoddart GL, et al. *Methods for the Economic Evaluation of Health Care Programmes,* 2nd ed. Oxford University Press; 1997.

Suggested Readings

Kass NE. Public health ethics: from foundations and frameworks to justice and global public health. *J Law Med Ethics.* 2004; 32:232–42.

Principles of the Ethical Practice of Public Health. New Orleans, LA: Public Health Leadership Society; 2002. Available at: http://www.phls.org/products.htm.

Nicosia N, Pacula RL, Kilmer B, et al. The economic cost of methamphetamine use in the United States, 2005. RAND Drug Policy Research Center. Santa Monica, CA: RAND Corporation; 2008.

Chapter 5 Review Questions

1. Describe how the values or principles underlying public health ethics differ from those that form the basis for bioethics.

A key difference between the underlying values that form the ethics for health care versus public health is whether the focus is on the individual or on the balance of benefits and risks among the individual, the environment, and the community.

2. Explain what a professional code of ethics is and how it is used by someone in that profession.

A professional code of ethics explicitly states the underlying values that a practitioner in that profession is expected to use. It can serve as a guide for professional decision-making in matters that have an ethical component and provide society with a description of how ethical issues will be framed and considered by that profession.

3. List the steps to take for working through an ethical dilemma.

(1) Identify the ethical issue and who is affected by it;

(2) Collect data and information about the issue;

(3) Frame the issue in a manner that makes underlying values explicit;

(4) Consider various options or responses and consider their potential impact;

(5) Implement the chosen response or option; and

(6) Evaluate the process of decision making as well as the effectiveness of the implemented option.

4. Explain why an economic decision should consider immediate and downstream costs and results.

To determine the true cost of a program or policy, it is important to consider upfront costs and all additional resource use created by the implementation of the program or choice. Options that appear to cost less up front may not be as effective as more costly options. That lack of effectiveness will likely produce additional costs later. To be as fully informed as possible, it is helpful to know about the future or downstream costs as part of the total financial picture. A full analysis will also weigh the outcomes or benefits against the cost.

5. List the steps to take for comparing two or more options on an economic basis.
  (1) Frame the question and determine which type of analysis will be conducted and which perspective will be used;
  (2) Identify relevant alternatives to be compared and their associated costs and downstream events they may cause;
  (3) Determine the monetary value of the costs and appropriate measurements for the outcomes;
  (4) Perform an initial analysis comparing the alternatives. Determine which option produces the greatest total benefit without the additional costs becoming greater than the additional benefit;
  (5) Test the robustness of the initial analysis by a sensitivity analysis; and
  (6) Interpret results of the analyses and select the most cost-effective option.

Applying Your Knowledge

1. **It is important to remember that each practitioner in health care or public health may have a set of values that are not in complete alignment with their professional ethics. Consider the ethical dilemma of the pharmacist who refuses to fill an emergency contraception order because it conflicts with his or her personal beliefs. How would this issue be viewed as a health care dilemma? A public health dilemma? Use the codes of ethics to frame the issues and the steps in solving an ethical dilemma to organize your discussion.**

2. **Look in the literature for an economic study of a public health intervention. Discuss how the authors applied the steps in conducting an economic analysis and interpret their results. Would their results apply to your community?**

PART two

Concepts and Tools of Public Health Policy

In this part of the book, the reader is exposed to the tools of public health. Chapter 6 describes all the factors that affect the health of a community that go beyond the patient factors we focus on in pharmacy. Because communities reflect their populations, Chapter 7 looks at practical approaches to cultural issues in public health. Chapters 8 and 9 provide complementary discussions about improving health and preventing disease, respectively. Chapter 10 looks at epidemiology, the science of public health, which is used to describe health and disease in populations; Chapter 11 focuses on methods to describe populations in terms of their health. The last chapter delineates the steps used to identify public health issues and appropriate interventions in a community.

Throughout this section, detailed case studies are used to provide examples and demonstrate applications of the various tools and methods of public health inquiry and intervention. After completing the chapters in this section, the reader should be able to recognize public health activities in his or her community and interpret results of program evaluations or research in which these methods are used.

CHAPTER 6

Determinants of Health

Learning Outcomes

1. Within an ecological framework, define health determinant.
2. Explain how the interaction of a person with his or her environment can positively or negatively affect health.
3. Identify health determinants at the level of the individual, the community, the state or nation, and at the global level.
4. Describe primary care and essential medications.
5. Define life expectancy and infant mortality rate.

Introduction

Public health is aimed at improving health and preventing illness. This chapter describes those factors, known as health determinants, which influence health and prevent illness. The chapter begins with a case study of two residents in one urban area but who live in different countries (one in the United States and the other in Mexico); the residents and their families experience some similar and some different health issues. The purpose of this chapter is to describe some of the differences and similarities in health between the two countries and then to explore why the differences or similarities exist. First, indicators are described that can be used to compare the health of the two populations; then, population health determinants are identified and compared between the two countries.

Health determinants are systematically examined by levels; the first level is that of the person, the second level is the community in which the person lives, the third level is the state and national environment, and the fourth level is the global environment. Because factors in the environment are considered in addition to individual health issues, this approach is considered an ecological perspective of public health. In general, the ecological approach is much broader and examines many factors outside the individual that might be related to health. The chapter ends with a discussion about the implications of an ecological framework in identifying health determinants for the role of pharmacists in public health.

Health in the Context of the U.S.–Mexico Border

The United States and Mexico share a border for 1952 miles along the U.S. states of Texas, New Mexico, Arizona, and California and the Mexican states of Tamaulipas, Nuevo Leon, Coahuila de Zaragoza, Chihuahua, Sonora, and Baja California. The border region shares environmental, social, economic, cultural, and epidemiological features and a population that lives and works on both sides of the border.[1] Americans commute to work in the assembly plants (known as maquiladoras) on the Mexican side of the border, while Mexicans commute to work in fields, restaurants, and hotels on the American side of the border. However, residents can have different health issues depending on their residence on one side of the border or the other.

CASE STUDY 1

Differences in health across the U.S.–Mexico border

Joe — an average person in the United States

Joe is a 36-year-old, overweight male who lives with his wife and two children. Joe works for a local wholesale food distributor; he earns about $42,000 a year. Joe's wife also is employed as a clerk in a local store, but her earnings are about minimum wage. However, she will be able to work more this year because both children will be in school. Joe and his wife both graduated from high school; his wife was going to go to college, but decided to get married instead. Joe's parents are both living. Although Joe's father has heart disease, he takes several medications and watches his diet. Joe's parents visit in the winter, but they live primarily in the Midwest. Joe doesn't worry much about his health or even the well-being of his family because they seem fairly healthy, and he has insurance through his job if they need it. His children get the usual childhood illnesses, colds, and flu, but otherwise they have been in good health.

Joe lives in Nogales, Arizona, which is on the border between the United States and Mexico. Joe's house is small as it has only two bedrooms. The house is older so its wiring has a tendency to go out, and the house continually needs repairs. Other than those minor problems, Joe and his family like the house and where they live. The family can look across the border into Mexico from their back patio and enjoy crossing the border to eat.

Jose — an average person in Mexico

Jose is a 26-year-old male who is married with two small children. The family is expecting another child. Jose works in an assembly plant and earns about $11,000 (in U.S. dollars) a year; his wife does not work in a salaried position, although she helps in her mother's herbaria when she is able. Jose and his wife both completed school through the sixth grade; neither was able to attend high school as the fees were too great. Jose worries about both his wife and his unborn child because he remembers his aunt and her baby who both died during childbirth. He worries about his other two children too; they are small for their age and have a tendency to develop diarrhea or respiratory infections, even though they usually recover quickly. Jose's father died when he was 50 from a heart attack. His mother is living but she has diabetes. Jose and his family, including his mother, have access to health care provided through his work site.

Jose lives in Nogales, Sonora, Mexico. Jose's house is small and is built part way up the side of a hill. Jose and his family can look out their front door to the north and see the border wall separating Mexico from the United States and the houses on the hills of Nogales, Arizona. Although Jose does not know Joe, he can see Joe's house up on the hill across the border wall in Arizona. Jose's wife likes to shop for groceries in Nogales, Arizona, because most of the groceries are cheaper, especially milk.

Indicators of Population Health

Individuals can be asked directly how they would rate their health—poor, fair, good, or excellent—and the rating seems to be a good indicator of overall health. Generally, individuals who rate their health lower also are more likely to experience disability or death. However, because data on self-rated health status is not available and would be very difficult to obtain, different indicators of population health are needed. To describe the health of a population, indicators such as **life expectancy, infant mortality rate, mortality rate, morbidity,** and **incidence** of disease are frequently used. Each indicator provides somewhat different information about the health of the population, so multiple indicators are often used.

Life expectancy

Life expectancy is the average number of years that a person can expect to live at a given age, usually birth, based on current death rates. Life expectancy is the simplest indicator of population health. Life expectancy is strongly affected by the infant mortality rate; that is, excessive deaths among infants will reduce life expectancy in a population much more than excessive deaths among older adults.[2] Consequently countries with high infant mortality rates will have low life expectancies, and countries with low infant mortality rates will have high life expectancies.

Infant mortality rate

The infant mortality rate is the number of deaths of infants less than 1 year old per year.[2] The number is reported per 1000 live births so that infant mortality rates can be compared between states or countries. Infant mortality appears to be particularly sensitive to health-related conditions and is often used as an indicator of the overall health of a population.[3] For example, Niger, a country in Africa, has an infant mortality rate of 112.4 per 1000 live births and a life expectancy of 56.9 years, while Iceland has an infant mortality rate of 2.9 and a life expectancy of 81.8.[4]

Mortality rate/maternal mortality rate

Mortality rate is the most common indicator of population health because it is a readily available one. The mortality rate

Two primary indicators of population health status

- Infant mortality, the number of deaths of infants less than 1 year old, is a sensitive indicator of the overall health of a population because infants are especially vulnerable to the effects of disease, poor nutrition, and poor physical environment.

- Life expectancy probably is the most direct indicator of population health; presumably, the average number of years that members of a population live is related to their overall health.

describes the number of deaths that occur for a specific population, typically per 100,000 residents.[2] For example, in 2000, Bolivia reported 256 deaths due to cancer per 100,000 residents, while Denmark reported 167.[4] Mortality rates are usually standardized; that is, they are adjusted so the rate compares populations with the same age distribution. Otherwise, a death rate might be much higher just because of a greater number of older people in one population than another. Median age, the age at which half the population is older and half younger, is often used to indicate the relative ages of populations.[4] For example, the median age in Guatemala is 18.2 (half of the population is less than 18), and the median age in Italy is 42 (half of the population is older than 42). Maternal mortality rate is a specialized rate that indicates the number of deaths associated with childbirth per 100,000 women.[4]

Morbidity

Morbidity, the level of disease in a population, also can be used to describe the health of a population.[2] The percent of the population with diabetes is an important indicator of health. For example, the United Arab Emirates reports that 19.5% of its population has diabetes while Mexico reports that 10.6% has diabetes.[4] Overall morbidity, that is, the amount of disease or disability present in a population, seems to be the best indicator of population health but the measurement of overall morbidity is difficult to gauge and unavailable for most populations.

Incidence of disease

Incidence refers to the number of new cases of a disease in a population within a specified time period.[4] Incidence could compare the number of new cases of flu the first week of school with the number of new cases in the second week to determine if that number is increasing or decreasing. Incidence usually is reported per 100,000 population. For example, South Africa reports an incidence of tuberculosis of 600 per 100,000 population, while the United States reports 10.5.[4]

 CASE STUDY 1 (*continued*)

Population health indicators for Joe and Jose

Joe, an American citizen, and Jose, a Mexican citizen, live within sight of each other on the U.S.–Mexico border; both Joe and Jose would rate their own health as excellent. However, they and their families have had somewhat different experiences with health issues. Joe is overweight. Jose's children have been sick more with infectious diseases such as respiratory infections and diarrhea than have Joe's children. Jose's father is no longer living, while both of Joe's parents are alive. Additionally, Jose's aunt died with her baby during childbirth. If they and their families are average, then the population of one country may, on average, be healthier than the population of the other country.

To ascertain relative population health, indicators for the United States and Mexico can be compared (see Table 6.1). Note that the median age of the U.S. population is 10 years older than the median age of the Mexican population. Life expectancy for Joe in the United States at 75.6 years is a bit more than the life expectancy for Jose in Mexico at 73.7 years. The difference is similar for women. The overall mortality rate is somewhat higher in Mexico than the in the United States; the rate is lower for women in both countries. However, the maternal mortality rate is about six times greater for Mexico than the United States and the infant mortality rate is about twice as high. Children under the age of 5 also are more likely to die of diarrhea and pneumonia in Mexico than in the United States. The proportion of U.S. women that are obese is greater than the proportion in Mexico; however, the proportion of the population with diabetes is about the same.

Based on the data shown for the two countries, you can conclude that the average person lives somewhat longer in the United States and that obesity is likely a greater problem in the United States than in Mexico. Morbidity associated with diabetes is similar in both countries. However, maternal mortality and infant mortality are greater in Mexico so women and infants are more likely to die. Children also are more likely to die from diarrhea and pneumonia. Given the increased incidence of tuberculosis, residents of Mexico may be more likely to experience infectious disease than in the United States. In the remainder of the chapter, the factors or health **determinants** that might explain these differences are described.

Table 6.1

Population Health Indicators: United States and Mexico

Indicator	United States	Mexico
Median age[a] (years)	36	26
Life expectancy (years)	77.5	75.3
Men	75.6	73.1
Women	80.8	77.6
Mortality rate (per 100,000)[b]	550.9	631.0
Men	623.1	742.1
Women	485.7	529.3
Maternal mortality rate (per 100,000 live births)	14	83
Infant mortality rate (per 1000 live births)	6.8	15
Causes of death, children under 5 (%)		
Diarrhea	0	5
Pneumonia	1	8
Morbidity (% of population)		
Obesity (women)	35.3	22
Diabetes	10	10.6
Incidence, infectious disease (per 100,000)		
Tuberculosis	5.8	16

[a]Median age refers to the age at which half the population is older and half is younger.

[b]Mortality rate is for a standardized population, which means the populations have the same age distribution.

Sources: 1. Pan American Health Organization. Country Health Profiles: United States of America. Available at: http://www.paho.org/English/DD/AIS/cp_840.htm. Accessed September 24, 2008. 2. Pan American Health Organization. Country Health Profiles: Mexico. Available at: http://www.paho.org/English/DD/AIS/cp_484.htm. Accessed September 24, 2008. 3. World Health Organization. Mortality Country Fact Sheet 2006: Mexico. Available at: http://www.who.int/whosis/mort/profiles/mort_amro_mex_mexico.pdf. Accessed September, 24, 2008. 4. World Health Organization. Mortality Country Fact Sheet 2006: United States of America. Available at: http://www.who.int/whosis/mort/profiles/mort_amro_usa_unitedstatesofamerica.pdf. Accessed September, 24, 2008.

The Determinants of Health

Background

The contemporary ecological approach to identifying health determinants likely originated with the **Declaration of Alma-Ata** in 1978. The Declaration was the outcome of a conference sponsored by the World Health Organization to identify a range of approaches for addressing priority health needs and the fundamental determinants of health. The declaration extended **primary care** from the medical model to include a wide range of factors, including social and economic; activities of civil organizations, including public health activities undertaken by local residents; and a concern for fairness in access to health care.[5]

The ecological approach was supported by the publication of a book by McKeown, *The Role of Medicine*, in 1976.[6] The conclusion from his work was that medical care had relatively little influence on extending the life span in the 20th century and little relationship to reduction of disease, especially infectious disease. McKeown concluded that factors such as nutrition and improved living conditions, improved sanitation, availability of clean water, and improved housing had a much greater impact on overall health than on medical care. The book by Beaglehole, *Public Health at the Crossroads: Achievements and Prospects*, is a recent version of a similar argument that includes a discussion of whether public health should focus more on the environmental determinants of health—pursue an ecological approach—or continue to focus on medical causes of poor health.[2] The discussion below of the determinants of health draws heavily on the Alma-Ata Declaration and McKeown and Beaglehole.

Determinants of health

The conditions or factors associated with health are known as health determinants. Determinants can be internal to the person, for example, the person has immunity to a particular type of virus, or the determinants can be external to the person in the environment where the person lives and works. Numerous physical factors in the external environment have been associated with health such as clean water, sanitation services, adequate food supplies of nutritious foods, easily accessible primary health care, and safe streets. Additionally, a number of social factors in a person's environment are associated with health. Examples include availability of education, adequate resources to provide the necessities of life, availability of support for vulnerable population groups such as children, and lack of violence.

The person–environment interaction

The person–environment interaction is central to the ecological approach to health.[2] Positive interactions result in health or the maintenance of health, while negative interactions result in illness and a decrement to health. For example, if a person can obtain clean water to drink, his or her health is maintained; if the water is contaminated and results in disease, then he or she can experience an illness that negatively impacts health. Therefore, the focus of an ecological approach to health is the description of environmental conditions that promote health or, conversely, those conditions that cause disease.

The person–environment interaction

The person–environment interaction is central to the ecological approach to health, and involves:

- Positive interactions with the environment that improve health; and

- Negative interactions with the environment that are detrimental to health.

Conceptual Framework

To systematically investigate the type of person–environment interactions that can affect health, the framework shown in Figure 6.1 will be used. In this framework, the person who has characteristics that can affect health is seen as the center of the environment with multiple levels of health determinants in the surrounding area.[5,7,8] At the person, or individual level, health determinants are those personal characteristics that are related to health (e.g., immunity to measles).

The determinants in the level next to the individual are the conditions in

Figure 6.1—Framework for Describing Health Determinants
The individual person is the first level displayed with individual characteristics that are related to health. The second level is the community, and it represents the individual's immediate external environment. Many community factors represent the community version of the personal factor, for example, educational systems are the community version of educational attainment. The third level is the level of the state/nation; an example is health insurance that enables the community to maintain clinics and individuals to use them. The fourth level represents global factors and includes factors that cross international borders, for example, infectious disease or pollution and public health organizations.

Source: Adapted from Susser M, Susser E. Choosing a future for epidemiology: II. From black box to Chinese boxes and ecoepidemiology. *Am J Public Health*. 1996; 86:674–7; and McLeroy KR, Bibeau D, Steckler A, et al. An ecological perspective on health promotion programs. *Health Education Quarterly*. 1988; 15:351–77.

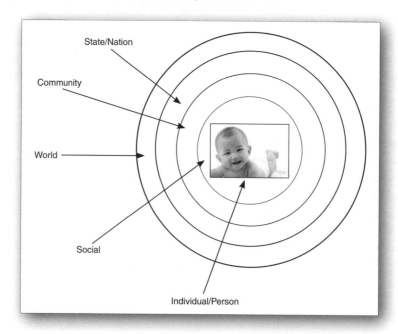

the person's immediate environment that influence his or her health and include factors like availability of clean water and nutritious food. This level refers to the community in which the person lives and works or where the person will have daily contact with multiple aspects of his or her environment. Characteristics of the community can directly affect how people behave, the types of experiences they have, and the activities in which they engage.

The second and third levels of determinants are more indirect and typically involve state or national governments or events that occur distant from the person. State and national governments affect the type of services and health care available to residents through funding of services or through regulations governing health care facilities and other services.

In the following section, each level of health determinants, beginning with the individual level, is defined and examples are provided. Many examples come from comparisons between countries because the greatest differences are evident at an international level and because data are available for such comparisons.

Determinants of health at the individual level

Determinants at the individual level may represent physical, social or psychological characteristics, and behaviors of the individual. These characteristics cannot be separated from the individual; however, they may be inherited (e.g., genetic characteristics) or acquired (e.g., level of education). Examples of determinants of health at the individual level are shown in Table 6.2.

Table 6.2
Individual Level Health Determinants

Determinant	Examples of Effect on Health
Physical	• Genetic susceptibility to breast cancer • Immunity protects against specific diseases • Low level of physical fitness increases likelihood of back injury
Socioeconomic status (SES)	• Poverty has been identified as the "greatest single killer" by WHO • Lack of economic resources is related to other factors that affect health (e.g., adequate nutrition)
Educational attainment	• Maternal educational level is strongly related to children's health • Increased education is associated with behaviors that improve health (e.g., smoking cessation)
Psychological factors	• Childhood abuse or neglect increase likelihood of poor health as an adult • Stress is associated with multiple diseases including cardiovascular disease, cancer, and other chronic diseases
Behaviors	• Behaviors with negative impact on health (e.g., smoking) • Behaviors with positive impact on health (e.g., regular exercise)

Source: Adapted from Beaglehole R. *Public Health at the Crossroads: Achievements and Prospects*, 2nd ed. West Nyack, NY: Cambridge University Press; 2004; McKeown T. *The Role of Medicine: Dream, Mirage, or Nemesis?* London, England: Nuffield Provincial Hospitals Trust; 1976; and Riley JC. *Rising Life Expectancy: A Global History*. New York: NY: 2001:200–19.

Physical

Both inherited and acquired individual characteristics are shown in Table 6.2. An individual may inherit genetic characteristics that are related to health; for example, a person may inherit a susceptibility to breast cancer or to obesity and diabetes. Genetic heritage often explains why some individuals may be healthier than others but does not explain differences between population groups because, on average, the genetic characteristics of groups tend to be similar.[2] Acquired physical characteristics related to health include level of physical fitness and amount of body fat. A low level of physical fitness increases the risk for injury and disability, while excess body fat increases the risk of developing diabetes.

Socioeconomic Status

Socioeconomic status (SES) has a powerful relationship to health; on a global scale, more deaths are associated with poverty than with any other single factor. As described in Table 6.2, the World Health Organization (WHO) has identified poverty as "the greatest single killer."[2] In human societies, economic resources are required to obtain the necessities of life—food, shelter, clean water, and a safe environment. Children are particularly vulnerable to the effects of poverty because they are dependent on others. Comparison of infant mortality rates for rich and poor countries illustrates the effect of SES on children. Sierra Leone in Africa has the highest infant mortality rate (160.3 per 1000 live births) and ranks eighth lowest for individual income. Norway has the fifth lowest infant mortality rate (3.3 per 1000 live births) and has the third highest individual income.[4]

Educational Attainment

Educational attainment also is associated with health. Populations with more education consistently have a higher life expectancy than populations with less education.[2] The relationship of education to health holds even within a population with a similar level of income; more educated individuals have, on average, better health. Additionally, health literacy, an aspect of education, is related to health. Health literacy or the ability to understand and implement health information[9] obviously affects how well an individual can take care of him- or herself. In addition, the health status of infants and children is related to the educational status of their mothers. For example, in Nigerian villages where health care services are limited, children whose mothers lack education are 2.5 to 4 times more likely to die than children of educated mothers.[10]

Psychological Factors

Psychological factors also are related to health; persons who have experienced childhood abuse or neglect are more likely to experience some health problems, for example, depression as an adult. Traumatic experiences can result in post-traumatic stress disorder (PTSD) and associated disorders such as substance abuse. Stress also is related to health, particularly if individuals do not have the skills or support to deal with the stress. Children are particu-

Poverty and education as determinants of health

Poverty is associated with more deaths than any other single factor; however, education can mitigate the effects of poverty. For example, children with mothers who have more education, even in an impoverished environment, are more likely to survive than children with mothers who have less education.

larly vulnerable to the effects of stress because they must rely on others to recognize the signs and to obtain help for them.

Behaviors

Behaviors, particularly those that compose lifestyle, are associated with health status. In contrast to genetic characteristics, behavior is generally assumed to be under the control of the individual. As shown in Table 6.2, behaviors that constitute a healthy lifestyle, such as exercise and healthy eating, have a positive impact on health. Other behaviors, for example, smoking and reckless driving, can increase risk for diseases like lung cancer or heart disease or physical injury and disability. For Americans, behaviors have become an important factor affecting their health; smoking contributes in excess of 438,000 deaths in the United States every year, more than any other preventable cause of death.[11]

[CASE STUDY 1 (continued)

Determinants of health at the individual level—Joe and Jose

Joe and Jose both have individual characteristics that might affect their health. Joe is overweight, which is a health disadvantage. Jose has American Indian ancestry so he may have a genetic susceptibility to developing diabetes, also a health disadvantage. Both Joe and Jose are paid average salaries for their country; however, when expressed in U.S. dollars, Joe is being paid considerably more than Jose even though groceries are more expensive in Mexico. Joe has greater economic resources than Jose so socioeconomic status should give Joe more of a health advantage than Jose. Joe has a health advantage related to education because he completed high school, and Jose only completed the sixth grade. Jose has a disadvantage relative to stress; Jose worries more about the well-being of his family, and he worries about how they will be able to buy what they need. Neither Joe nor Jose smoke; Jose quit because he didn't want to smoke around his children, but he is exposed to smoke at his work site. Both men drink beer but only moderately. Joe could improve his health status by changing his exercise habits and diet. Overall, Joe appears to have a health advantage over Jose at the level of individual characteristics primarily because of his higher income and higher level of education.

Determinants of health at the community level

Community level determinants of health are the physical and social characteristics of the community, many of which represent the environmental correlate of the individual level determinant of health. For example, the individual health determinant is level of education, and the community level determinant is availability of schools. The assumption is that community members are much less likely to attain higher levels of education if there are no schools or poor schools in the community. Selected community level determinants of health and examples of each determinant are shown in Table 6.3.

Economics

Economics is listed first under community level determinants to emphasize its relationship to poverty and the strong relationship between poverty and life expectancy. Globally, most poverty results from unemployment or underemployment;[2] therefore, the availability of employment with adequate salaries in a community will affect the health of the residents. As shown in the example in Table 6.3, aside from the simple ability of the individual or the household to afford the necessities of life, an employed populace

Table 6.3
Community Level Determinants of Health

Determinant	Examples of Effect on Health
Economics	• Availability of employment enables residents to buy the necessities of life • Economic base is sufficient to provide services
Food supplies	• Malnutrition resulting from inadequate amount of food • Malnutrition resulting from consumption of food with low nutritional value • Overnutrition resulting from a wide availability of inexpensive, calorie dense foods
Water and sanitation	• Diseases such as typhoid, hepatitis, diarrhea, and cholera that are transmitted through contaminated water are prevented • Waste water disposal prevents hookworm, diarrhea • Garbage disposal prevents vector borne (e.g., rat) diseases
Housing	• Adequate space prevents airborne diseases (e.g., flu, TB, meningitis) and reduces indoor air pollution • Presence of rats and mice resulting from structural defects • Bird flu resulting from chickens kept in house
Physical environment	• Poisoning (e.g., with lead) resulting from pollution • Ability to maintain weight if exercise facilities are available • Risk of auto accidents is reduced with traffic control
Social environment	• Culture that supports healthy lifestyles • Exploitation of vulnerable populations (e.g., children and the elderly) is prevented • Fairness in the allocation of resources
Education and social services	• Schools and teachers are needed for children to be educated • Post-secondary educational institutions train young adults so that they can earn a living • Social services provide support to families who experience trauma or disasters
Local government	• Adequate local government is required to provide services (e.g., utilities and streets) • Plans and infrastructure required to respond to disasters • Competence to recognize community health issues and take action to address
Primary care	• Access to high-quality primary care reduces disability secondary to injuries • Access to basic medications enables control of conditions (e.g., hypertension, unplanned pregnancies) • Timely medical interventions prevent mortality and morbidity associated with late intervention (e.g., breast cancer)

Source: Adapted from Beaglehole R. *Public Health at the Crossroads: Achievements and Prospects*, 2nd ed. West Nyack, NY: Cambridge University Press; 2004; Anderson ET, McFarlane J. *Community as Partner: Theory and Practice in Nursing*. Philadelphia, PA: Lippincott Williams & Wilkins; 2004; McKeown T. *The Role of Medicine: Dream, Mirage, or Nemesis?* London, England: Nuffield Provincial Hospitals Trust; 1976; and Riley JC. *Rising Life Expectancy: A Global History*. New York: NY: 2001:200–19.

pays taxes that can be used to build schools and hospitals as well as provide health care and other facilities that are related to health. If economic resources are diverted from public services for other uses that do not benefit the community (e.g., as in corruption), then the health of the community will be negatively impacted.

Food Supplies

Malnutrition resulting from either the quantity or quality of food available to community residents is related to health (see Table 6.3). Residents must be able to obtain adequate quantities of food to supply their energy needs. Globally, being underweight is the single most powerful factor affecting disease burden.[2] Underweight or malnutrition reduces the ability of an individual to survive infections, which contributes to reduced life expectancy in less developed countries. Overnutrition and poor quality diet are related to the epidemics of obesity, diabetes, and cardiovascular disease characteristic of developed countries such as the United States where one third of the adult population is obese.[12]

Water and Sanitation

Water is a necessity of life because people must have water to live; the related health issues are whether adequate water supplies are available and whether the water is clean. If water is contaminated, then residents will become ill. Related to the ability of a community to provide clean water is its ability to provide sanitation services and prevent contamination of water supplies. Garbage disposal also affects health because garbage may result in diseases, for example, malaria associated with vectors like mosquitoes. Virtually 100% of the population has access to safe water and sanitation in developed countries like the United States; in developing countries where access is much less, unsafe water, sanitation, and hygiene constitute the sixth leading cause of disease.[2]

Housing

Housing can have substantial influence on health. A lack of housing means that the person has no shelter to protect him or her from the weather, insects, or from other people and animals. Housing without adequate structures and ventilation expose residents to the effects of smoke, and is the eighth leading cause of disease in developing countries.[2] Problems with vermin (e.g., rats, mice) secondary to structural defects are an issue for many residents of impoverished neighborhoods, regardless of whether it is in the United States or in a developing country. Keeping livestock inside the home can allow animal diseases to be transmitted to humans. The contemporary concern is that chickens living in homes will allow the development of bird flu that can be transmitted from human to human.

Physical Environment

The physical environment of the community can directly affect the health of residents. If pollutants are present, residents will be exposed, and that exposure will increase their risk for developing cancers. If no outdoor recreational facilities are available, residents will be less likely to engage in physical activity and obesity is likely to be a problem. Safe streets and pedestrian walkways are required to allow residents to conduct their business without exposure to excessive traffic hazards. Adequate drainage is required to prevent flooding during storms.

Social Environment

The community's social environment, which is primarily how residents interact with one another, can affect health. A culture that supports and promotes healthy lifestyles will enable residents to engage in adequate levels of physical activity and encourage them to consume healthy foods so that their risk for lifestyle diseases is reduced. The social environment related to how community members treat vulnerable residents, for example, the elderly, can affect their health. Permitting scams or other exploitation of elderly residents reduces their ability to provide for necessities and consequently affects their health.

Education and Social Services

At the community level, education provides the facilities and personnel required to teach residents. Post-secondary educational institutions are needed to train young adults so that they can earn a living. In the 21st century, a well educated pool of workers is needed for economic development. Social services are required for residents who experience trauma such as domestic violence or child abuse so that they can go on to live productive lives and not suffer health problems associated with trauma.

Local Government

Local government is required to provide services—water, sanitation, and streets— required for functional healthy residents. Local government must have the ability to recognize the influence of local conditions on the health of residents and to take the actions required to address them. In other words, the government must be competent.

Primary Care

Access to high-quality primary care is one of the determinants of health. If residents cannot obtain care for minor conditions, for example, an infection such as strep throat then the disease can cause death or disability. Prompt high-quality treatment also is required for injuries, or the person can become disabled or die. Access to basic or essential medications is part of adequate primary care; medications are needed to treat acute conditions such as infections and to prevent other conditions such as strokes, resulting from untreated hypertension, as well as to promote health through preventive care such as contraception. Access to essential medications is one of the components of primary care identified by WHO at the Alma-Ata conference in 1978.[5]

Essential medications:

- Meet the priority health care needs of the local population;

- Are affordable and effective; and

- Are readily accessible (i.e., available near where people live and work).

Determinants of health at the community level—Joe and Jose

Although both Joe and Jose have their own houses, their living situations are different. Joe has good services, water, electricity, phone, sewer, garbage service, heat, and a structurally sound house. Jose has services but they are limited; he has electricity but no phone, and he has water but it is not safe to drink. His house is not connected to the sewer but has a rudimentary septic system. Jose has no garbage service; to get rid of his garbage, Jose either burns it or puts it in a plastic bag and then tries to find someplace to dispose of it. Further, there is no heat in his house and the house has structural defects that cost too much for him to repair. They have a problem with rats and mice entering the house due to its structural defects.

A greater variety of food supplies is available to Joe than Jose. Joe can go to the local supermarket, which is part of a regional chain, and purchase the foods he needs. However, he has to be careful with the family's spending so they don't buy too many fruits and vegetables. Jose purchases food from a family-owned neighborhood grocery store. Few fruits and vegetables are available, and most foods are relatively expensive so Jose's wife shops in Arizona when she can. The physical environment is somewhat similar; both towns have few sidewalks and lots of traffic. Transportation is a big problem for Jose because he does not own a car so the family must take a bus or walk where they want to go.

Jose has the advantage with respect to access to primary care; his health care, and that of his family, is provided at a small clinic in the assembly plant where he works. Waiting times are short, and all services are covered by a combination of government and employer financing. Joe has health insurance, but some services are not covered. For other others, there is a substantial co-pay and he and his family typically have to wait a long time whenever they visit the clinic.

Education is more accessible to Joe and his family; Jose's children probably will not be able to attend high school. On both sides of the border, post-secondary education is a problem. People interested in working in management or professional positions on either side of the border must leave the community to attend school.

Based on the discussion of the community level determinants of health, they seem to offer at least a partial explanation for the differences in health experiences between Joe and Jose. Jose has problems with basic services such as contaminated water and lack of heating for his home that are likely related to the diarrhea and respiratory infections his children experience. The differences in the relative cost of food for each household are likely related to the difference in their nutritional status; Joe is overweight, while Jose's children are somewhat small for their age. Jose clearly lives in conditions that are less healthy than Joe's circumstances, and Jose has fewer resources to address his problems such as lack of money and limited education.

Determinants of health at the state and national level

Community level determinants of health were described as the correlates of individual level characteristics that are related to health (e.g., individual poverty, community economics). The individual–community interaction results in a health consequence for the individual—the individual is exposed to contaminated water and becomes ill with diarrhea. Determinants of health at the state and national level act indirectly to influence health by providing resources or through laws and regulations (see Table 6.4). If the state

Table 6.4

State and National Level Determinants of Health

Determinant	Examples of Effect on Health
Communication networks	• Television and Internet accessibility for all residents allows education of the public on health issues (e.g., the importance of exercise) • Highway systems allow transportation of foodstuffs and other supplies required for a healthy life • Air travel permits emergency evacuation of injured persons
Government	• Competent elected officials who can recognize a health issue and use government to respond to them (e.g., vegetables contaminated with *E. coli*) • Passage of laws or regulations that protect the health of residents (e.g., regulations related to the safety and efficacy of medications)
Public health system	• Surveillance activities identify disease outbreaks quickly and prevent spread of disease (e.g., measles) • Assurance that preventive services (e.g., immunizations) are provided • Collection of the data needed to recognize a new disease (e.g., HIV/AIDS) or a new threat to health (e.g., contaminated water) • Proposal of laws or regulations that promote the health of residents
Health insurance/health systems	• Government that assures disadvantaged groups have access to services either through providing services or insurance • Laws or regulations that assure all residents have access to high-quality primary care (e.g., through licensing of pharmacists and other health care practitioners)

Source: Adapted from Beaglehole R. *Public Health at the Crossroads: Achievements and Prospects*, 2nd ed. West Nyack, NY: Cambridge University Press; 2004; McKeown T. *The Role of Medicine: Dream, Mirage, or Nemesis?* London, England: Nuffield Provincial Hospitals Trust; 1976; and Riley JC. *Rising Life Expectancy: A Global History.* New York: NY: 2001:200–19.

has laws and regulations governing water and sewer systems, then the state will indirectly determine whether a resident will be exposed to contaminated water. The state also can provide resources (e.g., tax monies) to communities without adequate resources to assist them in installing water and sewer systems.

Communication Networks
State and national governments typically have a great deal of influence on how residents can communicate. The U.S. government in the 19th century believed communication was essential to democracy so the federal government devoted substantial resources to the development of telegraph systems, rail systems, and the postal system. Communication systems can impact health through the ability to transport the necessities of life to areas of need (i.e., food supplies can be shipped quickly to areas where food was destroyed by fire or floods) and by enabling residents to obtain information and education. In the 21st century, government policies related to the Internet (free) have greatly impacted the type and amount of information available on health-related topics.

Government

Like local governments, elected officials at the state and national level must be able to recognize health issues and have the skills to address them. In a developed country like the United States, government is expected to respond in the event of a disaster by providing aid to victims and economic resources for rebuilding. Legislative bodies can pass laws to encourage healthy behavior or to prevent one person from harming another, for example, laws against smoking indoors and speed limits on highways.

Public Health System

One role of a competent government is to establish a public health system. In a public health system, one of the most important activities is surveillance. This system collects data on certain diseases so that they can determine if the health of a population is threatened. A national system is important because only a few cases of a disease may occur locally; when data is combined from across the country, it can be determined if a threat to health covers a larger area. Cases of diarrhea or death resulting from contaminated meat or vegetables that can occur in widely separated locales could not be identified without a national system.

Health Insurance/Health Systems

One way that state and national governments influence health is through residents' access to health insurance or health services, especially primary health care. Governments have several ways of meeting this need; some governments provide health care to all residents in the country, some provide insurance to residents, and some provide subsidies so that residents can buy their own insurance. In the United States, the federal government subsidizes private insurance and provides some insurance to poor residents in addition to the elderly, and provides health care services to military personnel and veterans.

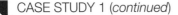

CASE STUDY 1 (continued)

Determinants of health at the state and national levels—Joe and Jose

Despite living in different countries, the communities in which Joe and Jose live have similar issues with the state and national governments for their respective states and countries. The communities are remote from both their state capitols and their national capitols so that community needs tend to be neglected. On the U.S. side of the border, state and national governments expect Nogales, Arizona, to pay for utilities, law enforcement, fire protection, and hospital services even though the services are being used to carry out state or federal objectives. The extra cost to the community reduces the resources available for services to residents so that Joe may have less access to educational programs and to recreational facilities. In Nogales, Mexico, because the community is so remote from the state and national capitols, fewer resources are allocated than in other communities. Again, this situation affects the services that are available to Jose and his family; they have fewer social services available and fewer medical services. For most care beyond primary care, Jose and his family must travel to another city. Thus, even though state and national government offices are remote from the communities, they affect the environment which then affects Joe and Jose and their families.

Determinants of health at the global level

Determinants of health at the global level, like determinants at the state and national levels, act indirectly to affect the health of an individual by influencing some aspect of the community related to health, for example, the availability of food or, more directly, by serving as a source of disease. Examples are shown in Table 6.5.

Communication Networks

Global communication networks can improve or harm health. Communication networks that enable most of the global population to learn about health issues and how to prevent them and to have access to health technology that cures disease or alerts other population groups to disease threats can improve health. Communications networks such as air travel can facilitate evacuation of populations in danger, but also can harm health by allowing highly infectious diseases with high mortality rates such as SARS to spread quickly from one part of the world to another.

Public Health Organizations

At a global level, public health organizations are needed to identify and respond to global health threats. The primary organization for addressing global health issues is WHO, the agency within the United Nations that is responsible for leading initiatives on global health, providing technical support to countries, and monitoring and assessing health trends.[13] Other organizations such as the Red Cross are needed to respond to the effects of disasters and violence.

WHO also is concerned with access to essential medications.[14] One goal of WHO in the 21st century is cooperation with pharmaceutical companies to assure the global availability of essential medications. Although access to medications for treatment of HIV/AIDS, malaria, and tuberculosis has improved, other essential medications often are not available. Data show that medications available in the public sector meet only one third of actual needs. Medications in the private sector meet two thirds of the need but are more than twice as expensive as medications available in the public sector, which makes them essentially unavailable to poor people.

Violence

War is the form of violence that probably has the largest impact on population health. The direct effects of war can result in killing and maiming large numbers of people, but war also affects the ability of the involved population to obtain food, water, and housing. War also prevents people from being employed and from sending their children to school. Terrorism and drug-related violence are additional threats to the health of populations. Violence can indirectly affect populations remote from the scene of the outbreak by disrupting food supplies, facilitating the spread of disease, and placing burdens on other countries for the care of refugee populations.

Global Environmental Change

Global environmental change resulting from climate fluctuations, primarily global warming, has implications for health. The most obvious changes are in the spread of diseases, such as malaria, from more tropical areas to the more temperate areas so that a disease like malaria could become common in countries like the United States where it is currently very rare. Climate change results in more weather-related disasters, for example, strong hurricanes, extensive flooding, and drought. Also included in global environmen-

Table 6.5

Global Determinants of Health

Determinant	Examples of Effect on Health
Communication networks	• Television and Internet accessibility to all residents allows education of the public on health issues (e.g., the importance of exercise) • Highway systems allow transportation of foodstuffs and other supplies required for a healthy life • Air travel permits emergency evacuation of injured persons
Public health organizations	• Organizations (e.g., WHO) that enable multiple countries to address a global health threat (e.g., bird flu, HIV/AIDS) • Organizations (e.g., WHO) that suggest standards for health care (e.g., essential medications)
Violence	• War injures local residents as well as interferes with their ability to obtain the necessities of life • War diverts resources from health-promoting activities, including health care services and education • Terrorism and gang violence results in injury and death
Global climate change	• Changes increase the number of weather-related disasters (e.g., hurricanes, floods, droughts) • Spread of diseases formerly restricted to tropical areas to more temperate zones (e.g., malaria)

Source: Adapted from Beaglehole R. *Public Health at the Crossroads: Achievements and Prospects*, 2nd ed. West Nyack, NY: Cambridge University Press; 2004; McKeown T. *The Role of Medicine: Dream, Mirage, or Nemesis?* London, England: Nuffield Provincial Hospitals Trust; 1976; and Riley JC. *Rising Life Expectancy: A Global History.* New York: NY: 2001:200–19.

Table 6.6

Summary of Health Determinants by Level

Individual	Community	State/National	Global
Physical characteristics	Economics	Communication networks	Communications
Socioeconomic status	Food supplies	Government	Public health organizations
Educational attainment	Water and sanitation	Public health system	Violence
Psychological factors	Housing	Health insurance and health systems	Global climate change
Behaviors	Physical environment		
	Social environment		
	Education & social services		
	Local government		
	Primary care		

Source: This is a summary of the information provided in Tables 6.2, 6.3, 6.4, and 6.5.

tal changes are environmental disasters such as the Chernobyl nuclear reactor incident in which radiation was released into the surrounding area and traveled through weather systems to Europe from the former Soviet Union or the Bhopal disaster; toxic chemicals from a chemical plant were released into the surrounding area.[2]

The four levels of health determinants are summarized in Table 6.6. Included under each level are the primary categories of health determinants related to population health.

CASE STUDY 1 (continued)

Determinants of health at the global level—Joe and Jose

Global determinants affect both Joe and Jose, particularly as they relate to the relationship between the United States and Mexico. Joe works for a distributor who buys produce from Mexico and ships it to grocery stores all over the United States. Jose works in an assembly plant that receives parts from a Japanese manufacturer and assembles the parts into equipment that is shipped all over the world. The presence of the produce distributors and the assembly plants means that there is a great deal of truck traffic through both towns and across the border. The border represents a major factor affecting life in the community as a large number of people pass through the towns and numerous border patrol agents as well as immigration and customs agents work in the town. Unemployment is high in Nogales, Arizona, usually between 15 and 20%, because people coming to the area are seeking employment. Another international factor that affects both Joe and Jose and their families is the drug trade. The presence of drug cartels in the area means safety is jeopardized and, because of the huge amounts of money involved, corruption of government officials is a problem.

The presence of the international border, the high volume of both person and vehicular traffic, and law enforcement issues do create health problems for the communities. The large number of immigrants brings with them any infectious diseases that they might have, including tuberculosis and hepatitis. The law enforcement issues associated with the border divert funds from the county health department, which means fewer resources are available for health department activities or other services provided by the city and county governments (e.g., construction of sidewalks).

Overall, Joe seems to have a health advantage by living on the north side of the border; he has greater economic resources, more access to healthy foods, and he and his family have a very low risk of developing the diarrhea and respiratory problems or of being exposed to other infectious diseases like tuberculosis. The health risks that Jose and his family experience seem primarily related to the difference in their living conditions. Jose and his family have relatively poor utility services at their home and they do not have heat in their house, which increases their risk of diarrhea and respiratory problems. The differences in health between Joe and his family and Jose and his family seem to depend a great deal on whether they live north or south of the border; thus, efforts to address the differences would need to be directed at their environment or living conditions.

Implications for Pharmacists' Roles in Public Health

The ecological approach to identifying health determinants implies that pharmacists have multiple roles in public health: a role associated with medications, a role associated with assuring conditions in which medications are effective, and a role in assuring conditions in which individuals can be healthy.

Roles for pharmacists in public health

Within an ecological framework, pharmacists have three possible roles in public health; the role associated with:

- Improving individual health through the use of medications;

- Assuring living conditions in which medications are effective and used appropriately; and

- Assuming responsibility as a citizen to assure healthy living conditions.

Role associated with medications

The role of pharmacists associated with medications begins at the individual level and involves improving individual health by preventing disease and disability. This role is familiar to pharmacists. By assuring that individuals obtain their immunizations, susceptibility to many diseases, including measles, mumps, tetanus, hepatitis, and pneumonia, is decreased. The risk of negative outcomes for many chronic diseases, including hypertension and diabetes, is reduced by use of appropriate medications. At the community level, the primary public health issue for pharmacists in the medication role is the availability of medications and pharmaceutical care. At the state and national level, the primary concern is promotion of policies, laws, or regulations that assure safe and effective medication and that allow pharmacists to engage in activities like medication management. At the global level, pharmacists participate in identifying essential medications and collaborating with industry to assure that essential medications are available at affordable prices.

Role assuring conditions for effective medication use

The pharmacist also has a role associated with assuring conditions for effective and appropriate medication use. At the individual level, medications are often more effective when they are used in a context of a healthy lifestyle, for example, medications to treat diabetes are more effective if the individual also controls his or her diet and exercises. The combined approach results in a better outcome for the individual, which is the goal of pharmaceutical care.

The pharmacist's role at the community level is to advocate for improving conditions that enhance medication effectiveness, for example, facilities for exercise and a source of healthy foods. Additionally, the pharmacist's role is to avoid inappropriate use of medications. For example, effective treatment is available to treat diarrhea in children but most childhood diarrhea can be prevented by supplying clean water. Therefore, the pharmacist advocates for an improved water supply and participates in related public health activities to assure that treatment for diarrhea is not used as a substitute for supplying clean water. The combination of effective medication therapy with appropriate public health interventions can act synergistically to improve the health status of a population.

At the state, national, and global levels, the pharmacist's primary role is to advocate for and support policies, regulations, or laws that assure the availability of essential medications and the appropriate use of medications.

Role in assuring healthy living conditions

Pharmacists have traditionally restricted their role to those directly associated with medications. An ecological approach to health as envisioned by the Alma-Ata Declaration also defines a role for the citizen, including pharmacists, in assuring healthy living conditions in the community where they live or work. All able citizens should have some responsibility for community health, but especially pharmacists because they are highly educated and they have expertise in health. Therefore, pharmacists are expected to participate in public health activities, including those with no connection to pharmacy, as part of their responsibility as citizens. Additionally, pharmacists can increase their impact on the health of their communities by expanding their role to include public health activities not directly related to medications.

Chapter 6 Summary

Health determinants are factors that are associated with health which, from an ecological perspective, include living conditions as well as health-related factors within the individual. The factors are viewed as levels: the individual level, the community level, the state and national level, and the global level. Individual level factors can be inherited (e.g., a susceptibility to cancer) or acquired (e.g., body fatness). Community level factors are those in the immediate environment of the individual and include characteristics of the community. Economics, the educational system, and the health care system are examples. State and national factors are primarily policies, laws, and regulations that promote health at the community level such as laws controlling pollution or establishment of hospitals. Global factors include factors that extend across community, state, and national boundaries; some examples include infectious disease, pollution, and natural disasters as well as organizations for addressing global health issues.

Within an ecological framework, pharmacists can have multiple roles in public health: roles associated with the use of medications, roles associated with assuring conditions for effective medication use, and roles in assuring healthy living conditions.

References

1. Pan American Health Organization. United States–Mexico Border Area. Available at: http://www.paho.org/. Accessed September 24, 2008.

2. Beaglehole R. *Public Health at the Crossroads: Achievements and Prospects*, 2nd ed. West Nyack, NY: Cambridge University Press; 2004.

3. Aschengrau A, Seage III GR. *Essentials of Epidemiology in Public Health*. Sudbury, MA: Jones and Bartlett; 2003.

4. The Economist. *Pocket World in Figures,* 2008 edition. London, England: Profile Books, Ltd.; 2007.

5. Anderson ET, McFarlane J. *Community as Partner: Theory and Practice in Nursing*. Philadelphia, PA: Lippincott Williams & Wilkins; 2004.

6. McKeown T. *The Role of Medicine: Dream, Mirage, or Nemesis?* London, England: Nuffield Provincial Hospitals Trust; 1976.

7. Susser M, Susser E. Choosing a future for epidemiology: II. From black box to Chinese boxes and eco-epidemiology. *Am J Public Health*. 1996; 86:674–7.

8. McLeroy KR, Bibeau D, Steckler A, et al. An ecological perspective on health promotion programs. *Health Education Quarterly*. 1988; 15:351–77.

9. National Center for Environmental Health: Childhood Lead Poisoning. Lead Health Literacy Initiative. Available at: http://www.cdc.gov/nceh/lead/resources/LeadLiteracy/LeadLiteracy.htm. Accessed September 9, 2008.

10. Riley JC. *Rising Life Expectancy: A Global History*. New York: NY: 2001:200–19.

11. Centers for Disease Control and Prevention. Smoking & Tobacco Use: Fact Sheet. Available at: http://www.cdc.gov/tobacco/data_statistics/fact_sheets/adult_data/adult_cig_smoking.htm. Accessed September 24, 2008.

12. Centers for Disease Control and Prevention. Obesity and Overweight: Introduction. Available at: http://www.cdc.gov/nccdphp/dnpa/obesity/. Accessed September 24, 2008.

13. World Health Organization. About WHO. Available at: http://www.who.int/about/en/. Accessed September 24, 2008.

14. World Health Organization. Essential Medicines. Available at: http://www.who.int/topics/essential_medicines/en/index.html. Accessed September 24, 2008.

Suggested Readings

Cairncross S, Hardoy JE, Satterthwaite D, eds. *The Poor Die Young: Housing and Health in Third World Cities*. London, England: Earthscan Publications; 1990.
This text is a powerful description of the effects of poverty on health. The discussion is somewhat academic but, because it is academic, substantial data is provided to support the authors' arguments.

McKeown T. *The Role of Medicine: Dream, Mirage, or Nemesis*? London, England: Nuffield Provincial Hospitals Trust; 1976.
This is the original publication that challenged the role of medical care in increasing life expectancy during the 20th century. A classic in public health, this text provided much of the foundation for the ecological approach to health.

Mann CC. *1491: New Revelations of the Americas before Columbus*. New York, NY: Knopf; 2005.
This description of the Americas before Columbus describes the central role of disease in the European settlement of the Western Hemisphere. It is a fascinating nonacademic book for anyone interested in the relationship between disease and civilization.

Riley JC. *Rising Life Expectancy: A Global History*. New York, NY: Cambridge University Press; 2001.
This broad discussion focuses on the factors that have resulted in a greatly increased life expectancy at the beginning of the 21st century. It explores the effects of public health and medicine as well as economic factors, nutritional factors, households and individuals, and literacy and education.

Chapter 6 Review Questions

1. Define health determinant and give an example.
A health determinant is a factor within the individual or in his or her environment that is associated with health. Environmental factors affect the individual's health when he or she interacts with the specific factor. Example: The community has adult education classes on healthy lifestyles; by attending the classes, a community resident

learns how to improve his or her lifestyle.

2. **Describe an example of an activity that a person could engage in that represents a positive person–environment interaction and an activity that represents an example of a negative person–environment interaction.**
A wide variety of responses are possible; the person does not have to control the interaction.

Positive interaction: A person attends classes on healthy lifestyles.

Negative interaction: A person eats in a restaurant where other people are smoking.

3. **Using the four categories of health determinants—individual, community, state/national, and global—match the appropriate category to the examples of health determinants listed below.**
Categories: (a) Individual   (b) Community   (c) State/national   (d) Global

_____ Subsidy paid to employers for health insurance (c)

_____ Water and sewer systems (b)

_____ Poverty (socioeconomic status) (a)

_____ Radiation release in a neighboring country (d)

_____ Factory with well paying jobs (b)

_____ Educational attainment (a)

_____ Access to essential medications (b)

_____ Law prohibiting indoor smoking (c)

4. **The infant mortality rate provides an indication of population health because:**
(a) Infants usually compose a very small portion of the population.

(b) Infants are sensitive to adverse conditions such as poor nutrition or contaminated water.

(c) Infant mortality has a stronger effect on life expectancy than adult mortality.

(d) More data is available on infants than on older adults.

(e) (a) and (c)

(f) (b) and (c)

Choice (f) is correct.

5. **Identify three criteria for a medication to be considered *essential*.**
Three criteria for essential medications are (1) the medication must meet a priority health need of the local population; (2) the medication must be readily available; and (3) the medication must be affordable or effective or both.

1. Imagine that you have the opportunity to complete a rotation in _____ (select either another state of the United States or another country). You are very excited about this opportunity and want to learn as much as you can about the health issues in the country as well as about pharmacy practice.
   (1) Where might you find information about the health of the population?

   (2) What indicators of health do you think are most relevant for the area?

   (3) What type of community characteristics would you look for to identify health issues in the country?

   (4) Can you identify any factors at the global level that might affect the health of the state or nation where you are completing your rotation?

2. Imagine that you are working in a pharmacy (if you work in a pharmacy, use that pharmacy; if you don't, use a pharmacy close to where you live) and one of the patrons who frequently comes to the pharmacy is obese as are her two children and her husband. Identify two individual characteristics of the person and two community characteristics that might be contributing to their problem with obesity.

3. Look up the web page for either the state health department or county health department for the area where you attend school. Identify four of their activities that are related to health.

4. The CIA (Central Intelligence Agency) uses the infant mortality rate as an indicator of political instability to help it identify where the next political crisis might occur in the world. The use of a population health indicator such as infant mortality seems unrelated to politics; explain why the CIA might be interested in the infant mortality rate.

CHAPTER 7

Cultural Competence in Public Health

■ ■ ■

Learning Outcomes

1. Define cultural competence.
2. Differentiate cultural and linguistic competence.
3. List and give an example of the three components of cultural competence.
4. List and describe two types of knowledge and give an example of each that practitioners need to address cultural issues.
5. List three characteristics of a practice site that would indicate the site addresses cultural issues.

Introduction

Public health interventions require acceptance by residents of the community, for example, educational programs; use of products like medications; behavior changes such as smoking cessation; environmental modifications including provision of safe water, nutritious foods, and safe highways; and immunization programs. Acceptance is more likely if the public health program is compatible with local values and beliefs and addresses concerns of specific population groups. In this chapter, the concept of cultural competence in public health is explored to address the concerns of community residents that might be related to culture. The chapter begins with a case study involving a patient who has been diagnosed with active tuberculosis (TB) infection. Then definitions of culture and cultural competence are provided; cultural competence and linguistic proficiency are differentiated within the context of the public health issues, and associated cultural issues, related to the treatment of TB. The importance of cultural issues and implications for health disparities in the United States are described. The role of interpreters and translators is defined and described. Then the relevance of Title VI of the Civil Rights Act (to providing interpreters or translation) is delineated as well as the CLAS standards. Because most students or practitioners will need to teach themselves about a new culture at some point in their practice, a framework for understanding how to learn cultural competency using attitudes, knowledge, and skill is described. The last section of the chapter discusses specific strategies that students or practitioners can use to increase their cultural competence.

Public Health Issues in the Context of Contagious Disease

Two aspects to the treatment of a person with a **contagious** disease are explained: the first is cure, usually with antibiotics, to improve the health of the individual. However, when the disease is contagious, a second aspect to the treatment is curing the disease in the individual to prevent its spread to other people. Prevention of the spread of the disease is a benefit to the community in which the sick person resides, and thus becomes a public health issue. Identifying individuals with the disease, providing treatment, and preventing spread of the disease in the community are responsibilities of the county health department. To the extent that these activities are related to the local **culture**, culture must be considered for treatment and prevention to be successful.

A fictitious case study involving a patient who has been diagnosed with active tuberculosis (TB) infection will be used to illustrate some cultural issues associated with the treatment of a contagious disease. TB is not only contagious but infectious and is caused by the *Mycobacterium* tuberculosis bacteria that typically results in lung disease; it is usually spread through aerosol droplets when a person who has untreated TB coughs or sneezes, and a person close to him or her inhales the bacterium. However, the bacterium can attack any part of the body including the kidney, spine, or brain. Persons with weak immune systems, for example, infants and small children, older adults, and persons with HIV/AIDS or those being treated for cancer, are particularly susceptible to TB.[1,2] On a global scale, women of reproductive age are more likely to die of TB than any other infectious disease. TB also is the leading cause of death among people with HIV/AIDS.[2] Since the treatment of TB involves multiple medications and prolonged regimens (a minimum of 6 months), the cultural issues associated with treatment include incorporating therapy into daily life and changing behaviors. These lifestyle issues are particularly relevant to pharmacists.

CASE STUDY 1

Cultural issues associated with the treatment of tuberculosis

Maria is diagnosed with TB

Maria is a 33-year-old female who has just been told that she has active TB. Maria's family immigrated to a U.S. community of about 30,000 people when Maria was a child; consequently, Maria is bilingual. Tuberculosis (TB) is a problem in Maria's country of origin. Because persons who live in poor, crowded conditions are at higher risk for TB, there is a stigma associated with having TB. To them, TB implies that you are poor, ignorant, and dirty. People do not want to admit that they have TB; if they do, they try to hide it from their family and friends.

As Maria drove to the health department clinic where TB patients were treated, she thought about her uncle who had had TB in her home country. Maria remembered that her grandparents had been very upset and had blamed her uncle for getting TB; they were sure that he had gotten it from going off to work in a mine, which they had not wanted him to do, and living in a house with 10–12 other miners. Maria was glad that her parents were not in town right now. They had gone home to visit, and Maria was using their car while they were gone. Maria still hoped that when she went to the clinic, the doctor would tell her that her chest problem wasn't TB.

The directions to the clinic said turn right at the stop sign; Maria turned and immediately saw the big sign identifying the County Health Department Tuberculosis Control Clinic. Maria cringed and thanked her lucky stars that her mother was out of town. She certainly didn't want to go into the clinic, but she went ahead anyway.

Maria at the county tuberculosis control clinic

Maria was greeted by a receptionist who spoke the local version of Maria's native language, which meant that English words were often mixed into the conversation. The receptionist was very nice; she asked Maria about her two children and then helped her to complete the paperwork for the visit and immediately put her in a room to see the doctor. The nurse came and quickly took her blood pressure, asked Maria why she was there today, made notes in the chart, and left. It seemed a long time before the doctor came. When he did, he greeted Maria and then quickly went on to tell Maria that she had active TB infection. She was told that she could give the infection to her children and other family members so she must begin taking medications for TB right away. Again, Maria cringed—not only did she have a dreaded disease, but she might give it to her children! The doctor told her other things that she needed to know about taking medications—that the medications would not cost her anything and how to keep from infecting her children, but Maria didn't hear much. She took her prescriptions, and went to get her medicines. Maria thought that if she got the medicine and took it right away, she wouldn't have to tell her parents that she had TB when they came home.

Maria went to the pharmacy window in the clinic, and picked up her medications. The pharmacist said that she needed to talk to Maria about her medications. When the pharmacist took the vials out of the bag and began showing them to Maria, she cringed. In big red letters on the vials were the words County Tuberculosis Clinic. The pharmacist began telling Maria about her medications and that it was important to take them; again, Maria did not hear much because she was trying to figure out how she could keep her family from seeing that she was taking medicine for TB. As Maria left the clinic, she thought that she knew what to do—she would just remove the labels from the vials.

Basic Concepts in Culture and Cultural Competence

Conceptual definitions of culture and cultural competence

Culture

Culture is often defined as a pattern of learned beliefs and behaviors shared among members of a group. Culture can proscribe communication styles, roles and relationships, and how men and women interact.[3,4] A simple way of thinking about culture is to consider behaviors that parents teach a young child, for example, what to wear, how to greet an adult, and what constitutes good manners when you are a guest. Children also learn how to interpret events from their parents and grandparents; for example, children watch how other family members act when a relative dies and, through cues like this, learn what it means to be a member of a family or perhaps a member of a particular community. Parents also teach children what to do if they have a cold, when to see a doctor, which foods are considered nutritious, and what types of exercise are appropriate. The belief that chicken soup is good for you if you have a cold or are sick is an example of a health belief related to culture (Figure 7.1). The use of chicken soup to treat colds and other

Figure 7.1—The belief that chicken soup is good for you when you are sick is an example of a culturally based belief.

Source: www.CartoonStock.com.

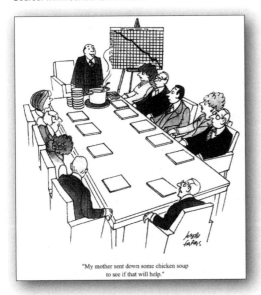

"My mother sent down some chicken soup to see if that will help."

■ ■ ■

Culture and cultural competence

Cultural heritage is obtained from a specific group. Because everyone belongs to some type of group, everyone has a cultural heritage that influences his or her beliefs and behaviors.

Culture is influenced by the local environment so that there cannot be a universal culture.

Cultural competence is different than professional competence. Consequently, health care providers can have one type of competence without the other.

ailments began in the Jewish community, but now has a broadened appeal in many other cultures including American. Because individuals do not usually remember learning these basic beliefs and behaviors, they often have difficulty describing their own culture.

Culture is typically associated with ethnic or national identity. For example, specific cultures are associated with Mexico, Western Europe, and Japan. However, culture is also learned as part of socioeconomic status, gender, occupation, religion, education, and community or geographic region.[3,4] For example, the English-speaking African American from Chicago may have little knowledge of the culture of the English-speaking African American living in an agricultural area in the Mississippi Delta, even though they speak the same language and have the same skin color. In an analogous manner, the culture of Western-style medicine, including public health, differs from that of the lay person or of traditional healers.

Cultural Competence

Cultural competence means having the **attitudes**, knowledge, and **skill** to establish organizational policies for the provision of services that are respectful and responsive to the needs of the community. Health care providers or organizations that are culturally competent are those that accept and respect cultural differences, continually seek to learn about culture and its effects on health, and adapt their service models to obtain the best possible outcome.[3,5] Competence implies having the capacity to recognize the cultural beliefs, behaviors, and needs of the community and being able to address those needs.[6]

Maria's cultural concerns

Maria probably is typical of many patients; she did not think about how the beliefs and behaviors that she had learned from her parents, grandparents, and the community might affect her ability to obtain effective medical care. Maria's primary concerns were making sure her children didn't get sick and not bringing disgrace on her parents.

In a similar manner, the staff at the county clinic did not seem to be aware of how their culture and the culture of Western medicine might be perceived by a patient from a different culture. The staff prided themselves on their ability to be efficient and to provide medical care based on the best scientific evidence as well as being caring and willing to work with poor patients. The staff members were proud of their clinic and their facilities; they wanted everyone to know about their facility so they made sure a sign identified it and the medication labels showed the clinic's name.

Linguistic proficiency versus cultural competence

Linguistic Proficiency

Linguistic proficiency refers to the ability to speak and write in a specific language. For example, the most proficient speakers and writers in English would be able to speak and write at the level of post-graduate university studies, whereas the least proficient might not be able to write in the language at all and have very limited ability to communicate orally. A person may be able to speak proficiently, but not be able to compose sentences and write in the language or even to read in the language above an elementary level.

Association of Language with Ethnic or National Identity

Language, like culture, is typically associated with ethnic or national identity. Persons from Mexico are expected to speak Spanish, persons from the United States to speak English, and persons from Japan to speak Japanese. Proficiency in a language is also community specific. For example, Spanish is spoken in Spain, Puerto Rico, Cuba, Mexico, Central America, and most of South America. However, different dialects are spoken in each country so that confusion can result even for two people speaking Spanish. But the culture of each country varies widely, and local circumstances can further modify the language. Residents of the border area between the United States and Mexico may speak primarily Spanish but incorporate many terms from the dominant American English culture into the local language, sometimes described as Spanglish. Linguists prefer the term code-switching to refer to the use of more than one language in conversation. Therefore, a person who learned Spanish in New York from Puerto Rican parents may not be an expert in the language of a small town on the U.S.–Mexico border.

Language proficiency versus cultural competency

- Language proficiency is related to one's ability to speak and write a specific language.

- Cultural competency is related to one's ability to address beliefs and behaviors learned from membership in a social group.

- Language proficiency can facilitate learning a new culture, but it does not automatically guarantee cultural competency.

CASE STUDY 1 *(continued)*

Language and cultural issues collide at the tuberculosis clinic

Even though Maria was born in another country, she grew up and attended school in the United States. So Maria was proficient in two languages: English and the language of her country of origin. Several staff members at the clinic also were proficient in both languages. The receptionist greeted Maria in her native language, and the pharmacist printed the directions about how to take the medications in her native language as well as counseled her in that language. Yet a cultural misunderstanding occurred because the staff at the clinic did not comprehend what having TB meant to Maria within her culture.

Importance of cultural issues in the United States

Culture, Race, and Ethnicity

Race and **ethnicity** are personal characteristics that are associated with culture; however, use of the terms is somewhat problematic. Race usually is considered to represent the biological characteristics of a group of people with the implication that a person from one race is biologically different than a person from another. To the extent that differences in race represent genetic heritage, differences in groups of people may mean they are more susceptible to certain diseases (e.g., sickle cell disease). However, identifiable biological differences tend to be small and the idea of distinct human races reflects more on the ideas behind the classification scheme than on any real differences.[7]

Ethnicity refers to a person's ancestry. The U.S. Census Bureau has defined ancestry as "... a person's ethnic origin or descent, roots, heritage, or the place of birth of the person, the person's parents, or their ancestors before arrival in the United States." The U.S. Census Bureau now uses a two-step approach to describing the race and ethnicity of population groups in the United States. One question on ethnicity asks if the person considers him- or herself Hispanic, and one question on race has 13 categories, most of which reflect national origin.[8] In this chapter, the basic census approach to race and the census definitions of race will be used. If the issue is ethnicity, then reference will be made to national origin.

Diversity of Population Groups in the United States

The 2000 census indicated that the total population of the United States was 281,421,906 (in 2006, the total population passed the 300 million mark).[8] The 2000 census collected data on self-identified race for Whites (any resident having origins in Europe or the Near East), Black or African American (having origins in Africa), American Indian and Alaska Native (having origins in the original peoples of North or South America), Asian (having origins in the Far East, Southeast Asia, or the Indian subcontinent), Native Hawaiian or Other Pacific Islander (having origins in Hawaii or other Pacific Islands), and some other race. The statistics showed that most people (75%) considered themselves to be White, 12% considered themselves to be Black or African American, and about 4% Asian. The remaining 9% considered themselves to be "other" or "more than one race." The diversity of the U.S. population changed from the 1990 to the 2000 census as illustrated in Figure 7.2. In a separate question, respondents were

Figure 7.2—Changes in Diversity from the 1990 to 2000 Census

Source: This figure is available at http://www.census.gov/population/cen2000/atlas/censr01-104.pdf.

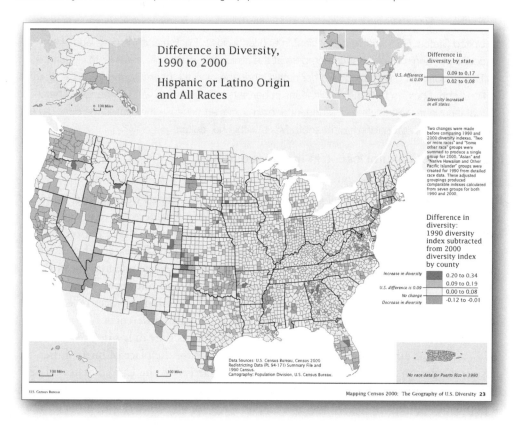

asked if they considered themselves to be Hispanic or Latino; about 12.5% of the total population responded yes. The minority prevalence by county based on the 2000 census is illustrated in Figure 7.3.[9] When primary language is considered, about 18% of people (48 million) speak a language other than English at home and half of them report that they do not speak English very well.[10]

Health Disparities between Population Groups

Health disparity refers to the difference in life expectancy and health status among ethnic and racial population groups. As a group, Americans are healthier than they have ever been and live longer, but the nation's health status will not be as good as it could be until all segments of the population have similar life expectancy and health status. The disparity in health between American populations who consider themselves White and populations of other origins is well documented. Differences have been described in access to care, life expectancy, and morbidity.[10,11] For example:

- Adults who do not speak English at home are more likely to say that their health care providers sometimes or never listened carefully or spent enough time with them than English speakers.
- Infant mortality rates are twice as high for African American and American Indian populations compared to White Americans.
- Maternal mortality is four times higher for African Americans as for White Americans.
- American Indians and Alaska Natives are 2.3 times more likely to have diabetes.
- The median age at death for American Indians living in Arizona is 59 years compared to 79 for non-Hispanic Whites.[12] The median age at death for

Cultural diversity in the United States is related to health disparities:

- On the 2000 census, at least a quarter of the U.S. population considered themselves to belong to one of five minority racial categories.
- Health disparities (i.e., poorer health status and reduced life expectancy) have been documented for most of these minority groups.

American Indians in Arizona is about the same as for residents of Ghana, a country in Central Africa.[13]

Figure 7.3—Minority Prevalence, United States by County, 2000

Source: This figure is available at http://www.census.gov/population/cen2000/atlas/censr01-104.pdf.

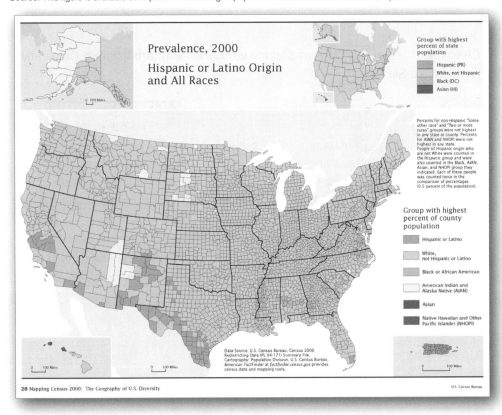

Cultural and language differences must be addressed if disparities in health status are to be reduced. The issue is evident when considering language differences; if the health care provider cannot communicate effectively with the patient and vice versa, it will be very difficult to develop a care plan that the patient can understand and that is consistent with cultural practices.

 CASE STUDY 1 (*continued*)

Brainstorming on cultural characteristics at the tuberculosis clinic

The staff at the clinic realized that they had focused too much on the technical aspects of care and not enough on the cultural aspects when Maria returned to the clinic experiencing side effects from her drug therapy and explained that she had removed the labels from the medication vials because she was ashamed to have TB and didn't want her family and friends to know. At the next staff meeting, some time was set aside to brainstorm on the cultural characteristics of the current services and the characteristics that might be more acceptable to the minority population.

The results of the brainstorming session are summarized in Table 7.1. Most of the staff was surprised to learn that patients might prefer a more personal interaction and that patients appreciated the staff asking about their children. Although most of the staff had heard stories from other providers that sometimes patients with TB were not allowed to return home, most of the staff had not realized that many patients were very ashamed to have TB and might decline treatment in an attempt to avoid the accompanying shame. Staff did recognize that both patients and providers were concerned about the well-being of children. At the end of the meeting, the staff felt that they could make several changes in their services to be more culturally compatible with the minority population.

Table 7.1

Characteristics of the Current Service versus Characteristics of a Culturally Responsive Service

Service	Cultural Values	Characteristics of Service
Current service	(1) Efficiency is highly valued (2) Technical aspects of care are highly valued (3) Disease is believed to be a universal problem (4) Professional status means that one does not encourage personal relationships with patients	(1) Staff does not want to waste time in small talk but get right to the problem and its solution (2) Staff makes sure that the treatment procedures and plans conform to best practice (3) As long as patients can understand that they need to take medications as directed, language is not an issue

Continued

Table 7.1 *Continued*

Service	Cultural Values	Characteristics of Service
Culturally responsive service	(1) Interpersonal relationships are highly valued (2) Welfare of children is a primary concern (3) Providers who try to speak the language are greatly appreciated (4) Pictorial and verbal modes of communication are preferred	(1) Patients like to have a personal greeting and have the provider ask about their families (2) Concern for children needs to be included in care plan (3) All providers need to learn to greet patients in their native language (4) Language interpretation and translation services are needed (5) The signs to the county clinic and the medication labels should be changed, if possible

Cultural competence and interpreter services

Interpreters versus Translators

A critical component of cultural competence is the use of the appropriate language if the provider and the organization do not use the same language as the patient. If the language is not shared between the provider and provider organization and the patient, then **interpreters** and **translators** are necessary. Interpreters work with spoken language; they convey what a person has said in one language to a second person in a different language in a spoken format. In contrast, translation involves written documents; translators render a document written in one language into a document written in a second language.[14] Both types of services are required in a health care organization that serves a multicultural, multilingual population.

Title VI of the Civil Rights Act of 1964

Title VI of the Civil Rights Act of 1964, the federal legislation dealing with discrimination, specifically addresses the need for interpreter and translator services. Title VI regulation prohibits the conduct of programs using federal financial assistance from discriminating on the basis of race, color, or national origin. Not providing interpreter services or using ineffective methods for persons with limited proficiency in English is a violation of the act. The act also addresses the use of written language.[15]

Interpreter Models: A Comparison of the Advantages and Disadvantages

The advantages and disadvantages of several models of interpreter services are summarized in Table 7.2. Bilingual providers represent the ideal solution if they have been trained as interpreters. However, providers, even though they speak the same language as the patient, may not share the same culture so that cultural issues remain. Regardless of the method selected, all interpreters need to be trained so that they have appropriate skills and vocabulary as well as understand the ethics of interpretation.

Table 7.2

Advantages and Disadvantages of Interpreter Models[a]

Interpreter Model	Advantages	Disadvantages
No interpreter	Reduced short-term cost to the provider	Considered unacceptable; may trigger response from the Office of Civil Rights; adverse events resulting from misunderstandings are likely
Family and friends	Readily available and speak local dialect; however, use only if specifically requested by the patient	Support role conflicts with interpreter role; may not have requisite medical knowledge; having children interpret disrupts parent–child relationship
Bilingual non-clinical staff	Readily available; no additional cost to organization	Not trained as interpreters; usually lack requisite medical knowledge; may know the patient
Professional on-site (staff) interpreters	Reliable; trained in ethics and requisite vocabulary; readily available	Expensive and may not be available in all languages needed
Telephonic and remote interpretation	Available through professional language services; readily accessible	Can be expensive; may lack knowledge of local culture and local idioms
Bilingual providers	Ideal solution if trained to interpret	Bilingual provider may share language but not culture; may not be trained as an interpreter; may retain status issues from originating country

[a]Adapted from Downing B, Roat CE. Models for the Provision of Language Access in Health Care Settings. Available at: The National Council on Interpreting in Health Care. 2002. Available at: http://www.xculture.org/NWRC_Med_Interp_Resource_Guide.php. Accessed September 5, 2008.

Use of family members as interpreters, especially children, is problematic. Family members often do not have the requisite medical knowledge to interpret; additionally, they may censor the information based on their relationship or as they perceive their role in supporting the patient. All the above concerns apply to using children as interpreters. Using children as interpreters disrupts the parent–child relationship and, if the child misinterprets the information and the family member is harmed, the interpretation process may represent a traumatic event for the child. Therefore, family members should not be used for interpretation unless requested by the patient.

Similar problems can arise with using bilingual support staff. Often support staff are in positions that require little education so they may not have an appropriate vocabulary to interpret medical terms or may censor the information based on their limited understanding of the situation. Additionally, minority communities often are small; if the staff person knows the patient, there could be repercussions for the patient if the health problem is socially stigmatizing.

Language interpretation does not necessarily assure cultural interpretation or the ability to recognize and address cultural issues. Cultural interpreters from the minority community may be needed in addition to language interpreters. A cultural interpreter can provide insight into issues related to health care and health care professionals. Cultural interpreters seem to be particularly important when patients are from a minority community with limited education and limited economic resources as they are less likely to have familiarity with the dominant culture.

 CASE STUDY 1 *(continued)*

Different models of interpretation at the tuberculosis clinic

The staff at the county health department reviewed the different models of interpretation for their clinic. They had two primary population groups: the white population and the minority population, and they realized that they had been using the bilingual support staff model. Whenever staff had problems with interpretation, they would call on the receptionist. When they considered what they should do, the staff immediately rejected the no interpreter model and the family member model. The telephonic interpretation program seemed like more than they needed since they had only two population groups. They did not have bilingual professional staff, although the pharmacist had some knowledge of the language. After deliberation, the staff decided that the best solution was to offer interpreter training to the receptionist and upgrade her position description.

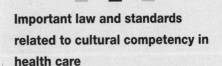

Important law and standards related to cultural competency in health care

Title VI of the Civil Rights Act of 1964 requires service providers to assist patrons with language.

CLAS Standards specify standards for cultural competence, language access services, and the organizational supports required for culturally competent health care.

CLAS Standards

The Office of Minority Health of the U.S. Department of Health and Human Services has published standards for providing culturally and linguistically appropriate services known as the **CLAS Standards**. CLAS is the acronym for Culturally Linguistically Appropriate Services. The CLAS standards, summarized in Table 7.3, address three areas: (1) culturally competent care (three standards), (2) language access services (four standards), and (3) organizational supports for cultural competence (seven standards). Note that more standards are devoted to organizational support than to either language access or clinical care. Hence, the standards emphasize the role of the organization in the provision of culturally competent care. Note also the specific prohibition related to the use of family and friends as interpreters unless the patient specifically requests it.[16]

Table 7.3

Summary of CLAS Standards for Culturally and Linguistically Appropriate Services[a]

Standard Group	Description of Standards
Culturally competent care	(1) Assure that all patients receive respectful care compatible with their cultural health beliefs
	(2) Implement strategies to have a staff representative of the source population
	(3) Assure that all staff receive education and training in the provision of culturally appropriate services
Language access services	(4) Provide language assistance services at no cost to the patient at all points of contact during all hours of operation
	(5) Provide notices verbally and in writing about the availability of language services
	(6) Assure the competence of the language assistance; *family and friends should not be used to provide interpretation, except by request of the patient*
	(7) Provide patient materials and signage in commonly encountered languages
Organizational supports for cultural competence	(8) Promote a written strategic plan for culturally and linguistically appropriate services
	(9) Conduct self-assessments of CLAS-related activities
	(10) Collect data on race, ethnicity, and spoken and written language
	(11) Maintain a current epidemiological profile of the source population
	(12) Develop collaborative partnerships with communities
	(13) Maintain a conflict and grievance resolution process
	(14) Make CLAS-related activities available as public information

[a]CLAS Standards are summarized from the original document; the original standards are available from Department of Health and Human Services, Office of Minority Health. National Standards on Culturally and Linguistically Appropriate Services (CLAS) in Health Care. Final Report; 2001.

 CASE STUDY 1 (*continued*)

CLAS standards at the tuberculosis clinic

The staff at the tuberculosis clinic reviewed the CLAS standards to determine if their clinic met them; they concluded that they performed at a minimal level on most standards but did not meet all. For example, they believed that they provided respectful care to everyone but they weren't sure, after the label incident, that the care was compatible with the minority population's cultural beliefs. Also, they did not have a formal training program; to date, training had been informal and often did not occur until an issue arose. The staff felt that by upgrading the receptionist's position and training her to interpret, they were currently addressing the issues related to access to interpretation. However, they felt that they needed to provide signage in appropriate languages and the signage needed to respond to cultural concerns. With respect to the organizational supports, the staff decided that they wanted to develop a document that provided a demographic and epidemiological profile of the population. (The pharmacist suggested that the next pharmacy student completing a rotation at the clinic could help with developing the profile.) The staff also wanted to develop a formal collaborative partnership with the community through an advisory committee so that they would have a way of identifying and addressing cultural issues.

A Framework for Learning Cultural Competence

In this section, a framework is presented that will assist in developing cultural competence. The framework is based on the issues described above related to recognizing cultural differences, respecting those differences, and adapting services to improve outcomes. However, the framework organizes the components of cultural competence and presents them in a manner that should enable a student or professional to take concrete steps toward becoming culturally competent.

The three components of cultural competence—attitudes, knowledge, and skill[4]— are shown in Figure 7.4. The components are shown as a pyramid with attitudes forming the base, knowledge as the middle layer, and skill at the apex. In the following sections, each component will be defined and their relationship to cultural competence described.

Figure 7.4—Components of Cultural Competence

Adapted from Betancourt JR. Cross-cultural medical education: conceptual approaches and frameworks for evaulation. *Academic Med.* 2003; 78:560–9.

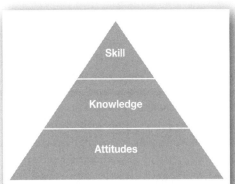

Attitudes form the foundation of cultural competence; without enabling attitudes, practitioners would not bother to learn about culture. Knowledge forms the core or middle layer. To be culturally competent, a practitioner needs to have specific knowledge about how the local culture affects health outcomes. Finally, at the apex is skill—the ability to use knowledge to adapt health services for meeting the needs of the local population.

Attitudes

Attitudes are defined as beliefs related to cultural issues and their relationship to health. Attitudes can act as barriers or enablers to providing culturally competent care. Attitudes are shown as the foundation of the pyramid based on the premise that, without enabling attitudes, the individual will not bother to learn about culture or how services might be modified to improve health outcomes. Thus, without enabling attitudes, there is no pyramid and no cultural competence.

Attitudes as Barriers to Cultural Competence

Here are a few examples of attitudes that act as barriers:

- Health care services, including public health services, are universal and do not need modification to accommodate cultural differences;
- This is the United States, and everyone should become part of the dominant culture; and
- "I don't have any culture; therefore, the services I offer are neutral with respect to culture."

Attitudes that Enable Development of Cultural Competence

Enabling attitudes are those that facilitate learning about other cultures and developing an appreciation for differences in culture. Examples of enabling attitudes include:

- Curiosity, that is, the desire to learn about others;
- Respect, that is, having consideration for the other person and that he or she might have different beliefs and values than yours;
- Empathy, that is, being able to appreciate where the person is coming from; and
- Wanting the best outcome possible for an individual or for a population group. A focus on outcomes enables one to actively explore cultural differences that might interfere with obtaining a good outcome and to identify those cultural differences that might improve outcomes.

CASE STUDY 1 *(continued)*

Enabling attitudes at the tuberculosis clinic

The staff at the county TB clinic generally had enabling attitudes; they respected all patients treated at the clinic, and they wanted to provide high-quality care with the best outcome possible for each patient. The staff was generally open to learning about the local culture and frequently ate at cafes where ethnic food was served. The biggest limitation in their attitudes appeared to be their general belief that health care services were universal and that culture wasn't a big issue with respect to health care. But they were willing to learn. As soon as cultural issues became evident, they began discussing what they could do to improve their services.

Knowledge

Knowledge of Specific Cultural Beliefs

Knowledge forms the core of the pyramid; without knowledge about a specific culture, it is impossible to build skill. Note that knowledge is specific to a particular culture and requires that the provider know specific facts. For example, the belief about which method of administering a medication is best can be culturally based. One cultural group may believe that the best method of administration is the simplest method, while another culture may believe that injections are more potent than oral medications. Hence, parents may readily have their children vaccinated if an injection is used but be unwilling to have their children receive oral vaccine. If the population group is a disadvantaged minority, they may believe that the dominant culture is purposely providing them with a less expensive and inferior product, the oral medication, rather than the more expensive injection.

Community-Specific Cultural Knowledge

Knowledge about culture also means one is able to recognize that culture is community specific and that skin color and language may be related to culture, but they do not determine culture. Therefore, the English-speaking rancher from Montana may have little knowledge of the culture of the English-speaking professor at an urban university even though they speak the same language and have the same skin color. Acknowledging community-specific differences is important, but it should also be noted that people who speak the same language and have enabling attitudes will find it easier to learn about one another's culture.

Cultural knowledge of staff at the tuberculosis clinic

The staff at the county TB clinic had substantial knowledge about the minority culture; they were familiar with the social stigma associated with having TB and had heard stories about TB patients not being allowed to return home after being hospitalized for it. The staff also recognized that the minority population valued children and family. The staff had general knowledge of the primary religion and religious holidays as well as ethnic foods. Additionally, the staff was aware of the respect that the minority population had for health care professionals and that patients generally accepted any proposed treatment without comment.

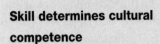

Skill determines cultural competence

Skill is taking action to address cultural issues; without action, inappropriate policies and procedures continue and adverse effects on health continue.

Skill

Skill forms the apex of the pyramid, indicating that the person or the organization has the ability to modify services to accommodate cultural differences so that outcomes will be improved. Skill forms the action component of cultural competence and implies that enabling attitudes and knowledge about the culture do not, by themselves, constitute cultural competence. Certainly outcomes are not improved if no action is taken to respond to a cultural issue.

Skill is probably the most difficult aspect of cultural competence to develop. Role models or examples are needed to learn skill. If one is associated with professionals who are actively developing policies and procedures to address cultural issues, they will develop skill. Having someone present to discuss how they have addressed cultural issues can help others learn the skill. Finally, experience is needed; that is, one must perform the task to develop skill.

Modification of services to address cultural issues at the tuberculosis clinic

For the staff at the county TB clinic, it appears that they generally had enabling attitudes and knowledge about the culture but lacked a systematic approach to modifying their services to address cultural issues. When the staff met to brainstorm about the label incident and how they could address the issue, they were beginning to develop skill. For example, they immediately took action to address the issue of not having formal interpreter services available. They also talked about what they could do to address the label and signage issues.

Learning Cultural Competence

The issue for persons providing health care or working in public health is how to become culturally competent. One study has shown that most providers develop cultural competence through self-initiated learning.[17] Respondents indicated that they had learned little about care for cultural minorities in their professional program and that their knowledge of different cultural groups was obtained by working in a multicultural practice site. Further, given the number of different cultures that a practitioner is likely to encounter in the United States, practitioners are almost certain to obtain new cultural knowledge after training or when they change practice sites. In this section, strategies for learning cultural competence are described.

The goal of this section is to provide a systematic approach to learning cultural competence that can be used in a practice setting, either in public health or a clinic. Methods for learning the three components of cultural competence—enabling attitudes, knowledge, and skill—are described and then other issues related to learning, such as reflection and structure, are discussed and options for addressing them described.

Develop enabling attitudes

The objective of training related to the development of enabling attitudes is to become aware of the influence of culture on health status and on the outcomes of care provided to individuals or populations. This approach is based on the assumption that all practitioners want the best outcomes possible for their patients or for the target community. Enabling attitudes typically are developed through sensitivity training and awareness training.[4]

Sensitivity Training

Sensitivity training usually involves having participants reflect on culture, racism, classism, sexism, and so on. These discussions can be related to a case example. Participants are provided with a description of the case (verbal or videotape), then asked to identify the issues and how the issues affected outcomes either for the patient or for the target population.

Awareness Training

Awareness training can be accomplished by having participants obtain population level information, often census information and vital statistics, to describe the target community. The target community can be described relative to ethnic composition, gender ratio, economic and educational status, religion, languages spoken, and health status. In particular, differences in health status between the community and the health status of the general U.S. population should be identified.

Obtain specific knowledge about the target population

Framework for Learning about Culture

Specific knowledge refers to facts and examples that describe the culture of the target population. A framework for learning about the culture of the community is shown in Table 7.4. Items related to history, language, religion, food, dress and social rules, folk medicine, beliefs about health and illness, and the use of **Western biomedicine** are included in the table. To learn about the community, obtain information on each of the items listed. The table could be used like a table of contents; pictures and notes related to each of the items can be collected.

Methods for Obtaining Information

The methods that can be used to collect the information include the use of key informants, media, and publicly available data. Key informants are residents of the community who have knowledge and insight into community issues;[18] related to culture, they would be residents who have consciously developed their ability to describe the local culture. Information on culture can be obtained from individual patients too.[19] Additional

Table 7.4

A Framework for Describing Community Culture Related to Health

Item	Description	Example
History—especially immigration patterns and originating countries	The target community may be an old community with few recent immigrants or a new community with many recent immigrants	Major population groups of the target community on the U.S.–Mexico border consists of persons of Mexican ancestry or European ancestry who have lived in the community for generations as well as recent immigrants from Mexico and Anglos from other areas of the United States
Language—primary languages spoken, literacy level and local dialects	Language use is strongly influenced by educational level; groups in the United States who are well educated will be fluent in English; groups with limited education may have limited literacy in their native language and speak limited English	The primary language for 90% of the population is Spanish; however, English terms are used for some conditions and behaviors. Further, many residents have low literacy in both Spanish and English
Religion—the dominant religion and major religious holidays; relationship between religion and secular parts of society	This category includes both official or general descriptions of the religion and local practices, particularly as they relate to health	Our Lady of Guadalupe is a central component of Mexican political and religious culture; healing rituals also may involve Our Lady of Guadalupe
Food—traditional foods, especially those used for celebrations	This category includes general dietary habits as well as beliefs about what should be eaten when ill	Tamales are traditionally given as gifts and served at Christmas; making tamales is a family activity
Dress and social rules	Of particular interest to health care providers is how professionals are expected to dress and greet patients	Dress for professionals is more formal than the usual American—MDs will wear shirts and ties with a white coat, nurses wear white dresses and often caps; greetings are exchanged with everyone whenever another person enters the room
Folk medicine	This category is associated with the use of home remedies, for example, teas or healing rituals and over-the-counter medications	Curanderos (traditional healers in Mexico) are often consulted; widespread use of herbal remedies and teas; consultation with a curandero may be recommended by other family members
Beliefs about health and illness	Belief system does not have a disease orientation to health; rather consider a broad range of causes of illness, for example, fear or emotional distress	Chubby children, particularly boys, are considered healthy; a boy who is slim may be considered neglected
Use of Western biomedicine	This category includes the social norms related to the use of home remedies and when to consult a Western-style medical practitioner	Consulting a physician for prenatal care is not customary; Western-style medical care is thought to be necessary only for the delivery

sources of knowledge include books, magazines (bilingual magazines are available in the southwest), information on the Internet, movies, and TV programs. Children's books also can be a good source of cultural information. Finally, ask questions.

Knowledge of the Culture of Western Biomedicine

Knowledge of the culture of Western biomedicine also is important to being able to work across cultures. Western European–American biomedicine has its own set of concepts, values, and beliefs.[11] Several aspects of Western medicine that might conflict with beliefs of other cultures are shown in the box below. For public health, the belief in individual responsibility is particularly relevant. This belief is frequently identified as the rationale for government not to become involved and has been used to oppose non-smoking bans and fluoridation of public water supplies as well as the case for not taxing junk food.

The culture of western medicine and public health

Western medicine has its own culture, which is often overlooked when discussing culture and health. Values and beliefs that may conflict with local cultures are:

- The view that society is based on individuals. Individual action and independence are highly valued; therefore, individuals are thought to be responsible for their health. Hence, public health measures may be seen as an infringement on individual liberty rather than a way to improve the health of the population.

- The view that illness belongs to medically derived categories. Illness is conceptualized as having a discrete cause that is biologic, behavioral, or environmental; consequently, lay beliefs related to other causes, for example, spiritual ones, are ignored.

- The assumption that there is only one system of medicine—Western medicine. If there is only one system of medicine, then the only treatments that are relevant are those derived from Western medicine. A common outcome of this belief is the failure of health care providers to ask about or to discuss other methods of treatment.

- The view that patients must fit the system rather than the system adapting to the patient. Services are provided through clinic settings rather than in the home. Home-based services related to family planning or mental health services may be much more acceptable to some groups.

Knowledge of Your Own Culture

Finally, practitioners will want to have knowledge about their own culture. Practitioners who are able to recognize and describe their own beliefs related to health and illness and other characteristics of their culture will be better able to explore other cultures and will enable them to talk with others about cultural issues. To learn about their own culture, practitioners can work through the framework described in Table 7.4 for their home community or their community of origin. Family members, particularly grandparents, can be excellent sources of information on culture. Another method of identifying the cultural characteristics of one's own culture is to interview persons from other cultures. Persons from other cultures often notice aspects of the culture that members of the same culture may not recognize.

Learn the skills to address cultural issues

Obtain Experience at a Culturally Competent Practice Site

Probably the best method to obtain skill—that is, the ability to take action to address cultural issues—is to obtain experience at a practice site with the organizational characteristics delineated in the CLAS standards. For example, such a practice site would:

- Provide orientation or training in cultural and linguistic competence for the populations they serve;
- Collect data on race, ethnicity, spoken, and written languages;
- Maintain a current demographic and epidemiological description of the populations served;
- Have collaborative relationships with the community (e.g., advisory boards); and
- Supply information to the public on how they provide culturally and linguistically appropriate care.

Use Guided Reflection

Guided reflection is one method that can facilitate this type of learning. Within an academic setting, most students may participate in guided reflection when discussing case studies; the group facilitator asks questions to focus the discussion on specific aspects of the case. However, that type of formal structure may not be available at a practice site. One suggestion might be to have a regularly scheduled meeting dedicated to sharing experiences and information related to cultural competence issues. Also, most sites already have journal clubs that could be used to review articles about culture and cultural competence.

Establish a Structure for Learning

Most students probably do not think specifically about how structure is related to learning, but pharmacy curriculums are typically quite structured. Students attend regularly scheduled classes, laboratories, or discussion groups. Materials related to learning are provided. Again, something like a journal club could provide structure at a practice site. Keeping a diary or journal also would be a method for enhancing one's learning about culture, particularly if it follows the format shown in Table 7.4. Journal entries can serve as the basis for discussion at regularly scheduled meetings.

CASE STUDY 1 (*continued*)

Efforts to increase cultural competency at the tuberculosis clinic

The staff at the county TB clinic decided that they would meet at lunch every other week for five meetings as an initial effort to increase their cultural competency. Since the staff decided that the first thing that they wanted to accomplish was to increase their knowledge of the local minority culture, several of the initial meetings would involve staff members reporting on information that they had learned. They also would locate at least two guest speakers from the minority community and invite them to a meeting to give a presentation on culture. The staff had already decided that they would like to form a community advisory board so they would try to identify community members who could serve on the board. At the last two scheduled meetings, the staff would develop a formal plan for making their services responsive to the culture of the community.

Chapter 7 Summary

Cultural competence means having the attitudes, knowledge, and skill to establish organizational policies for the provision of services that are respectful and responsive to the needs of the population. In contrast, language proficiency is related to the ability to speak a specific language and does not denote cultural competency. Enabling attitudes include having respect for different beliefs and believing that culture has an important influence on the outcomes of health interventions. Knowledge involves knowing specific facts about the population group. Skill is the ability to take action to improve services that improve the needs of the target population group. In addition to knowledge of the target population, practitioners should have knowledge of their own cultural beliefs related to health and knowledge of the culture of Western medicine. Practice sites that address cultural issues will have a formal program for training practitioners to be culturally competent; they will have specific knowledge of the populations involved, for example, demographic and epidemiological descriptions; and they will have established collaborative relationships with the community through, for example, advisory boards.

References

1. Centers for Disease Control and Prevention. Questions and Answers about TB 2005. Available at: http//www.cdc.gov/tb/faqs/qa_introduction.htm. Accessed September 5, 2008.

2. Centers for Disease Control. Fact Sheets: Trends in Tuberculosis, 2005—United States. Available at: http://www.cdc.gov/tb/pubs/tbfactsheets/TBTrends.htm. Accessed September 5, 2008.

3. The National Alliance for Hispanic Health. *A Primer for Cultural Proficiency: Towards Quality Health Services for Hispanics*, 1st ed. Washington, DC: U.S. Department of Health and Human Services; 2001.

4. Betancourt JR. Cross-cultural medical education: conceptual approaches and frameworks for evaluation. *Academic Med.* 2003; 78:560–9.

5. Betancourt JR, Green AR, Carrillo JE, et al. Defining cultural competence: a practical framework for addressing racial/ethnic disparities in health and health care. *Public Health Reports.* 2003; 118:293–302.

6. U.S. Department of Health & Human Services. Cultural Competency-Basic Concepts & Definitions. Available at: http://www.med.umich.edu/multicultural/ccp/basic.htm. Accessed September 5, 2008.

7. Coons SJ. Reporting race and ethnicity in clinical studies and health services research. *Clinical Therapeutics.* 2006; 28:430–1.

8. U.S. Bureau of the Census. Main Page. http://www.census.gov/main/www/cen2000.html. Accessed September 5, 2008.

9. U.S. Bureau of the Census. Overview of Race and Hispanic Origin. 2001. Available at: http://www.census.gov/population/www/cen2000/briefs.html. Accessed September 5, 2008.

10. Agency for Healthcare Research and Quality. National Healthcare Disparities Report, 2005. Available at: http://www.ahrq.gov/qual/nhdr05/nhdr05.htm. Accessed September 5, 2008.

11. Kagawa-Singer M, Kassim-Lakha S. A strategy to reduce cross-cultural miscommunication and increase the likelihood of improving health outcomes. *Academic Med.* 2003; 78:577–87.

12. Arizona Department of Health Services. Differences in the Health Status among Race/Ethnic Groups, Arizona, 2005. Available at: http://www.azdhs.gov/plan/report/dhsag/dhsag05/pdf/measures8.pdf. Accessed September 5, 2008.

13. The Economist. *Pocket World in Figures*, 2007 edition. London, England: Profile Books Ltd.; 2007.

14. Cross Cultural Health Care Program. Introduction to Interpreting. Available at: http://www.xculture.org/BTGIntroMedInterp.php. Accessed September 5, 2008.

15. Downing B, Roat CE. Models for the Provision of Language Access in Health Care Settings. Available at: The National Council on Interpreting in Health Care. 2002. Available at: http://www.xculture.org/NWRC_Med_Interp_Resource_Guide.php. Accessed September 5, 2008.

16. Department of Health and Human Services, Office of Minority Health. National Standards on Culturally and Linguistically Appropriate Services (CLAS) in Health Care. Final Report. 2001.

17. Chevannes M. Issues in educating health professionals to meet the diverse needs of patients and other service users from ethnic minority groups. *J Advanced Nursing.* 2002; 39(3):290–8.

18. Murray SA, Graham LJC. Practice based health needs assessment: use of four methods in a small neighborhood. *BMJ.* 1995; 310:1443–8.

19. Cuellar LM. Teaching students the rationale for providing culturally competent care. In: Cuellar LM, Ginsburg DB. Preceptor's Handbook for Pharmacists. Bethesda, MD: American Society of Health-System Pharmacists; 2005:254–62.

Suggested Readings

Alvord LA, Van Pelt EC. *The Scalpel and the Silver Bear*. New York, NY: Bantam Books; 1999.
This is a story of a Navajo surgeon who combines Western medicine and traditional healing to benefit herself and her patients.

Caudle P. Providing culturally sensitive health care to Hispanic clients. *Nurse Practitioner*. 1993; 18:40–51.
This short, easy-to-read article presents the basics of Hispanic culture for health care practitioners.

Cross Cultural Health Care Program. Introduction to Interpreting. Available at: http://www.xculture.org/BTGIntroMedInterp.php. Accessed September 5, 2008.
This is an excellent resource for materials and information related to cross cultural health care.

Fadiman A. *The Spirit Catches You and You Fall Down: A Hmong Child, Her American Doctors, and the Collision of Two Cultures*, 1st ed. New York, NY: Farrar, Straus & Giroux; 1998.
This is a poignant account of well-intentioned health care practitioners, community advocates, a Hmong child who has seizures, and her parents. Everyone tries to do what is best for the child from their perspective without addressing others' concerns.

Shorris E. *The Life and Times of Mexico*. **New York, NY: WW Norton & Co.; 2004.**
This cultural history of Mexico is written in English but told from the Mexican perspective.

U.S. Department of Health & Human Services. Cultural Competency-Basic Concepts & Definitions. Available at: http://www.med.umich.edu/multicultural/ccp/ basic.htm. Accessed September 5, 2008.
This government web site related to cultural competency is an excellent resource for information and materials related to cultural competency.

Chapter 7 Review Questions

1. Define cultural competence using the three components: attitudes, knowledge, and skill.
Cultural competence is (1) having the attitude that culture is important to health, (2) continually seeking to learn about the cultures of patients, and (3) taking action to adapt services to their cultural needs.

2. For each item below, match the appropriate type of competence.
(a) Linguistic proficiency   (b) Cultural competence
(c) Both linguistic proficiency and cultural competence

_____ Tends to be associated with ethnic background or national identity (c)

_____ Represents the type of knowledge that one would learn from their grandparents (b)

_____ Uses grade completed in school as an approximate measure (a)

3. List the three components of cultural competence and provide an example of each.
Attitude—respecting other people's beliefs is an example of an enabling attitude; the belief that health care is universal and personal beliefs don't matter is an example of an attitude that acts as a barrier.

Knowledge—knowing that it's valuable having a family member accompany the patient to a clinic visit is an example of specific cultural knowledge.

Skill—having the ability to work with a patient of a different culture to adapt the medication regimen to his or her needs is an example of skill.

4. List two types of knowledge and give an example of each that practitioners need to address cultural issues.
Any two of the three types of knowledge listed would be correct:

(1) Specific knowledge related to the culture of the population being served; for example, that one does not pat a child on the head.

(2) Knowledge of the cultural aspects of Western medicine; for example, that efficiency is highly valued.

(3) Knowledge of one's own culture; for example, that professionals are expected to dress more formally than patients and that more formal dress denotes respect to patients.

5. **Identify three characteristics of a practice site that would indicate it addresses the cultural needs of patients.**

Any of three of the four characteristics described would be correct:

(1) The site provides an orientation to new employees on cultural and linguistic competence.

(2) The site had data that describes the populations that they serve.

(3) The site has a formal collaborative relationship with the community, for example, an advisory board.

(4) The site provides information to patients on the cultural and linguistic adaptations of services that are available.

Applying Your Knowledge

1. **Select a persona from the list below. The persona should be as different from you as possible. Now imagine that you are that person and you are calling the director of a recreational facility in your neighborhood. This is a new facility built for families with the goal of increasing physical activity; it was built with tax dollars, but there is a membership fee. You have the money for the membership fee, but when you went to register you were told that there were no more memberships available. You are calling the director to complain.**

   In your new persona, describe your feelings. Do you believe the director's reason for denying your membership? Why or why not? What could the management of the facility do to be more sensitive to your feelings? Do you think that other residents of the neighborhood with a background similar to yours feel the same way?

   Persona List (if you are female, your persona is male; if male, then your persona is female):

   (1) African American, works as a custodian, did not graduate from high school

   (2) Asian, recent immigrant, professional in country of origin, limited English, currently living on assistance from church

   (3) White American, recent immigrant from another part of the United States, now working in a new job with a national chain of retail stores but took a cut in pay to move here

   (4) American Indian, family has lived in the area for generations, works as an accountant

(5) Hispanic, second-generation American, goes to community college while working at a fast-food chain

2. A pharmacy student has just begun working at the same pharmacy where you work. This pharmacy serves a significant minority population. What would you suggest to the new employee to get to know the culture of the neighborhood/community?

3. You are currently working with a community coalition in a metropolitan area on the East coast to address the needs of young families. A significant minority group is living in the community, many of whom do not speak English and who have had little education, even in their country of origin. Because they tend to have large families, this minority group may require educational materials that are appropriate to their circumstances. Another member of the coalition says that they know a pharmacist who recently moved to the community from the West and whose country of origin is the same; they are sure that this pharmacist would gladly translate the educational materials. What are your concerns with this situation?

4. A friend tells you that she is doing volunteer work at the local food bank, which provides emergency rations for community residents. The food bank has an advisory board representing different groups in the community, and your friend is asked to attend one of their meetings. Also the food bank requires all employees, even if they are volunteers, to attend a class on cultural competence; they require that people working there know basic facts about the population served. Your friend is upset with these requirements and asks you why she has to do this: "Why can't I just hand out the food?" she says. How would you respond?

Health Promotion

Learning Outcomes

1. Define health promotion.
2. Describe how the determinants of health are related to health promotion interventions.
3. Identify the three types of knowledge provided by health education.
4. Differentiate among individual, community, and state or national level health promotion interventions.
5. State the rationale for providing health promotion interventions through community pharmacies.

Introduction

One goal of public health is to improve health, that is, to increase the well-being of residents of a community, state, or nation. This chapter describes the types of interventions that can be used to improve health or well-being through use of a case study about Kim, a fictitious pharmacy student. Kim is the subject of a campaign to improve health who becomes an advocate for modifying health-related environmental characteristics. The chapter begins by briefly reviewing the determinants of health, which will serve as the foundation for the activities described later as health promotion interventions. Three important components of health education—awareness knowledge, how-to knowledge, and knowledge of principles—are described, and their relationship to health promotion is delineated. Health promotion interventions are described at the individual level, community level, state or national level, and at the global level. The chapter ends with a discussion of why community pharmacies are ideal locations for conducting health promotion interventions.

Physical Activity in the Context of Modern Lifestyles

Lifestyles in the United States are characterized by consumption of excess calories and lack of physical activity. In fact, more than half the U.S. population does not obtain the minimum amount of exercise recommended by the Centers for Disease Control and Prevention (CDC). Consequently, approximately one third of adults are obese (BMI > 30).[1,2] Because lack of physical activity is thought to be the primary causal factor for obesity,[3] **interventions** are needed that initiate lifestyle changes, including increased physical activity for weight maintenance as well as weight loss.[1,4] Physical activity also promotes health and wellness, even for individuals who have a normal BMI; it reduces stress, improves fitness, and increases bone strength. Therefore, actions by the individual to increase his or her physical activity or actions by communities to increase physical activity of residents can improve the well-being of the population as well as reduce the incidence of disease associated with sedentary lifestyles.

CASE STUDY 1

Life as a pharmacy student and maintaining a healthy weight

Background

Kim is a 24-year-old female pharmacy student in her second year of the professional pharmacy program. Kim's weight would be considered normal for a person of her height; her BMI is 25. However, Kim has a history of weight problems and has been overweight most of her life. When Kim was 19 and a sophomore in college, her weight was so high that she was considered obese; her BMI was 30. The summer before Kim began pharmacy school, she decided that she did not want to be obese and went on a strict diet until she lost enough weight for it to be considered normal.

Maintaining her weight in the normal range has not been easy for Kim. Kim's mother is obese, has had high blood pressure for about 10 years, and was recently diagnosed with diabetes. Kim's father is a heavy equipment operator, is overweight (his BMI is 28), and also has high blood pressure. Kim became used to meals that consisted of potatoes, meat, a small amount of a vegetable, and sometimes a salad as well as dessert. For variety and when the family was busy, they relied on fast food from nearby restaurants. When the family went out to eat, they liked to eat in steakhouses. After Kim left home to attend the state university and became responsible for her own meals, she ate a lot of pizza and burgers with fries—partly because pizza and burgers were easy to get. Several places in the student union sold pizza or burgers in addition to restaurants operated by national burger chains or pizza chains just off campus.

Kim's current lifestyle

Kim's current lifestyle is dominated by school; she spends a lot of time sitting in classes, studying late at night, or surfing the Internet. Kim continues to manage her weight by strict dieting and counting calories. She usually goes without breakfast and packs her lunch for school so that she can count calories. If necessary, Kim will skip dinner to keep from gaining weight. Kim now lives off campus and drives to school every day. Kim lives in a large apartment complex, but the complex is new and has no grocery stores or other shopping areas nearby. Kim needs to drive to get groceries; when she feels that she can afford the calories, she gets a latte. Kim does not participate in any type of sports or recreational activities so her lifestyle would be considered sedentary (i.e., no regular exercise). Kim has not thought much about making an effort to exercise. Neither of her parents had an exercise program, and Kim is rarely ill so exercise does not seem important considering her school demands.

Determinants of Health

The determinants of health, defined as those factors associated with health, will be reviewed briefly. Determinants of health can be characteristics of the individual, for example, age, or they can be characteristics of the external environment, for example, clean air. (See also Chapter 6.) When discussing the determinants of health, the external environment is central because of the individual's interaction with his or her environment and the effects on one's health. The external environment can be separated into the immediate external environment, usually considered the community in which the individual lives, and the larger external environment in which the community is embedded including the state, nation, and globe.

Individual level determinants

Numerous factors are associated with health at the individual level. Physical factors such as genetic characteristics or body weight, either underweight or overweight, are related to health. The most powerful individual level factor related to health is probably socio-economic status. In fact, poverty has been identified by the World Health Organization as the "greatest single killer." Educational attainment and health literacy are related to health because more educated people can expect to be healthier in general, and persons with a high level of health literacy are able to better understand and implement health information. Individual behaviors also are related to health; such behaviors as not smoking or driving safely are clearly related to health.

Community level determinants

The individual–community interaction results in a health consequence for the individual. Individuals who live in a community that has clean water, healthy foods, sanitation services, and housing accessible to its residents will have healthy residents. Economic resources also affect health because residents who have access to well paying employment can provide for their health-related needs. The social environment is related to health; to be healthy, residents need a safe environment and access to education and social services as well as to primary care, including essential medications. Because many community determinants are provided by local government, it must have the ability to provide the services and to take actions to promote health.

State/national/global level determinants

State, national, and global level health determinants tend to act indirectly to influence the health of the individual. State and national governments can assure that resources are available for healthy living and can promulgate laws and regulations that promote health. At the global level, factors like communication networks can promote health by making fresh fruits and vegetables available throughout the year at a reasonable price.

Health Promotion

Health promotion defined

In this chapter, **health promotion** is defined as actions affecting one or more deter-minants of health that enable people to maintain or improve their physical, mental, or social well-being. The opposite of health promotion is to wait until an individual becomes ill or injured and then take actions (i.e., seek medical care) to restore health. Consider the use of seat belts. Many people who use seat belts may have a high level of physical, mental, and social well-being. Using a seat belt helps them maintain a high level of well-being because they are less likely to be injured in minor accidents or to receive life-threatening injuries in more severe accidents. The seat belt example also illustrates that health promotion allows persons who have, for example, a chron-ic disease like diabetes, to maintain their current level of health by reducing their exposure to additional threats.

■ ■ ■

Health promotion versus medical care

The primary focus of health promotion is to maintain or improve current levels of well-being.

In contrast, the primary focus of medical care is to restore health in response to illness or injury.

Health promotion within an ecological framework

Within an ecological framework, the person–environment interaction is the key to health; positive interactions result in health or the maintenance of health, while nega-tive interactions result in illness or a decrement in health. Physical activity is an example of a positive interaction. Individuals can modify their behavior so that they engage in a reasonable amount of physical activity by using walking paths or bike paths in their community. In this case, the individual is engaging in a health-promoting activity that is enabled by the availability of paths for walking or biking. In contrast, if there are no in-door smoking regulations in a community, people are exposed to second-hand smoke in their environment or a negative person–environment interaction. If people are allowed to smoke anywhere, then the environment can be seen as enabling the behavior of smoking.

Three strategies for health promotion include: (1) providing people with informa-tion that encourages them to engage in healthy behaviors or discourages them from en-gaging in behaviors detrimental to health; (2) modifying the environment to encourage positive person–environment interactions or discourage negative person–environment interactions; and (3) providing information related to health promotion while, at the same time, modifying the environment to encourage healthy behaviors.

Role of Education in Health Promotion

Health education is defined as any activity intended to produce changes in knowledge or ways of thinking that facilitates skill acquisition or behavior change related to health.[5] Health education first became popular with the lay public in the early 1800s. Books were published for the lay public that provided information on physiology and anatomy as well as diagnostic information. However, before the 20th century, little specific knowledge was available about how to promote health or prevent disease. The knowledge that was available often provided little benefit or sometimes even harm. For example, general cleanliness was considered good for health but no one specifically understood how diseases could be transmitted via water or prevented by using clean water. As knowledge of how to prevent disease has developed, health education related to avoidance of specific diseases, for example, diarrheal diseases, is available. Health education has become very important, particularly for persons living in poor environmental conditions or without easy access to medical care.

Knowledge components of health education

Knowledge is central to health promotion. For an individual or community to engage in health promotion activities, they must have the requisite knowledge about the activity and its relationship to health. Because education is concerned with the transmission of information and creation of knowledge, health education is a major component of health promotion activities. Health education should provide three types of knowledge: awareness knowledge, how-to knowledge, and knowledge of underlying principles.[6] All three types of knowledge have been identified as necessary to either change behavior or modify the environment.

Awareness

Awareness knowledge is simply knowledge that a health issue exists.[6] Creating awareness typically is the first step in health promotion activities, and it is the objective of many public relations campaigns to improve health (Figure 8.1). Individuals and communities must have knowledge of the factors that are related to health before any

> ■ ■ ■
> **Knowledge components of health promotion**
>
> Three types of knowledge are needed for health promotion:
>
> - Awareness—knowledge that something (e.g., physical activity) is related to health;
>
> - How-to knowledge—development of skills to act on the awareness knowledge; and
>
> - Knowledge of principles—knowledge of what constitutes beneficial use as opposed to detrimental use.

Figure 8.1—Poster promoting W.I.C. (Women, Infants and Children)

Source: Reprinted from the Alabama Department of Public Health.

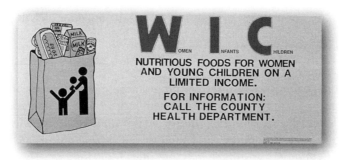

actions can be taken to improve and maintain health. Individuals who do not know that the consumption of fruits and vegetables is essential to good health will not be motivated to eat an adequate amount of them. However, awareness by itself does not assure that individuals or communities will take the actions needed to increase consumption of fruits and vegetables; they also need knowledge of how to use the information to change their behavior or their environment and an understanding of the principles underlying its use.

How-To Knowledge

How-to knowledge represents the skill component of using information about health.[6] If individuals plan to increase their vegetable and fruit consumption, they need to know where to obtain fruits and vegetables, how to store them to prevent spoilage, how to prepare and serve them, and perhaps how to encourage their children to consume them. How-to knowledge can be a neglected component in health education; pamphlets, posters, and TV advertisements may extol the benefits of consuming fruits and vegetables, but information on how to store fresh fruits or vegetables, recipes for preparation, or strategies for encouraging children to eat fruits and vegetables is often more difficult to obtain.

Knowledge of Underlying Principles

Knowledge of underlying principles also is required to enable individuals to use information on health promotion correctly.[6] If an individual does not understand the necessity of washing fruits and vegetables before consumption, the individual may wash the product in dirty water or not wash it adequately to remove the bacteria that produce disease. Individuals who want to eat more fruits and vegetables to improve their health also will need a basic understanding of the caloric consumption–health relationship or they might prepare all their vegetables with butter and cream sauces, which could lead to high caloric consumption and weight gain. Education on the underlying principles related to health is often neglected in health education campaigns or programs.[6]

Health Promotion Interventions

Interventions for health promotion are those activities intended to maintain or improve well-being and are directed toward everyone in a population group, including individuals who are currently healthy. Health promotion interventions also are directed at populations as defined by geographic or political boundaries such as all residents of a city or the residents of a state. The health promotion intervention is expected to benefit everyone in the population, regardless of current health status. Health promotion interventions are based on the determinants of health. Nutrition is known to be a determinant of health; therefore, health promotion interventions could be developed related to nutrition at the individual level, the community level, or at the state, national, or global level

Individual level interventions

Goals and Rationale

The goal of individual interventions in health promotion is to persuade individuals to live in a manner that maintains or improves their health based on the rationale that they can take actions, which will affect their health. Actions related to hygiene or safety are typically included in health promotion. Examples of hygienic actions include brushing one's teeth, taking showers, washing hands, wearing clean clothes, keeping one's living area clean, and using a tissue when sneezing (Figure 8.2). Examples of safety actions include using a seat beat, wearing a helmet when riding a bicycle, looking both ways before crossing a street, stopping for red lights, not driving after consuming alcohol, and not smoking.

Health promotion activities tend to have multiple effects rather than one specific effect. That is, a health promotion activity like exercising has multiple health-related **outcomes** such as developing muscle strength and bone strength; helping to maintain weight, enabling the individual to have good posture; taking pleasure in physical activity; or completing the tasks of daily living. Additionally, exercise reduces the risk of specific diseases such as cardiovascular disease, obesity, and diabetes.

Figure 8.2—Poster for Health Promotion at the Individual Level
Source: Reprinted from Centers for Disease Control and Prevention. Available at: http://www.cdc.gov/healthyswimming/posters.htm#Wash

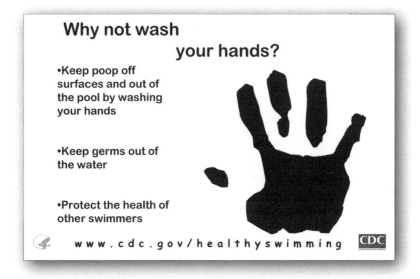

Target Population

Health promotion interventions, including a focus on the individual, usually are aimed at broad population groups that may be defined by geographic or political boundaries. For example, all school children in a school district attend health classes at their schools. All patrons of grocery stores belonging to a particular chain are exposed to posters or pamphlets advocating the consumption of five servings of fruits and vegetables a day. Campaigns to avoid drinking and driving typically are aimed at the entire population, even residents who do not drink, based on the assumption that nondrinkers can influence the actions of their friends and family who do drink.

Assumptions of health promotion at the individual level

Health promotion interventions at the individual level are based on the assumption that individuals can take actions (e.g., wash their hands) that will positively affect their health.

Interventions

Interventions for health promotion at the individual level are likely to include a large educational component to encourage individuals to engage in activities that maintain or improve their health. Health classes in elementary schools are examples of health promotion interventions. Children are taught why to brush their teeth twice a day, how to brush their teeth, and why brushing their teeth is good for them, which are the components of health education described as awareness, how-to knowledge, and principles knowledge. The intervention may involve keeping a chart and awarding gold stars to children who brush their teeth every day for a week.

Encouraging people to wash their hands is another example of a health promotion intervention. Some restaurants place posters in their restrooms reminding employees that they must wash their hands before returning to work. Children are taught how to wash their hands and reminded to wash them before meals and after using the restroom.

Health promotion interventions often involve safety. Campaigns to encourage children or adults to wear helmets when riding bicycles are examples of health promotion. Again, the intervention likely will rely heavily on education. Posters are displayed where residents are apt to see them. Education on wearing a helmet is probably a part of health education classes in schools and perhaps the subject of advertisements on television or in print media. The most effective educational campaigns will include a message to create awareness of the need to wear a helmet, the correct way to wear the helmet, and ways the helmet protects the head. Personal stories about helmet safety can be quite persuasive and demonstrate how the helmet allowed an individual to avoid head injury.

Outcomes and Evaluation

The primary outcome of health promotion is the proportion of the population engaging in appropriate healthy behaviors such as washing hands, consuming five servings of fruits and vegetables a day, using seatbelts, or not smoking. Health promotion campaigns could be evaluated by conducting a survey before and after the campaign to determine if the proportion of the population engaging in specific activities has increased. Indirect measures also provide data, for example, a campaign to increase hand washing might monitor the amount of soap used based on the assumption that increased soap use indicates increased hand washing.

CASE STUDY 1 *(continued)*

Kim's health promotion interventions, individual level: 5k walk/run

Kim herself became the target of a health promotion intervention. The recreation center at the university decided to improve the level of physical fitness among students. A pharmacy student who worked at the campus rec center conducted a survey of pharmacy students and several groups of other students; he found that about 30% of students surveyed got no exercise at all. So the rec center decided that they would sponsor a 5k walk/run. They identified several local merchants who were willing to help sponsor the event as well as the rec center and the student council. Because the group wanted students who currently did not engage in physical activity to participate, they emphasized how much fun the event would be and offered small prizes to anyone completing the 5k as well as opportunities to win raffle prizes. Several of the raffle prizes were free consultations with a trainer at the rec center.

Kim was aware of the 5k walk/run, but didn't think much about it until her friend and classmate started talking about it. Several more classmates talked about participating, so they all signed up for the event. Since Kim felt quite out of shape, she decided to start training for the event by walking at least a mile 3 times a week. When Kim and her friends completed the 5k event 6 weeks later, Kim decided that she would like to try a 10k and run at least part of the way. Kim began training for a 10k by walking and running intervals for 2 miles 3 to 5 times a week, depending on her exams. Kim began to feel a lot less stressed, and she felt good from getting the exercise.

Community level interventions

Goals and Rationale

The goal of health promotion at the community level probably is best described as creating an environment that enables residents to be healthy. If an individual is to be able to wash his or her hands or keep a clean house, that person must have access to clean water. If the individual is to live in an environment that is smoke free, then corresponding laws or policies must assure public areas are smoke free.

Target

The target of health promotion interventions at the community level probably is best described as community infrastructure and policies or laws related to health.

Interventions

The determinants of health described at the community level identify those aspects of the community which would be the subject of a health promotion intervention. The most obvious infrastructure determinants of health probably are water supplies, sanitation, food supplies, the physical environment, and the availability and accessibility of schools as well as primary care, including pharmacies. Interventions could be aimed at developing any part of the infrastructure or at improving the existing infrastructure. For example, a primary care clinic might be available, but residents in certain areas may have limited access due to the lack of public transportation. The intervention then would involve changing bus routes or establishing some type of public transportation.

Policies or laws are the other primary venue for health promotion activities at the community level. Laws requiring children to attend school and programs to prevent truancy could be considered health promotion interventions. Laws and policies related to safety are another example. Traffic laws that establish penalties for running red lights and driving on the wrong side of the road are laws that promote health. Housing ordinances that require houses built in the community to be connected to the sewer or to meet certain standards are health promoting.

Assumptions of health promotion at the community level

Community level interventions are based on the assumptions that:

- An individual's immediate environment can enable or inhibit that person's ability to engage in healthy behaviors; and

- The immediate environment contains factors (e.g., clean air) that promote health or factors (e.g., polluted air) that are detrimental to health.

The formation of community coalitions is one way to promote the adoption of laws or policies by local government that will promote health.

Health education is important for community level interventions as well as for individual level interventions. Community leaders, including members of the local government, and local residents need basic awareness of health issues and information on addressing them before they will undertake infrastructure development or pass laws or institute policies that promote health. Fluoridation of water supplies is an example. Local government is not likely to undertake fluoridation if they do not know that it benefits health, and local residents may not permit fluoridation if they do not understand its value in promoting health. Therefore, substantial educational campaigns related to a particular health promotion intervention may be needed even for interventions involving community infrastructure or laws or policies.

Outcomes and Evaluation

The primary outcome of community level health promotion activities is the proportion of the population that lives in a safe environment and has access to clean water and sanitation, easy access to healthy foods, no exposure to pollutants in the physical environment, adequate housing, and availability of schools, social services, and primary care. Community services can be evaluated by examining the proportion of the population with access to services or to a clean environment.

CASE STUDY 1 (*continued*)

Kim's health promotion interventions, community level: bike and walking trails

Kim's friend was a member of a local organization advocating for bike and walking trails. The organization was trying to convince the county government to construct bike and walking trails along several highways in the county. Several highways were heavily used by cyclists and runners but there were no trails, so they were forced to ride or run in the traffic lane. Kim attended a meeting of the county supervisors with her friend and other members of the organization. A member of the organization gave a presentation about the importance of the trails in preventing injuries or accidental deaths for residents who rode bikes or ran along these highways. The presenter showed pictures of the dangerous areas and provided some statistics about how many people rode bikes or ran along the two highways. After the presentation, several supervisors asked questions. Two of the supervisors were very opposed to the proposal, and stated flatly that it wasn't the county's responsibility to provide walking or bike trails. Several other supervisors liked the idea, but didn't know where they could find funds for building the trails. The board voted to investigate the possibility and consider it again at a later meeting.

This was Kim's first experience with advocating for change in the community that should improve residents' health; she was disappointed that the board of supervisors didn't adopt the proposal. However, Kim's friend told her that advocating for this kind of change takes time and would probably require numerous meetings. At their next meeting, the organization's members decided that they would meet with individual supervisors to explain their concerns and identify who they could count on to vote for the proposal.

State and national interventions

Goals and Rationale

The goal of health promotion interventions at the state and national level is probably best represented by resource allocation or laws or regulations that enable local governments to modify infrastructure or require the government to provide health-promoting services. However, state or national governments also may conduct educational campaigns aimed at individuals through TV advertisements or the Internet or through distribution of educational materials. The focus in this section, though, will be on resource allocation or laws and regulations.

Target

The target for health promotion interventions involving resources or laws typically is local government or local organizations, possibly a community coalition or a community health center involved in promoting health.

Interventions

A typical intervention for a state government or the U.S. federal government is providing funds for health promotion through grant programs. The local government or community organization develops a grant proposal and submits it to the government agency administering the grant program. The grants are reviewed, and funds are awarded. One advantage to a grant program is that it requires the grantee to describe how he or she will use the funds and assures that the grantee knows how to develop the infrastructure or the program.

> ■ ■ ■
>
> **Assumptions of health promotion at the state level**
>
> State level interventions are based on the assumptions that:
>
> - Allocating funds can enable communities to develop infrastructure that promotes health; and
>
> - Proposing laws or regulations can enable communities to deter individuals or groups from acting in ways that are detrimental to the health of residents.

State legislatures may directly allocate funds to communities for infrastructure development. Improvement of roadways, including the addition of sidewalks or walking trails, often are funded with a combination of money from state, federal, and local governments. Both the federal and state governments may provide some services that are health promoting, for example, the formation and maintenance of parks and recreational areas.

The government, at both the state and federal levels, also may pass laws or regulations that are health promoting. States pass laws regulating traffic on roadways and fines for speeding, and they maintain a highway patrol to enforce the laws. The federal government passes regulations requiring states that use federal funds to meet requirements related to roadway design and for laws regulating use. Seat belts are another example. States pass laws related to seat belt use, and they decide how they will enforce the law. However, the federal government has laws and regulations related to the installation of seat belts in vehicles.

Outcomes and Evaluation

The outcomes of state and federal involvement in infrastructure development or passage of laws related to health promotion are infrastructure and laws that support health promotion. A grant program may be evaluated by calculating the number of communities that did not have a specific service such as fluoridation before the program began, then calculating the number after the program. States and the federal government also collect data on highway accidents or similar data to evaluate the outcomes of governmental efforts to promote health.

 CASE STUDY 1 (continued)

Kim's health promotion interventions, state level: funding for safety improvement

Several weeks later, Kim's friend told her that a group from the local organization proposing the trails was going to the state capitol to meet with legislators. One of the members of the organization was a social worker who knew several of the legislators; one legislator was also an avid cyclist. The group decided that they should meet with the legislators to find out how to influence any proposed legislation that would provide some funding for safety improvement.

Kim visited the legislators with her friends. The meetings were interesting, but they did not seem to accomplish much. The legislators listened and they seemed impressed that students were involved in the effort, but they made no commitments. Kim felt discouraged, but the social worker felt encouraged; he said that they had started to educate the legislators and the county supervisors about the issues. He thought they should continue to follow up with them and provide more information and also persuade others to contact both groups. The social worker thought that it would take several years to actually get bike and walking trails.

Global level interventions

Global health promotion probably is best exemplified by treaties or agreements among nations related to the safety of food and products, for example, children's toys. The United States establishes agreements with its trading partners to assure that food products imported into the United States are safe for consumption. Regulations also govern the amount of lead that is allowed in children's toys.

International health organizations such as WHO (the World Health Organization[7]) and PAHO (the Pan American Health Organization[8]) may act as advocates for interventions that promote health. Both organizations provide support for individual country efforts to promote health by providing data on health issues and by offering educational materials or even technical assistance.

The Role of Community Pharmacy in Health Promotion

Ideal locations for health promotion activities

Four characteristics of pharmacists and pharmacies make community pharmacies an excellent location for health promotion activities. The geographic location of pharmacies in neighborhoods is particularly important to promoting lifestyle change so that residents have easy access to the pharmacy. The pharmacy often is within walking distance, and the extended service hours increase the convenience of obtaining services. Hence to receive counseling on, for example, weight loss, the patient could walk to the pharmacy and consult with the pharmacist in the evening after work. In contrast, to receive the same counseling from a physician, the patient probably would need to take time off work, commute to a clinic which is likely distant from both the worksite and home, and wait until the physician was available to meet.

Pharmacists also have patient counseling skills. They frequently counsel patients about their medications, and pharmacists have a respected position among the public as health care professionals. Thus, pharmacists have the expertise to participate in health promotion activities, and they are ideally located to meet the needs of residents.

Ability to customize interventions for the neighborhood

Most pharmacists provide a great deal of individual education related to prescription medication; hence, pharmacists already have patient education skills. Because neighborhood residents visit a pharmacy frequently, the pharmacist can reinforce education, offer encouragement for behavior change, and provide support and subsequent education as needed. Pharmacists can tailor educational materials to the needs of the neighborhood. If the neighborhood includes a substantial proportion of Spanish speakers, materials can be provided in Spanish. If the literacy level is low, the education could be provided via videos. Pharmacists also are in an excellent position to refer residents to literacy programs, for example, English as a second language classes.

Pharmacists can assure that educational materials are available for the types of health issues relevant to residents. For example, if the pharmacy is located in the arid Southwest, educational materials on the importance of adequate hydration likely would be useful to residents. If the pharmacy is located in the upper Midwest, information on avoiding frostbite likely would be pertinent. Pharmacists also can tailor the educational materials to the needs of the neighborhood; for example, if smoking is an issue, materials on smoking cessation can be provided. Thus, community pharmacists and pharmacies are well positioned to engage in health promotion interventions.

Rationale for health promotion activities in community pharmacies

Community pharmacies are ideal locations for health promotion activities because of their:

- Geographic location in neighborhoods so that local residents have easy physical access;
- Extended service hours, which are convenient to local residents;
- Content expertise related to medications and experience with individual patients; and
- Respected position among the public as health care professionals.

Kim's health promotion interventions, neighborhood: sidewalks

Kim works part time in a community pharmacy during the school year, and works as much as she can during the summer. The summer after she participated in the walk/run and started training for the 10k, Kim noticed it was much easier for her to talk to patients about their need to exercise and even encouraged them with her own story. She told them she had been a "couch potato" a year ago and now was training for a 10k; she also talked about how much better she felt and how she had more energy and felt less stressed. Kim encouraged patients to just walk down the street and back in the beginning. Kim had assumed a new role with patients because now she was a positive role model for lifestyle, which is a role advocated by the American Association of Family Physicians.

Kim also became interested in the condition of sidewalks and streets in the neighborhood around the pharmacy; she was telling patients to walk, but she did not know if it was safe for them to walk in that neighborhood. Kim's friend told her about a paper tool that she could use to assess the walkability of the neighborhood (see Figure 8.3). It sounded strange to Kim, but she got her friend to help her and they walked around the neighborhood. Kim was surprised at how unsafe it was to walk. Because it was a new neighborhood, she had expected it to be a nice place to walk but found there were almost no sidewalks. Kim and her friend saw children riding their bicycles in the street and parents with strollers in the street. Kim did not see any older adults; perhaps the lack of sidewalks kept them from walking at all. Kim thought that she would recommend patients go to the park if they wanted to walk. She didn't want someone to be involved in an accident because she had recommended that they walk more.

Figure 8.3—Walkability Audit Tool[9]

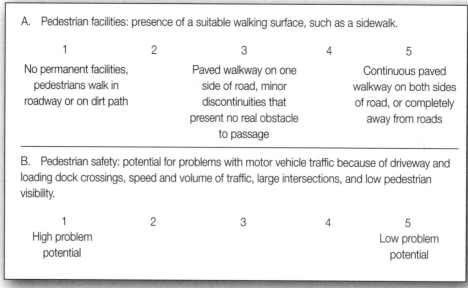

A. Pedestrian facilities: presence of a suitable walking surface, such as a sidewalk.

1	2	3	4	5
No permanent facilities, pedestrians walk in roadway or on dirt path		Paved walkway on one side of road, minor discontinuities that present no real obstacle to passage		Continuous paved walkway on both sides of road, or completely away from roads

B. Pedestrian safety: potential for problems with motor vehicle traffic because of driveway and loading dock crossings, speed and volume of traffic, large intersections, and low pedestrian visibility.

1	2	3	4	5
High problem potential				Low problem potential

Continued

C. Crosswalks: presence and visibility of crosswalks on intersecting roads. Traffic signals have functional "walk" lights that provide sufficient crossing time.

1	2	3	4	5
Crosswalks not present despite major intersections				No intersections, or crosswalks clearly marked

D. Maintenance: buckling pavement, overgrown vegetation, standing water, etc. on or near the path. Does not include temporary problems.

1	2	3	4	5
Major or frequent problems				No problems

E. Path size: useful path width, accounting for barriers to passage such as utility poles and signs mounted in the walkway.

1	2	3	4	5
No permanent facilities	<3 feet wide, significant barriers			>5 feet wide, no barriers

F. Buffer: space separating path from adjacent roadway

1	2	3	4	5
No buffer from roadway, or pedestrians walk in roadway			>4 feet from roadway	Not adjacent to roadway

G. Accessibility: ease of access for the mobility impaired. Includes handrails accompanying steps, ramps to accommodate wheelchairs, etc.

1	2	3	4	5
Completely impassible or no permanent facilities	Very difficult or dangerous		Universally accessible route available but inconvenient	Designed to facilitate universal access

H. Aesthetics: includes proximity of fences and buildings, noise, landscaping quality, and presence of pedestrian-oriented features such as benches and water fountains.

1	2	3	4	5
Uninviting				Pleasant

Continued

Figure 8.3—*Continued*

I. Shade: amount of shade, accounting for different times of day.

1	2	3	4	5
No shade				Full shade

Sum of High importance (A–C): _____ x 3 = _____

Sum of Medium importance (D–H): _____ x 2 = _____

Sum of Low importance (I): _____ x 1 = _____

Total Score: _____/100

Chapter 8 Summary

The determinants of health at the level of the individual, community, and state or nation are used as a foundation for describing health promotion. Health promotion is defined as interventions aimed at modifying a health determinant that will increase the well-being of a population. Health education is an important component of health promotion interventions because people must have knowledge that a specific factor, that is, a health determinant, is related to health. Then they must have knowledge of how to address the factor; they also need knowledge about the principles of the intervention to use that intervention appropriately.

Health promotion interventions can be implemented at the individual level, as exemplified by a campaign or event designed to increase physical activity; at the community level, as exemplified by efforts of a local organization to improve walking and cycling trails; or at the state level, as exemplified by efforts from the state legislature to obtain funding for the improvement of trails. Pharmacists can have a role at all levels of health promotion interventions, including efforts at influencing local or state government to improve the environment for residents to engage in health-promoting activities. This chapter demonstrates that health promotion inventions are very different than medical interventions, but they are an important component of public health if the well-being of populations is to be maintained and improved.

References

1. Centers for Disease Control and Prevention. Contributing Factors: Overweight and Obesity: An Overview. Available at: http:///www.cdc.gov. Accessed March 1, 2009.

2. National Center for Health Statistics. Prevalence of Overweight and Obesity among Adults: United States, 2003–2004. Available at: http://www.cdc.gov/nccdphp/dnpa/obesity/index.htm. Accessed March 1, 2009.

3. Slack MK. Interpreting current physical activity guidelines and incorporating them into practice for health promotion and disease prevention. *Am J Health-Syst Pharm.* 2006; 63:1647–53.

4. Trust for America's Health. F as in Fat: How Obesity Policies Are Failing in America. Available at: http://healthyamericans.org/reports/obesity2008/. Accessed March 1, 2009.

5. Tones K. Health education, behaviour change, and public health. In: Detels R, Holland WW, McEwen J, et al. eds. *Oxford Textbook of Public Health.* Volume 2. New York, NY: Oxford University Press; 1997:783–814.

6. Rogers EM. *Diffusion of Innovations.* New York, NY: Free Press; 2003.

7. World Health Organization (WHO). Available at: http://www.who.int/topics/health_promotion/en/. Accessed March 1, 2009.

8. Pan American Health Organization (PAHO). Available at: http://www.paho.org/Project.asp?SEL=TP&LNG=ENG&ID=145. Accessed March 1, 2009.

9. Centers for Disease Control and Prevention. Walkability Audit Tool. Available at: http://www.cdc.gov/nccdphp/dnpa/hwi/toolkits/walkability/Walkability_Audit_Tool.pdf. Accessed March 1, 2009.

Suggested Readings

Rogers EM. *Diffusion of Innovations.* New York, NY: Free Press; 2003.
Rogers presents a framework for the diffusion of innovations, presents the stages of diffusion, and discusses early adopters versus late adopters. Rogers also discusses the pro-innovation bias of diffusion research. While not appearing to be related to health, many of Rogers' examples are health promotion activities such as adopting pure drinking water in Egyptian villages and smoking cessation programs. The failure of populations to adopt innovations also is described. The book is clearly written with copious examples; it is highly recommended for a non-public health perspective on health promotion.

Unnatural Causes. DVD available at: www.unnaturalcauses.org. Produced by California Newsreel with Vital Pictures; 2008.
This program investigates health from the perspective of social, economic, and physical environments where people are born, live, and work. Surprisingly, the investigators find that conventional medical care, genes, and behaviors account for only 25% of the difference in mortality between neighborhoods in the same city. This film is very well done and thought provoking.

Chapter 8 Review Questions

1. **Define health promotion and provide an example.**
   Health promotion is an action that results in the improvement of an individual's well-being. An example would be training to participate in a run/walk.

2. **Conducting a class to teach new parents how to prepare vegetables for children is an example of health education.** _____ True _____ False
   True

3. **If members of the city council knew what aspects of their city are determinants of health, they could assure that council actions promote the well-being of residents.** _____ True _____ False
   True

4. **Match the level of intervention—individual, community, or state—to the example health promotion interventions listed below. There is one best answer.**
   (a) Individual   (b) Community   (c) State

   _____ The legislature passed a law that prohibits teens from driving a vehicle with other teens as passengers for 6 months after they obtain their driver's license. (c)

   _____ The city council required that each council district assess roadways for bicycle safety and write a report. (b)

   _____ The college of pharmacy placed posters that list the number of calories burned by climbing two flights of stairs next to the elevators of all the buildings in the health sciences complex. (a)

5. **The county health department decided to form a partnership with community pharmacies to promote the use of sunscreen because** _____.

   Any of the following would be acceptable:

   • They could reach most of the neighborhoods in the city through pharmacies.

   • Pharmacies sell sunscreens.

   • A majority of the local population is likely to patronize a pharmacy sometime during the week.

   • Patrons can talk to the pharmacist if they have questions about using sunscreens.

Applying Your Knowledge

1. Using the same walkability tool as Kim did to assess the neighborhood where the pharmacy in which she worked is located, assess your own neighborhood or campus of your school (or both).

2. Visit a community pharmacy and identify the products that are related to health promotion. Consider both OTC and prescription products.

3. Attend a city council meeting to determine if any of the factors considered determinants of health are discussed during the meeting.

4. Interview the fire chief or station chief to discover how they think that they affect the health of the community.

Disease Prevention

■ ■ ■

Learning Outcomes

1. Describe the continuum from perfect health to death and circumstances in which disease prevention and health promotion activities may be used.
2. List the three levels of prevention and describe the types of populations targeted at each level.
3. For each level of prevention, list the goals of interventions and the types of interventions used to reach those goals.
4. Describe types of primary, secondary, and tertiary interventions for disease prevention at each of these levels: individual, community, and national or international.
5. Give examples of activities performed by pharmacists that demonstrate involvement at the three levels of prevention.

Introduction

In the previous chapter, the idea of health promotion was presented. This chapter will cover a complementary concept called disease prevention. A review of the health-to-death continuum will show how disease prevention programs pick up where health promotion programs end. In the case study, colon cancer is used to illustrate the three levels of disease prevention—reducing the risk of developing cancer, detecting cancer early through screening programs, and treating the disease to cure it or to avoid complications or premature death. The chapter will conclude with examples that illustrate how this public health concept can be used to consider preventable risks from medication use.

The Continuum from Health to Death

As Figure 9.1 shows, every living individual falls somewhere on the continuum from perfect health to death. Disease was added as an intermediate state between health and death, even though some people live in relatively good health until the day they die. Disease prevention is concerned with the individuals who are most likely to develop disease or suffer an injury that causes poor health (**morbidity**) or premature death (**mortality**) because they are deemed to be preventable.

While **health promotion** activities are designed to maximize the health of a population (the left side of the continuum), **disease prevention** programs are used to minimize the risk of disease and premature death. Some overlap exists in program goals and activities of health promotion and disease prevention programs where health begins to transition into early disease.

Figure 9.1—The Health-to-Death Continuum

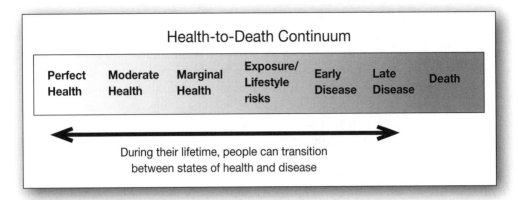

Not all premature deaths are preceded by disease. For example, death caused by an accident or injury may occur quickly. Therefore, the key concepts that will be considered in this chapter are whether a death is premature regardless of cause and, if the cause is known, whether it be prevented.

Disease Prevention Can Be Local or Global

Like health promotion, actions taken to reduce or eliminate preventable disease and death may occur at the individual, community, state, national, and international levels. While health care professionals tend to focus on interventions that target individuals (i.e., their patients), public health professionals take a broader view and aim to intervene at multiple levels for a more effective and enduring prevention effort.

Individual disease prevention

Disease prevention at the level of the individual person focuses on behaviors that put a person at risk of being exposed to a disease-causing agent as well as behaviors that deteriorate health. A person who is healthy is usually better able to resist disease and, if he or she becomes ill, is better able to recover fully. Interventions that are tailored to the individual are likely to be more effective. For example, an individual can reduce the risk of skin cancer by reducing his or her exposure to ultraviolet light through the use of sunscreens and barriers like clothing, hats, and shade. Individuals can also reduce the risk of premature death from skin cancer by examining themselves for changes in their skin and seeking medical care early when they detect a changing mole or other suspicious lesion. If they require treatment, they will receive individualized therapy and monitoring to eliminate the cancer or at least slow its progression.

Prevention as cornerstone of public health

Avoiding preventable disease, injury, and premature death is a cornerstone of public health philosophy and action.

Community disease prevention

Preventing disease at a community level may involve identifying populations in the community that are at risk of exposure to a disease because of where they live or work. Preventing exposure may involve removing contaminated soil, water, or buildings. It may also involve local ordinances to prevent behaviors that have harmful consequences. Prevention may include efforts to create areas where people can exercise safely or grow vegetables in a community garden. Communities may prevent disease through the involvement of groups of citizens in education or support groups for diseases, campaigns against violence or hate crimes, creation of public places for relaxation and interaction, or increased access to screening and early treatment services. For skin cancer, a community may provide education about the risks of cancer to ensure its residents know there is a risk. A community may build a cover over public pools to block the sun and allow swimmers to wear t-shirts over swimsuits and sunscreen in the water if the pool is outside. The community may strictly enforce regular checks of tanning salons to ensure the tanning beds are functioning well. The community may initiate a tree-planting program for schools and residential areas to increase shade. It may ensure that outdoor events are scheduled either in the morning or the evening when the risk of sunburn is lower.

State, national, and international disease prevention

State-level disease prevention efforts may include regulation of businesses and their disposal of wastes that may contaminate water, air, or soil. Laws may be created to eliminate or control sources of preventable injury or disease such as local non-smoking ordinances and restricting the sale of alcohol. States also control the licensing of health care professionals and their clinical sites, which can affect local access to the care needed to treat and recover from a disease.

At a national level, disease prevention may involve regulation of manufacturers that produce products used to prevent or detect disease. This regulation may include product packaging and advertisement as well as ingredients and preparation. Prevention may involve airing educational public service announcements on television and via the web as well as incorporating information about diseases into the storylines of popular television programs. Restrictions on advertising products that may be harmful such as alcohol and tobacco can also be considered a health promotion or disease prevention activity at the national level. Interstate activities that can negatively impact the health of residents of more than one state (e.g., air or water pollution) will also be targets for national prevention efforts. Funding for research to treat disease and return the afflicted to health is another way disease prevention is provided from a national level. Within the United States, mandates can be enforced that reduce the risk of injury or exposure to disease-causing agents. Examples of national programs to prevent disease include recalls of contaminated food or toys or unsafe medications.

Prevention at the international level is similar to that of the national level except it requires voluntary cooperation among the nations involved in the prevention ac-

> Prevention interventions may occur at many levels, from efforts aimed at individuals to efforts that are multinational. The most effective prevention programs usually involve interventions that span from individuals to communities and beyond.

tivities. For diseases that occur in most countries and toxic substances that cross borders, efforts to reduce exposure and improve recovery require all involved nations to develop interventions they can implement within their own borders.

 CASE STUDY 1

Preventing colon cancer and its complications

Incidence, prevalence, and death rates for colorectal cancer in the United States

According to the National Cancer Institute, colorectal cancer is the second leading cause of cancer-related death in the United States. In 2005, just over 48 new cases were reported of colorectal cancer for every 100,000 people, and approximately 25 people died per 100,000.[1] The incidence of colorectal cancer and **death rates** are evenly split among the genders, but tend to occur more frequently in adults over 50 years old and in African-American and White races. A 2008 report from the National Cancer Institute showed declines in overall incidence and death rates from all cancer for the first time in 10 years. Although the cancer incidence is declining, many people will be diagnosed and die from it each year. [2]

Cancers appear to have many factors that contribute to their development and affect how well a person will recover from the disease. As causes of cancer are understood through research, treatments can be refined to be more effective and less toxic. Prevention programs can target more specific causes to further reduce the **incidence rate**. Although the exact mechanisms involved in the development of colorectal cancer are not completely understood, some factors have been associated with an increased risk of developing it. They include age (over 90% of cases occur in those who are 50 years or older); history of inflammatory bowel disease; family history of polyps or colorectal cancer; poor lifestyle habits such as lack of exercise and a diet high in fat and low in fiber, vegetables, and fruit; obesity; and consumption of alcohol and tobacco.[3] Early detection and treatment can improve survival rates for this type of cancer.

NP as a typical high-risk patient

NP is a black male in his late 50s who has enjoyed a relatively healthy life in spite of his bad habits and unhealthy lifestyle. He tips the scales at 260 pounds, which is more than he should carry on his 5'9" frame. NP is the manager of a local department store, and spends most of his time in his office working on a computer, making calls, and keeping the books. He enjoys a couple beers in the evening when he watches TV and still smokes about one pack of cigarettes per day despite recent efforts to quit. His father died of colorectal cancer when he was 62, and his brother was recently diagnosed as having polyps.

NP takes medication for high blood pressure and high cholesterol, both of which seem to be working since his blood pressure and lab values are now in the normal range. Recently, he has been feeling more tired than usual; he has lost about 15 pounds over the past 4 months without trying; and he is experiencing some indigestion with embarrassing gas. He figures it is part of growing older, but a recent news story about colon cancer has him thinking he may have something else going on.

Levels of Prevention

Figure 9.2 shows how the three **levels of prevention** are related to the health-to-death continuum, health promotion, and to one another. Prevention activities can vary in terms of the populations they target, their goals, interventions used to prevent disease or its effects, and ways to measure the effectiveness of interventions. Leavell and Clark captured these ideas when they described the three levels of prevention as primary, secondary, and tertiary.[4] Today, these levels are commonly used to indicate the type of prevention intervention that a program will provide. These levels represent a progression of activities—preventing exposures or injuries, preventing new disease, and preventing complications or premature death.

As the levels progress from primary to tertiary, the population targeted becomes more specific; the interventions become more patient specific; the goals have higher stakes; and the success measured goes from exposures prevented to lives saved. Together, interventions across all levels of prevention will contribute to an ultimate goal of reducing or eliminating avoidable illness, injury, and premature death. Table 9.1 shows a grid of the three levels of prevention and their relative goals, target populations, and interventions. Each level is described in detail in the following sections.

Figure 9.2—Relationships among Health Promotion, Levels of Prevention, and States of Health and Disease

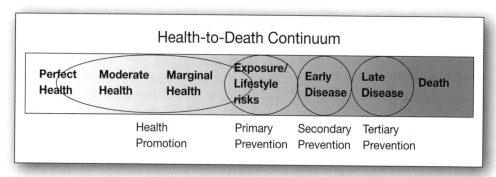

Table 9.1

Levels of Disease Prevention by Target Population, Goal, Rationale, Interventions, and Outcomes

Disease:

	Primary	Secondary	Tertiary
Population	General or At-risk	Exposed or early disease	Advanced disease or Complications
Goal	↓ new cases	↓ severity ↓ complications	↓ impact ↓ deaths
Rationale	↓ risk by exposure	Early identification allows earlier treatment	Minimize impact of disease on person
Interventions	Education Prophylaxis Health promotion	Screening Early treatment Access to care	Treatment Rehabilitation
Evaluation (Outcomes)	↓ incidence of exposure	↓ incidence of disease ↓ morbidity	↓ prevalence ↓ morbidity ↓ mortality

The three levels of prevention are primary, secondary, and tertiary. Their role in prevention begins at avoidance of exposures or situations that increase risk of disease; moves to early detection of exposures or disease; and ends with efforts aimed at returning the sick or injured person back to health, thereby avoiding long-term morbidity and premature mortality.

Primary prevention

Goals and Rationale

In **primary prevention**, the goal is to reduce the probability of developing a disease in a **target population**. Interventions focus on exposures and resistance based on the rationale that reducing exposure to diseases or toxic substances and fortifying the body so it can resist disease-causing agents or organisms can reduce the likelihood that a disease will develop.

Target Populations

Primary prevention programs may focus on the general population or a subset of the population with a higher risk of exposure or increased susceptibility to a disease, if exposed. For some common and widespread diseases, like influenza or heart disease, the subpopulation that is targeted by the intervention could be quite large. For other diseases with rare or limited incidence, the targeted population may represent a mere fraction of a percent of the total population. The key is that the target population will be defined by its risk of exposure to a specific disease or toxin or susceptibility to its effects.

Interventions to Reduce Exposure

One approach for primary prevention activities focuses on removing the risk of exposure to the disease-causing agent. For some infectious diseases, such as malaria, this may involve draining standing water where the mosquitoes that carry the disease-causing microorganism breed. If the mosquito vectors are eliminated, the risk of exposure to the microorganism is also eliminated. Other infectious diseases, like influenza, spread through inhalation of aerosolized viruses from unguarded sneezes or coughs and by touching contaminated surfaces and then touching the face. Reducing exposure for this disease would require isolating those who are sick and contagious from those who have not yet been infected. In large-scale outbreaks (i.e., **epidemics**), public places like theaters and schools have been closed in an attempt to reduce the spread of disease.

Primary prevention

Primary prevention is focused on reducing the risk of exposure to disease-causing agents and increasing the ability of a person or community to resist the development of disease if exposure occurs.

Interventions to Increase Resistance to the Disease

Another primary prevention intervention to reduce the risk of disease is to bolster a person's ability to resist development of a disease if exposed. This intervention may be accomplished through general improvement of health (e.g., health promotion programs), through interventions that bolster resistance to a specific disease (e.g., vaccines), or both. In the case of influenza, a trivalent vaccine can be used to develop antibodies specific to the three most likely virus strains. For a disease related to lifestyle risks, like type 2 diabetes, maintaining good health can reduce development of the disease by avoiding the risk factors directly related to it.

Outcomes and Evaluation

The outcome for primary prevention interventions is a reduction in the number of people exposed to a disease-causing agent; however, measuring exposure rate may be difficult for some diseases. Since the ultimate goal is a reduction in the number of new cases, that measure can also be used to determine the effectiveness of primary prevention interventions. Another potential measure of primary prevention effectiveness is a more global view of how quickly and how far the disease spreads in the community. Effective interventions should slow the spread and limit the number of populations affected.

Overlap with Health Promotion Activities

If primary prevention sounds a lot like health promotion, it is because many of the same methods are used in health promotion. To help distinguish between the two types of interventions, it may be helpful to think of primary prevention in terms of improving health to resist a specific disease and to think of health promotion in terms of improving and maintaining health in general. The distinction between the two terms is often blurred in many program descriptions, which tends to add to the confusion. The most important concept here is not whether an intervention is labeled correctly as either promotion or prevention, but whether the intervention is effective in reducing the number of new cases of disease.

CASE STUDY 1 *(continued)*

Primary prevention and colon cancer

NP's individual health improvement/risk reduction

NP searched the web for information about how to prevent colorectal cancer. He found reports that said one in three cases of cancer of any kind could be avoided if people exercised regularly, ate healthy foods, and kept their weight in the normal range. Based on what he saw, NP decided to join a gym and work out each morning before going to work. He also bought some high-fiber vegetables (e.g., broccoli, cauliflower, cabbage) and started eating them three times a day along with an apple and a banana. Within 2 days, he realized he needed to ease into this new way of eating. He went to the gym regularly the first week, and then slowly started skipping more and more morning workout sessions. After 1 month, he had stopped going to the gym and resumed his old eating habits.

NP heard that calcium and vitamin D were found to reduce the risk of cancer. When he searched the web, he also read that aspirin was recommended. He decided to try again to reduce his risks by taking aspirin and calcium supplements. While he was at it, he would also try to quit smoking ... again. This time, he would use the nicotine patches advertised on TV. Like his first attempts with better nutrition and exercise, NP started strong and then slowly began to forget his supplements and resumed smoking. Undaunted, NP decided to look for something else he could do to reduce his colon cancer risks.

Community-based education and awareness efforts

Unlike other cancers or diseases that have an association with environmental causes, the health department could not perform an environmental cleanup to reduce colorectal cancer. Instead, it focused on promoting healthy diets and exercise. In NP's community, the health department had prepared brochures and posters about colorectal cancer prevention, symptoms, screening methods, and treatment; the department distributed them to businesses and public places like the library. NP had been asked to post several posters in his store. The health department got a local television news personality to present a 30-second public service announcement about colorectal cancer awareness, and placed two large billboard signs of a happy colon dancing and singing with equally happy vegetables and fruit along the main thoroughfare in town. Every time NP saw these silly signs, he would resolve to try again to reduce his risks. Figure 9.3 shows potential primary prevention interventions for colorectal cancer that may apply to NP's case.

Figure 9.3—Colorectal Cancer and Primary Prevention Measures

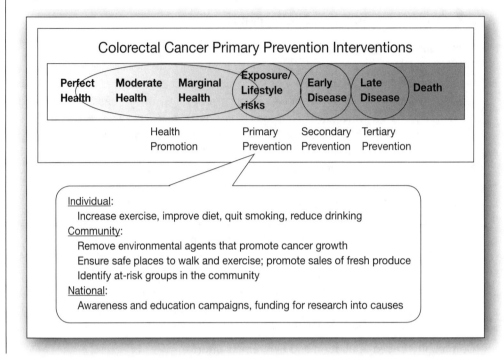

Secondary prevention

Goals and Rationale

After a group of people have been exposed to a disease-causing agent or organism, the goals of prevention becomes focused on reducing the likelihood that the exposure will actually result in the development of the disease and, if the disease *does* occur, reducing its severity and length of illness. Early identification of individuals who have either been exposed to a disease-causing agent or are in the early stages of a disease make it possible to provide treatments that can avoid, mitigate, or even reverse the disease development.

Target Populations

For a given disease, the target population for a **secondary prevention** program will be a subset of the original primary prevention group. This is because only a portion of the at-risk individuals will actually be exposed to a disease-causing agent or develop the early stages of a disease.

Screening to Identify Exposed Persons

Screening to detect an exposure or the presence of early disease is a hallmark activity of secondary prevention. The screening may consist of one or more laboratory tests if biological markers show exposure or early disease, but screening may also consist of a series of questions used to evaluate risk of exposure by exploring whether a person was in close proximity to a person or place that is a source of disease. Screening interviews are often used in large-scale outbreaks when no laboratory tests can detect exposure; the costs of lab tests for a large population is prohibitive; and early intervention is needed to prevent the development of full-blown disease. For example, in an outbreak of meningococcal meningitis, which is a serious bacterial infection of the central nervous system, exposure risk can be assessed by a series of questions that determine how close each person was to the sick person. This is important because antibiotics can be used to prevent the development of the disease if they are taken soon after exposure. At the community level, screening information may be used to identify local trends in disease occurrence and guide efforts to isolate or quarantine individuals to prevent further spread of the disease.

Screening to Identify Early Disease

Screening is also important for identifying whether a person is beginning to develop a disease. Many diseases have early biological markers indicating subclinical conditions of a disease that will progress if untreated. Blood pressure that is high across three separate readings indicates hypertension; serum hemoglobin A1c levels greater than 6% indicate glucose intolerance that may mean early diabetes; or elevated PSA levels may indicate prostate cancer.

Screening questions can also be used to identify early disease. For example, the American Diabetes Association uses a seven-item questionnaire to assess risk for diabetes.[13] (Au: no ref. 13.) Similar screening questionnaires can be found for a variety of diseases.

Interventions to Prevent the Development of Disease

Once people are identified as members of a target population through a screening process, interventions are used to prevent the development of disease. For infectious diseases and some toxic exposures, the intervention will include the use of **post-exposure prophylaxis (PEP)**. Medications used for PEP include some antibiotics, antivirals, vaccines, and decontamination agents. The key to effectiveness is timely administration of the PEP. The window of opportunity is short, usually measured in hours, between the time when a person is exposed and the time when the infection or toxic exposure develops fully. Examples of PEP include the use of ciprofloxacin or rifampin (antibiotics) for meningococcal meningitis prevention, *Varicella* vaccine for PEP for chicken pox, and atropine PEP for a toxic exposure to organophosphate pesticides.

For target populations with early chronic diseases like diabetes or heart disease, the secondary prevention interventions will be aimed at reducing the risk factors in an effort to slow the progression of the disease and its severity. For cancer, early intervention often improves survival rate because the tumor load in the body is still small and easier to eradicate.

■ ■ ■

Secondary prevention

Secondary prevention is focused on the detection of exposures and early disease through screening. It also attempts to arrest the development of disease through post-exposure prophylaxis and early treatment of disease.

Outcomes and Evaluation

Measures of success for secondary prevention activities include a reduction in the incidence (i.e., number of new cases) of disease, number of exposures or early disease detected and treated, and a reduction of the severity of disease if it cannot be completely cured.

Secondary prevention and colorectal cancer

Community-based health fair with screening

The health department organized a health fair at the local mall. Health care providers and students were invited to set up booths to provide information as well as offer free screening and advice to community residents. The goal of the fair was to screen individuals in the community for potential health problems so they could be referred to their primary care provider for further testing and care.

The pharmacy school had asked its students to participate, so they had two booths. One booth provided kits for testing for hidden blood in the stool, a colorectal cancer risk questionnaire, and information about colorectal cancer. The other booth provided hemoglobin A1c tests, a diabetes risk screening questionnaire, and information about type 2 diabetes. The colorectal cancer booth was visited by 50 people, of which 27 had high risk according to their risk questionnaire. The results of the occult blood in the stool test would not be known for about a week. All people were told to see their physicians for followup testing if their test found blood in the stools.

The health screening fair is held twice a year in the town. Ever since it debuted 6 years ago, the number of residents who attended and took advantage of the low cost or free screening services had grown from about 80 to over 400. The long-term results of these early screenings and the impact on diseases in the community would not be measurable for several more years.

Figure 9.4—Colorectal Cancer Screening Poster

Reprinted from CDC.

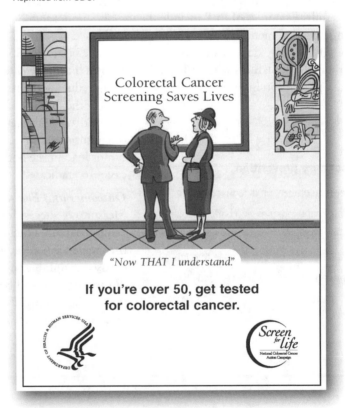

NP's screening results and steps to seek early care

NP was one of the 27 visitors who received the take-home stool test. His results, which arrived about a week later, were positive for small amounts of blood. After thinking about it for several days, NP finally decided to make an appointment at the clinic for followup testing. His colonoscopy was performed about 1 month later. During the procedure, two polyps were found and removed. One polyp was pre-cancerous; the other had more developed disease, so NP began discussing his options for treatment of early colorectal cancer. Figure 9.5 lists possible secondary prevention interventions for colorectal cancer that may apply to NP's case.

Figure 9.5—Colorectal Cancer and Secondary Prevention Measures

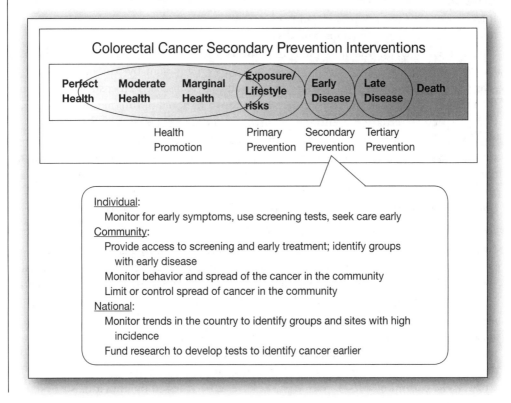

Tertiary prevention

Goal and Rationale

The goal of **tertiary prevention** is to reduce the mortality and morbidity associated with a disease and to return a person to a state of health that is as close to normal as possible. The rationale for interventions in tertiary prevention is to minimize the impact that a disease and its treatment has on a person.

Target Populations

In tertiary prevention, the target population is usually a small subset of the secondary prevention population. Individuals whose exposure to a disease-causing agent has results in disease and those in the early stages of a chronic disease who have progressed to more advanced stages are now at risk of disease complications, permanent disabilities, and death. They will be the focus of tertiary prevention efforts. Examples of tertiary prevention target populations would be people whose exposure to the influenza virus resulted in the flu or those whose poor glucose control progressed to a diagnosis of type 2 diabetes.

Treating to Cure and Avoid Complications or Death

> ### Tertiary prevention
>
> Tertiary prevention focuses on treatment of disease with the goal of returning a person back to health as well as reducing complications, long-term disability, and premature death.

Interventions for tertiary prevention work to reduce deaths, complications, and disability and to cure disease. For diseases that can be cured, such as infections and some cancers, the interventions employ treatments known to cure the disease. This intervention occurs on a patient-by-patient individual level. At the community level, tertiary prevention may be focused on ensuring access to the medical care needed to receive treatment. From a national or international intervention perspective, tertiary prevention may involve funding the research to find cures.

Examples of interventions at the individual level include the use of antibiotics to treat actual infection (not post-exposure prophylaxis to prevent infection) and control of blood sugars in a patient with diabetes to avoid permanent damage to the kidneys, eyes, and heart. For severe cases of influenza, treatment may be aimed at avoiding complications such as pneumonia as well as providing support to help patients recover.

Rehabilitation for Permanent Disability

Not all diseases can be completely cured. In some survivors, lasting effects may compromise a return to complete health. To maximize function and achieve a more normal lifestyle, rehabilitation is used as another component of tertiary prevention. Physical and occupational therapies are used to help individuals learn new ways to perform their daily routines. Examples of rehabilitation used to increase function include cerebral vascular accidents (strokes) and spinal cord injuries resulting in paraplegia or quadriplegia. At the individual level, the rehabilitation involves a series of sessions with therapists, use of devices to assist in performing routine functions, and changes in living areas and lifestyle. At the community level, public places have to be accessed by individuals who have limited mobility so they can continue to participate in the community.

Outcomes and Evaluation

For tertiary prevention programs, success is measured in terms of reductions in premature death due to the disease and number of survivors who develop complications. The number of cases cured, if possible, is a positive measure of success for a tertiary prevention program. At the community level, the effectiveness of programs may also be measured in terms of access to medical care and the ability of disabled persons to continue being active members of the community.

CASE STUDY 1 *(continued)*

Tertiary prevention and colon cancer

Community tertiary prevention efforts

Before NP ever entered treatment for his colorectal cancer, the community had begun efforts to improve the oncology services (i.e., cancer treatment) in the town. Over the previous 5 years, a new cancer center had been opened in one of the local hospitals and three oncologists had been hired along with numerous oncology-focused health care personnel, including three pharmacists. The Center boasted outpatient treatments with several inpatient beds for overnight therapies. In addition to treatment, the Center staff actively participated as a study site for phase II and III trials of new **antineoplastic medications** and radiation treatments. The closest bone marrow transplantation service was 300 miles away in a large metropolitan area that served patients from the surrounding area.

The state's American Cancer Society affiliate served as a source of support for patients and families during all phases of cancer, including treatment and end-of-life care. It had also been active in seeking financial support for cancer therapy to ensure all those who had cancer could afford to be treated. A local support group of colorectal cancer survivors met monthly in town, so NP had an additional source of support and resources when he was in the recovery phase of his treatment.

NP receives treatment

NP met with his physician and the oncologist to determine an appropriate course of treatment to hopefully put his cancer in remission or at least slow its growth. Surgical intervention to remove all suspicious areas in the colon and large intestine were followed by a course of chemotherapy to ensure eradication of any missed cancer cells and to reduce the risk of metastases (i.e., spread of initial cancer tumor cells to other parts of the body).

NP's chemotherapy was monitored by the oncology pharmacist, who watched for early signs of adverse reactions; usual signs that the medication was working; answered treatment questions; and adjusted the doses as needed for any changes in kidney or liver functions. Because antineoplastic medications (i.e., cancer drugs) still lack specificity, they affect rapidly dividing healthy cells as well as rapidly dividing cancer cells. The pharmacist provided the physician with recommendations for supportive medications and care that could reduce the side effects and help the normal cells recover more quickly. Figure 9.6 listed possible tertiary prevention interventions for colorectal cancer that could apply to NP's case.

Afterword

Three years after first being diagnosed and treated for colorectal cancer, NP has undergone annual screenings to ensure that the cancer has not returned. His prognosis for reaching the 5-year survival goal is very good. He has been actively exercising four times a week, and his consumption of vegetables and fruit is now up to four per day. He quit smoking about 8 months ago, although he will be the first to say that he has to try to quit smoking every day. He enjoys an occasional glass of wine or beer, but limits it to one glass. He has lost almost 40 pounds and was able to quit using his medications for blood pressure. His cholesterol is still elevated, so he continues to use his "statin." He is supplementing his diet with calcium and vitamin D, even though studies concluded that dietary sources were preventative. Recently, he was voted in as President of the local chapter of the American Cancer Society, and he is working on plans for a research fundraising campaign.

Figure 9.6—Colorectal Cancer and Tertiary Prevention Measures

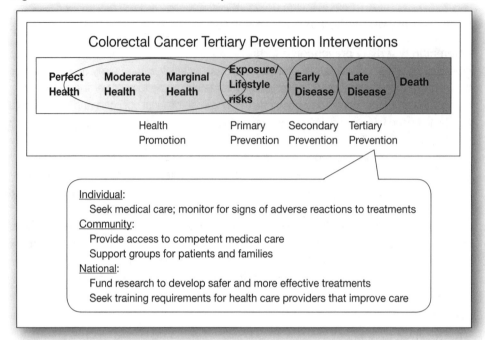

Pharmacists and Prevention

Pharmacists have been involved in prevention activities for years. Most of the interventions are conducted at the individual level and are best categorized as tertiary; however, examples of primary and secondary prevention activities and work at community and national levels abound. Primary prevention activities include vaccination, an area where pharmacists are becoming increasingly involved.[5] Pharmacists have also been very active in educational campaigns, often at community and national levels. An example of this primary prevention activity is Poison Prevention Week, which is a national project carried out through community-level activities such as school programs and public service announcements.

Pharmacists have increased their involvement in secondary prevention activities, which includes providing screening services and screening devices to facilitate early detection of a disease or exposure. These programs have expanded from individual on-demand screenings to community-wide screening or health fairs that are open to the entire community. At the national level, professional organizations support these interventions through continuing professional development and training programs that focus on developing the necessary techniques to perform the screenings. These organizations also assist with promoting reimbursement to ensure pharmacies can afford to offer the services.

Tertiary prevention activities at the individual level are the main area of intervention for pharmacists. Treating patients who are ill to help them regain their health or at least reduce the lasting impact of the disease is the focus of training and practice. Pharmacists are actively involved in ensuring that patients understand how to use medications safely to avoid preventable injury from medication errors. They can also monitor the patient to ensure that the treatment is working and not causing any new adverse reactions. At the community level, pharmacists may be involved in **health boards** or other groups that are seeking to improve access to services and decide which treatment services are most needed in the community. At the national level, pharmacists contribute to tertiary prevention by sharing their innovative practice ideas with others, participating in clinical research, advocating for their patients to ensure they have access to care, developing best practices guidelines based on evidence, and ensuring the competence of the practitioners in the pharmacy profession.

Chapter 9 Summary

In public health, the three levels of disease prevention share a common goal of reducing avoidable premature death and disability caused by disease, toxic exposures, or injuries. This chapter covered the goals, target populations, activities, and outcomes for primary, secondary, and tertiary prevention to see how they are related and how they address different aspects of disease risk. These levels of prevention were considered from individual, community, and international perspectives since disease prevention can have different foci depending on the perspective. Using colorectal cancer as the case study, the chapter also looked at various activities to reduce disease risks in individuals and communities. Many primary prevention activities mesh with health promotion activities, while many tertiary prevention activities align with the therapeutic goals commonly encountered in pharmacy. Increasing pharmacy participation in primary and secondary prevention activities will further strengthen public health efforts to reduce the incidence of disease and its impact on people and communities.

References

1. U.S. Cancer Statistics Working Group. United States Cancer Statistics: 1999–2005 Incidence and Mortality Web-based Report. Atlanta, GA: U.S. Department of Health and Human Services, Centers for Disease Control and Prevention and National Cancer Institute; 2009. Available at: http://www.cdc.gov/uscs. Accessed February 13, 2009.

2. Jemal A, Thun MJ, Ries LAG, et al. Annual report to the nation on the status of cancer, 1975–2005, featuring trends in lung cancer, tobacco use, and tobacco control. *J Natl Cancer Inst*. 2008; 100(23):1672–94.

3. Centers for Disease Control and Prevention. Cancer—Colorectal Cancer Risk Factors web page. Available at: http://www.cdc.gov. Accessed February 13, 2009.

4. Leavell HR, Clark EG. *Preventive Medicine for the Doctor in His Community*, 3rd ed. New York, NY: McGraw-Hill; 1965.

5. Hogue MD, Grabenstein JD, Foster SL, et al. Pharmacist involvement with immunizations: A decade of professional advancement. *JAPhA*. 2006; 46:168–79.

Suggested Readings

Peters S, Singla D, Raney E. Impact of pharmacist-provided osteoporosis education and screening in the workplace. *JAPhA.* **2006; 46:216–8.**

Hogue MD, Grabenstein JD, Foster SL, et al. Pharmacist involvement with immunizations: A decade of professional advancement. *JAPhA.* **2006; 46:168–79.**

Weitzel KW, Goode J-VR. Implementation of a pharmacy-based immunization program in a supermarket chain. *JAPhA.* **2000; 46:252–6.**

Chapter 9 Review Questions

1. **Describe how health promotion and disease prevention activities may complement one another.**

   In primary prevention, the goal is to prevent exposure to a disease-causing agent. If that is not possible, the goal then becomes improving resistance to the disease-causing agent so the body can defend itself. Being healthy is one mechanism that can improve the body's resistance to disease, so health promotion activities that improve health will complement primary prevention goals.

2. **Using type 2 diabetes as the disease, list the three levels of prevention and describe the types of populations that would be targeted at each level.**

   Primary prevention for type 2 diabetes focuses on individuals whose lifestyle puts them at risk of developing the risk factors associated with diabetes and those who have a family history that includes near relatives (i.e., parents or siblings) who have diabetes.

   Secondary prevention interventions target individuals who have the risk factors of obesity; poor glucose control; and symptoms of early disease such as thirst, frequent urination, or sugar cravings. This is a subset of the population targeted in the primary prevention interventions.

   Tertiary prevention targets individuals who have a diagnosis of type 2 diabetes and its complications. This is a subset of the secondary prevention target population.

3. **For an infectious disease like chicken pox, list the three levels of prevention and describe the populations targeted, goals of the levels, and the interventions often used to achieve goals. (To find out more about the disease, go the CDC web site [www.CDC.gov] and choose Chicken Pox.)**

   Primary prevention targets those individuals who are *at risk of being exposed* to the *Varicella* virus. The goals are to reduce the number of new cases of chicken pox by reducing the number of exposures. Interventions include isolation of people with chicken pox, vaccination for *Varicella*, and general health improvement.

Secondary prevention targets individuals who have been exposed to the *Varicella* virus and are now at risk of developing chicken pox. The goals are to reduce the number of exposures that progress to actual disease. Interventions include post-exposure prophylaxis administration of the vaccine and the use of an antiviral medication within the first 24 hours of the appearance of symptoms. Early disease is treated in a supportive manner, and patients are monitored for emerging complications.

Tertiary prevention targets the individuals who have a severe case of chicken pox as well as those who suffer complications from the disease or its treatment. The goals are to reduce premature death, long-term sequelae or complications, and permanent disabilities as well as to increase the cure rate. Medical treatment is the primary intervention (e.g., the use of medications).

4. **Describe individual, community, and national disease prevention activities that might be used for HIV/AIDS. (To find out more about the disease, go the CDC web site [www.CDC.gov] and choose HIV/AIDS.)**
Individuals can take actions to reduce their exposure to the virus, which is spread primarily through contact with infected blood and unprotected sex as well as sharing dirty needles that were used by an infected person. Such actions would include using clean needles, condoms, and latex or other gloves. Currently, no vaccines are available for preventing HIV. For those who suspect they have been exposed, they can get tested to verify exposure; cease activities that tend to spread the infection; and seek care to treat the infection in its early stages. Once the infection progresses to AIDS, the individual can adhere to the complex treatments to reduce progression of the disease.

The community can take primary prevention actions by providing access to clean needles and condoms and also reducing the risk of spreading through standard precautions in health care settings. Confidential screening tests may promote good secondary prevention and get infected individuals into treatment earlier. Ensuring access to the medications needed to control the disease would be an example of community-level tertiary prevention.

At the national level, efforts to increase research funding to find more effective treatments, cures, earlier identification of infected individials, and preventive vaccines are one type of intervention that could be classified as primary, secondary, and tertiary. Another tertiary intervention may be to provide more funding for treatment programs and to assist with the purchase of the medications. Efforts to support education campaigns would be a primary prevention action. National policies that support efforts to work towards global eradication of the disease would begin with tertiary actions to treat and reduce risk of spread and end with the elimination of the threat of infection, which would be considered a primary prevention action.

5. **Give examples of activities for pharmacist interventions at the primary, secondary, and tertiary levels.**

   Two examples of a primary prevention activity performed by pharmacists are vaccination and educational programs about poison prevention. Two examples of secondary prevention activities are screening for diabetes and providing post-exposure antiviral medication for patients with influenza. Two examples of tertiary prevention by pharmacists include ensuring patients take medications correctly to avoid medication errors and monitoring patients to identify potential adverse reactions or treatment failures as soon as possible.

Applying Your Knowledge

1. **Describe primary, secondary, and tertiary prevention activities related to safe medication use that a pharmacist can provide at the individual or community level.**

Epidemiology and Disease

Learning Outcomes

1. Define epidemiology and pharmacoepidemiology.
2. Describe the roles of epidemiology in public health.
3. Explain the meaning of epidemiological terms such as incidence, prevalence, epidemic, odds ratio, and relative risk.
4. Given data about a disease in a population, identify who has increased or decreased risk of illness or death.
5. Explain how epidemiology can promote more funding for research and programs that address a specific disease.

Introduction

Epidemiology is a collection of study designs and analysis methods used to describe disease behavior in a population so that preventive actions can be taken to reduce disease. This chapter will begin with a short introduction to epidemiology and its origin. One facet of epidemiology that focuses on medication use (i.e., pharmacoepidemiology) will be presented; examples involving medications and pharmacy services will be used throughout the chapter to illustrate concepts and study designs. To further describe epidemiological terms and study designs, a medication error case will serve as an example of a preventable cause of disease and explore various methods for describing the magnitude of the problem—who is affected by it, when it happens, and why it happens. The fictitious case will employ counts and frequency rates obtained through observation, measures of associations, inferences of causation, and experimental designs to test interventions created to reduce risk. The many roles of epidemiology will be presented at the end of the chapter.

Public Health in the Context of Medication Errors

Medication use can help patients feel better and return to a state of health. Medication can also create a number of risks, including death. The risks created by the use of medications have been dubbed drug-related problems (DRPs), which include problems created by using a medication that is not needed or not using a medication that is needed, taking an inappropriate product or dose, having an adverse reaction to the medication, and inadvertently creating drug interactions with other substances.[1] Many of the drug-related problems are caused by errors, which means they are preventable causes of injury and disease.

In addition to being preventable, medication errors have been responsible for sufficiently large numbers of injuries and death to make them a public health concern. In the United States, annual medication error related injuries and deaths have been estimated at 1.5 million and 7,000, respectively. At least a quarter of the medication-related deaths are preventable.[2] The medication-related death rate, including those deaths caused by errors, is somewhere between the fourth and sixth leading cause of death in the United States.[3]

Not all medication errors cause injury or death, therefore, confusion exists about what should be measured when studying this public health problem. It is generally agreed that most medication errors are caught and corrected before a patient is exposed to the medication so no harm is done. However, as long as errors are occurring, prevention is critical to avoiding the risk of one of those errors causing injury or death. Prevention requires understanding the problem; researchers have focused on the steps in the medication ordering, dispensing, and use process to identify where errors occur. For example, in one study, the most common types of errors were administering improper dose (41%), giving wrong drug (16%), and using wrong route (10%).[4]

Definition of medication error

Because of confusion about what constitutes a medication error, the National Coordinating Council for Medication Error Reporting and Prevention (NCCMERP) created the following definition:[5]

Disease, injury, and death may be caused by clinically used medications. Some of those injuries and deaths are due to medication errors. Because such errors are a preventable cause of injury and death, there is great interest in finding their causes so preventive measures can be implemented.

"A medication error is any preventable event that may cause or lead to inappropriate medication use or patient harm while the medication is in the control of the health care professional, patient, or consumer. Such events may be related to professional practice, health care products, procedures, and systems, including prescribing; order communication; product labeling, packaging, and nomenclature; compounding; dispensing; distribution; administration; education; monitoring; and use."

Medication errors as a preventable cause of disease

HC receives the wrong medication

HC is a relatively healthy young man in his mid-30s who had been feeling excessively tired and cold. He also seemed to be gaining weight in spite of his active lifestyle. His skin had been dryer than usual, and he noticed that he would get constipated easily. His physical exam showed a body temperature slightly below normal (97.1°F), dry skin, and an enlarged goiter. Lab work revealed that his thyroid stimulating hormone (TSH) level was 14.3 mU/L, which is much higher than the normal range. Sustained high levels of stimulating hormones indicate that the target organ, in this case the thyroid gland, is not responding in a normal manner. His level of free T4 was 0.5 ng/dL. HC was diagnosed with primary hypothyroidism.

Treatment began with oral thyroid hormone replacement that would be slowly increased until he had the right level to mimic a normally functioning thyroid gland. The plan was to begin with the lowest dose (25micrograms) daily for 1 month and then increase the dose by 25micrograms each month until the symptoms were gone and the lab values were in the normal range. Unfortunately, the handwritten prescription was difficult to read, used dangerous abbreviations and an unnecessary terminal zero, and resulted in an incorrectly filled and dispensed medication. HC had never used the product before, so he did not realize it was incorrect. The label was technically correct, but its inclusion of the zero led to the selection of an inappropriate strength tablet to fill the prescription (i.e., 200mcg tablet instead of 25mcg tablet). Figure 10.1 shows the prescription HC received and the label on the dispensed product.

Figure 10.1—Handwritten Prescription and Label Placed on Prescription Vial

Handwritten Prescription information:

L-thyroxine 25.0mg
Sig: ī po qox ī month
then īī po qod X ī month
#90 NR

levo-thyroxine, USP
200mcg

GenX Brand
Expires 02/01/15

Prescription vial label:

l-thyroxine 0.025mg

Take one tablet daily for one month,
    then take two tablets daily for one month.

No Refills   90 tablets

Impact of the error on HC's health

After taking the medication for 30 days, HC noticed some improvement in his symptoms. He followed the instructions to double the dose for the second month, as directed. Within 5 days of doing so, he began to notice a fine tremor in his hands and he had a hard time getting a good night's sleep. On a happier note, he noticed that his exercise efforts were paying off with some weight loss, but he could hardly stand the way his pulse seemed to race and how hot the workout room at the gym was when he was walking quickly. By the 10th day of the increased dose, he felt like his heart was going to leap out of his chest, so he called the physician to find out what was going on.

Epidemiology as the Scientific Basis for Public Health

Investigating diseases to find their causes in order to prevent them has been a key role for public health. This effort has been aided through the use of a scientific approach to investigation called epidemiology. Epidemiology is based on the belief that no disease occurs at random and that one or more factors cause a disease to occur. Once the cause(s) of a disease can be determined, the possibility of finding ways to prevent the disease increases.[6] The science of epidemiology has several important functions. It is used to monitor the level of disease in a community, investigate disease outbreaks, guide distribution of resources for disease treatment and prevention, and discover exposures that facilitate or mitigate the development of disease. These facets of epidemiology can be seen in its definition:[7]

■ ■ ■

Epidemiology is based on two key beliefs. First, a disease does not occur at random but results from one or more exposures or factors that facilitate its development and severity. Second, if the exposures or factors that cause disease can be determined, exposures and disease may be prevented.

"….the study of the distribution and determinance of health-related states or events in specified populations, and the application of this study to control of health problems."

Although the definition does not specify human populations, those populations will be the focus of the epidemiology discussed in this chapter. Figure 10.2 shows the relationship between exposure to causal or risk factors and the development of disease.

Figure 10.2—Exposure-to-Disease Timeline that Is the Basis of Epidemiology

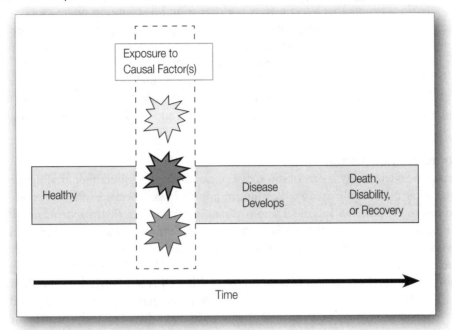

Origins and evolution of epidemiology

Modern epidemiology has its origins in the study of infectious disease where it was used to link disease outbreaks with the characteristics of affected populations and the communities in which they lived. Although earlier examples exist, Snow's use of epidemiology to identify the source of a Cholera outbreak in London in 1854 is often cited as a classic early example of modern epidemiology.[8] Concurrent with the development of epidemiology was the discovery of micro-organisms that cause infectious disease. It is no accident that as more became known about the microbial causes of infectious disease, the role of epidemiology as a tool for public health also grew.

During the 20th century, the capability of epidemiology to describe diseases caused by factors other than infectious microorganisms was realized. Some examples of how epidemiology was used to link factors and behavior to the development of disease include the tobacco use by physicians and subsequent development of lung cancer studies by Bell and Smith in the 1950s and the Framingham Heart Study that began exploring risk factors for developing cardiovascular disease.[9,10] The Framingham Heart Study continues to this day, making it one of the largest and longest scale epidemiological studies ever undertaken for exploring risk factors for a non-infectious disease. Formally begun in 1950 in a small community outside of Boston, the study has produced a wealth of information about cardiovascular disease risks that serve as a foundation for many of the guidelines used today to help people avoid heart and vascular disease through better diets, more exercise, not smoking, and maintaining a healthy weight. The study is currently looking at the third-generation of participants, which is allowing additional inquiry into genetic factors.[10]

More recently, epidemiology has been applied to investigation into non-biological or non-infectious factors that affect disease occurrence and distribution such as social epidemiology, political epidemiology, and environmental epidemiology. These fields are similar in that they apply epidemiological methods to the exploration of causes of disease but differ in the underlying theories used to guide identification of risk factors and interpret results. Epidemiology in all areas is aided by advances in knowledge in the biological, natural, and social sciences that are gained through research. Completion of the Human Genome Project, which mapped the human genetic codes, will impact epidemiological research for many years.

Pharmacoepidemiology

Pharmacoepidemiology is one of those disciplines that apply epidemiological methods to the study of clinically used medications in populations.[11] Because of its focus on medication use patterns and medication-related health impact, pharmacoepidemiology is of particular interest to pharmacists. Pharmacoepidemiology may be used to describe patterns of use or adverse reactions, compare actual use to guidelines or expected use patterns, determine factors that promote or inhibit use of medication, and link usage to health outcomes. Examples of pharmacoepidemiological studies include Phase IV studies (i.e., post-marketing surveillance studies used to detect rare adverse reactions), studies of protective effects not identified in smaller clinical trials, identification of sources of contaminated or counterfeit medications, and impact of medication on disease survival rates. It can also be used to study patterns and causes of medication errors and adverse drug events to determine whether they are random events or predictable events that can be prevented.[11]

> Pharmacoepidemiology is a subset of epidemiology that is concerned with medication usage patterns, adverse reaction distributions, and medication-related impacts on disease and health in a population.

Using Epidemiology to Understand Disease Outbreak in a Population

Pharmacists, like their health care counterparts, have been trained to consider the disease process within a patient and explore what may have caused it, how it will most likely progress if untreated, what methods of therapy are effective, and how to prevent it from happening again. In many ways, epidemiology does the same thing except it considers disease in an entire population not just a single patient. Epidemiology is used to answer questions about who, what, where, when, and how of a disease in a community.[12] Its methods can be applied to investigations of disease outbreaks, research into factors that increase and decrease risk of disease, evaluation of disease prevention programs, distribution of public resources to fight disease, and the formulation of public health policies.

1. What is it? (defining the disease)

When health officers in a community detect one or more people with an unusual set of symptoms, they may initiate a field investigation to determine what is happening and find ways to contain and control the outbreak. The process of investigating a disease begins with a case definition. A **case definition** will explicitly list signs and symptoms, lab values, location, population characteristics, and even timing for a case to be considered part of a disease investigation. Often the case definition will include criteria for determining whether a person has a suspected, probable, or confirmed case of the illness. Once a case definition is created, the epidemiological investigation can proceed to answer the following five questions about a disease outbreak in the community.[12]

2. How big is the outbreak?

In epidemiology, this question refers to measures of disease occurrence such as number of new cases, total number of cases, and number of deaths. By themselves, these counts of disease and death fail to convey a complete picture, so they are often combined into ratios with the total number of people who are in population or have been exposed to a known cause of disease serving as the denominators. For example, if 20 new cases of heart disease have arisen in a community, it is hard to tell if the problem is large or small unless we know that the population is 1,000 or 100,000. To better understand the size of the disease in a community, ratios that compare the number of sick to the larger population are used.

To better assess whether an outbreak is a problem, the disease rates can be compared to historical norms to determine whether the increase or decrease in disease occurrence has been unusual. If historical data do not exist, the rates may be compared to other populations with similar characteristics to see if the disease levels are different.

3. Who is affected by the disease?

Another piece of information to examine is the incidence and prevalence of the disease in different members of the community. To do this, information about individuals will be needed. In addition to demographic measures like age, gender, race, socioeconomic status, and occupation, an investigation may also seek information about prior behavior and disease status. If a pattern emerges with regard to characteristics or behaviors that seem more common in the group that develops the disease, two important things happen: one is the ability to focus resources on that subpopulation at highest risk of disease, and the second is the start of a hypothesis about potential cause of the outbreak if it is not already known.

Even if the cause of an outbreak is not known, identifying the populations affected can still lead to preventive actions. The classic example of this approach is Snow's work in the 1846 cholera epidemic in London. Through analyzing populations by their sources of drinking water, Snow eventually pinpointed the water company and one of its pumps as the source of the contaminated water. The pump handle was removed, and the number of new cholera cases declined dramatically. At the time, the microorganism that caused cholera was not known and many public health officials were focused on bad air or miasmas as the cause. When an outbreak of disease occurs today, the investigation will still look at characteristics shared by those who fall ill in order to pinpoint the source of outbreak. For example, when a food poisoning outbreak occurs in a community, field investigators will interview people who became ill to determine whether they consumed the same food product or ate the same meal at the same restaurant to pinpoint the cause.

4. Where is the disease located?

In addition to considering the characteristics of the populations in which a disease does or does not occur, investigation into an outbreak also needs to consider the environment in which the outbreak occurs and how it may affect the spread of the disease. Place may be described generically as rural or urban or specifically as a country, state, or city. Location information that is relevant to an investigation will depend on the disease under study. For some diseases such as cancer, exposures over many years may affect risk so investigators must look at where a person was born and raised, his or her occupations, and proximity to known high-risk sites over time.

In addition to historical exposures, travel to parts of the world where a disease is present can put a traveler at risk of exposure. Once exposed, the traveler may bring the disease home and expose others to it if it develops into a clinical case that can be transmitted. The global outbreak of severe acute respiratory syndrome (SARS) is an example of how travel can complicate efforts to identify the location of origin for an outbreak.

5. When does the disease occur?

Another aspect of any investigation into a disease in a community is determining whether the exposure or disease occurs at higher rates at specific times. Understanding the timing of disease may provide additional clues about potential sources of exposure to a causative agent. Timing measures include a determination about whether a disease occurs all the time at a consistently low level like diabetes, at regular intervals like influenza, or sporadically like HIV/AIDS. Some diseases like influenza are also called seasonal, since they appear at certain times of the year. Winter months are typically "flu season," and health officials expect to see an increase in cases during that time of year. In contrast, sporadic diseases occur at random with no set pattern.

Timing can help to uncover sources of a disease such as food poisoning. By comparing exposures within a certain amount of time of the development of symptoms, it is often possible to find a common source of contamination. Further study of the source is then used to confirm the presence of the offending microorganism or chemical.

6. Why does the disease occur?

The last question for epidemiological investigators to address is the identification of potential relationships between exposures to certain factors and the appearance of disease. Later, more definitive tests can be used to test whether an exposure leads to a different rate of disease. Most of the time, the exposure being tested is something that increases the chances of the disease developing, something that makes it more severe when it does develop, or increases the likelihood that a person will die. Identifying these exposures can lead to efforts to eliminate them or reduce their impact. It is also possible to have exposures that are protective and reduce the occurrence of disease in a population. Determining these protective factors is another important goal of an epidemiological investigation.

Epidemiology is used to learn more about diseases, their behaviors in a population, and their causes. It does this by first defining the disease and then answering five questions: How big is the outbreak? Who is affected? Where is it located? When does it occur? Why does it occur?

CASE STUDY 1 *(continued)*

Investigating HC's mysterious illness

Like any good clinician, the physician first takes care of HC to reduce his symptoms and then investigates the problem in a more global manner because he has had a couple of patients recently with the same problem. He wonders if something is going on with the medications or if this is all just a fluke and the cases are not related.

Based on HC's symptoms, he defines the problem as "acute onset hyperthyroidism of unknown cause." At first, he suspected the medication, but the prescription vial label was correct. Next he quizzed HC about how he takes the medication and found no indication that he was exceeding the prescribed dose of two tablets in the second month. He tells HC to stop taking the medication for 1 week, then go back to one tablet each day since he seemed to tolerate that dose and can get some relief of symptoms. He notes in HC's chart that the 25-microgram dose appears to be appropriate.

After HC left the office, the physician pulled medical charts for the other patients he remembered as having similar symptoms. He was ready to start the process of asking questions about who was affected with similar symptoms, how many were affected, when did those symptoms occur, where did affected patients receive care, and why was this happening?

He decided to begin his investigation into his outbreak of hyperthryroidism by finding patients who had had similar symptoms during the previous year to see if any similarities or trends could explain what was going on. His electronic medical database and charts had information about diagnosis, primary physician, lab values, current medication dose, and dates for events.

Measures of Disease Frequency and Distribution

The process used by epidemiologists has been described as count, divide, and compare.[12] Numbers of cases or deaths are counted and then divided by the number of people exposed or in the at-risk population to make a frequency or rate. Comparisons of the rates are used to determine whether a certain population appears to be at greater or lesser risk of a disease. Based on these comparisons, inquiries into potential risk factors can begin.

Disease frequency measures are used to describe disease rates in terms of comparisons to the whole population or the population that has been exposed to a risk factor. Several types of incidence, prevalence, and mortality rates are used. In general, these different types of rates vary by the period of time included in the count (1 day or 1 year) and the population used in the denominator (people who are at risk or the whole population). Descriptions of commonly encountered ratios are described here.

Prevalence

Incidence and prevalence are two measures of disease frequency commonly used in epidemiology. **Incidence** is defined as the number of *new* cases of disease in an at-risk population during a specific period of time, while **prevalence** will indicate the *total number* of disease cases in the total population at a given point in time. These values are often converted to either a percent or per 100,000 population to allow comparisons with others populations of different sizes.[6] Together, the measures provide valuable information about the scope of the disease in a population. When prevalence rates are greater than incidence rates, it implies that the disease persists for a length of time before being either cured or causing death.

Prevalence rates are calculated using counts of existing cases of the disease, regardless of how long a person has been ill as the numerator. As long as the disease exists within the time period specified, usually 1 year, a person is counted. The denominator is the count of the total population from which the people who became ill were initially found. Figure 10.3 shows the equation for calculating prevalence (P):

Figure 10.3—Prevalence Rate Formula

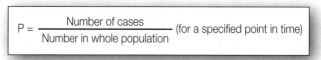

$$P = \frac{\text{Number of cases}}{\text{Number in whole population}} \text{ (for a specified point in time)}$$

For example, consider a chronic, long-term illness—diabetes mellitus. The number of people with diagnosed and undiagnosed diabetes in the U.S. population in 2007 was estimated at 23.6 million. This translates into a prevalence rate of 7.8% of the U.S. population with diabetes. The prevalence rate could also be written as 7,800/100,000 people had diabetes in 2007.[13]

Incidence
Incidence rates focus on the rate of new cases of disease in at-risk populations. There are two types of incidence rates used to do this. The **cumulative incidence rate (CI)** will compare counts of new cases to total population at risk for a specified period of time, such as 1 year. This calculation assumes that the entire population at risk is available to be counted at the start and end of the time period. Figure 10.4 shows the formula for calculating a cumulative incidence rate.

Figure 10.4—Cumulative Incidence Rate

Cumulative Incidence (for new cases in a specified period of time):

$$CI = \frac{\text{Number of new cases during a specified period of time}}{\text{Number of total population at risk}}$$

Continuing with the diabetes example, the number of new cases of diabetes in people aged 20–39 years during 2007 was 281,000. This figure can be used to calculate a cumulative incidence rate of 92.9/100,000 new cases of diabetes in the U.S. population 20–39 years old in 2007. (Note: The calculation used 302.6 million for total U.S. population.[13])

Because of situations where members of the at-risk population may not be included in the initial count or may "drop out" of the population before the end of the designated time period, a second type of incidence called the **incidence rate (IR) or incidence density (ID)** is used. Unlike the CI, the incidence rate uses information from all individuals regardless of how long they are in the at-risk population by using a person-time count in the denominator. Now the denominator will be the total amount of time each person spent in the at-risk population. Examples of person-time units are person-months or person-years (Figure 10.5).

Figure 10.5—Incidence Rate (or Incidence Density)

Incidence Rate (for new cases in a specified period of time):

$$IR \text{ (or ID)} = \frac{\text{Number of new cases during a specified period of time}}{\text{Total number of person-time when at risk}}$$

To illustrate this calculation, consider incidence of a severe life-threatening allergic reaction to an antibiotic. If the incidence compares the number of cases of severe reaction to the total population that used the antibiotic during a 1-year period, the calculation would severely underestimate the actual incidence. Suppose for 1,000 patients who use the antibiotic once during a year, three develop the life-threatening reactions. Cumulative incidence for 1 year would be 3/1,000 = 0.003 (or 0.3%). Because the danger of a severe allergic reaction exists only when the patient is taking the penicillin, which is between 7 to 21 days depending on the diagnosis, the actual time any one person spends at risk of a severe reaction is much less than 1 year. Assuming an average of 14 days of therapy, each person in the population would be at risk 2 weeks of the year and not at risk 50 weeks of the year. The ID calculation would begin with a calculation of time for each person to determine the fraction of the year spent at risk. This would be 2w/52w/ yr, which is 0.03846 year (or 3.85% of a year). These individual time periods are added to get the total person-year at risk for the whole population of 1,000. In this example, it is 38.46 person-years (0.03846 per person for 1,000 people). The ID is then calculated as 3 cases/38.46 person-years or 0.078 (7.8%) ID for a severe allergic reaction.

Mortality rates

In addition to measures of diagnosis rates, disease impact on a population can be measured by the results it produces—namely **morbidity** (long-term disability or disease) and **mortality** (death) rates. Just like incidence and prevalence rates, these counts are compared to a larger population to determine rates. For example, the age-adjusted death rate for colorectal cancer in the United States was 18.8 per 100,000 men and women per year based on data collected on between 2001 and 2005 for patients with colorectal cancer. The mortality rate in this example was age-adjusted because the distribution of death rates is unequal across the different age groups. Once data are age-adjusted through comparison to a standard population year, data from different years or groups can be compared. The calculation of age-adjusted incidence or mortality rates is beyond the scope of this text.[14] Mortality data are usually collected from death certificates.

Since 1999, causes of death listed on death certificates should be categorized with the **International Classification of Disease, 10th edition (ICD-10)**, which was created and now maintained by the World Health Organization (WHO) to standardize death rate counts around the globe. It should not be confused with the clinical version of the ICD-10 called the **ICD-10-CM** where the CM stands for "clinical modification." This second set of classifications, which will replace the current ICD-9-CM in 2013, is used in the United States to standardize diagnoses of disease in living patients. This clinically modified version is used primarily in clinical settings for diagnosis codes on billing forms, although it could be used to identify populations for the purpose of incidence and prevalence counts. The National Center for Health Statistics (NCHS) and Centers for Medicare and Medicaid (CMS) are responsible for maintaining and updating the ICD-9-CM and ICD-10-CM codes. Copies of both the ICD-10 and ICD-10-CM are located on the web sites of the WHO and CDC, respectively.

Endemic and epidemic

For diseases that usually occur at relatively constant low levels in a community (i.e., **endemic** diseases), a sudden increase in the number of new cases may indicate that an outbreak is occurring and steps are needed to stop the spread of disease. For example, if a county that usually has two or three cases of pertussis (whooping cough) each year counts 12 new cases in one of its cities, it will take notice of the sudden increase and investigate why this is happening. At some point, when the number of cases increases far beyond the usual level and begins to affect populations in neighboring counties, the outbreak will probably be classified as an **epidemic**. When diseases spread widely and include many countries and affect many people, they are called **pandemics**. For example, each winter, influenza outbreaks occur in the United States, and about every 3 years the number of pneumonia and influenza (P and I) deaths exceed the usual annual rate enough to classify the outbreak as an epidemic.[15] In 1918, the influenza outbreak involved multiple continents, millions of people, and was appropriately called a pandemic. For diseases considered eradicated in the United States such as smallpox and polio, the appearance of a single case is considered a **sentinel event** that is sufficient to get immediate attention of public health officials.

> Although counts of disease or death rates in a population provide some information, comparisons to larger populations produce a more informative ratio. Incidence (new cases), prevalence (total cases), and mortality (death) rates are commonly used to describe disease frequency.

CASE STUDY 1 (continued)

HC is not alone

Based on his initial exploration, the physician found that there were currently 200 patients at the clinic who had a diagnosis of uncomplicated, primary hypothyroidism (ICD-9-CM code: 244.9 hypothyroidism all causes and were using a thyroid supplement medication. Out of this total population, he counted 16 patients who had a diagnosis of one or more of the 20 hyperthyroidism episodes probably due to medication during the past year (ICD-9-CM code: 242.80 hyperthyroidism due to excessive medication). None of the patients had died. Out of the total population, 10 patients had moved away at some point during the year so he didn't have complete information for them. The cumulative incidence for 1 year was calculated at 16 cases/200 at risk = 0.08 or 8% of patients who had one or more hyperthyroid episodes in the preceding year.

Based on when the 10 patients left during the year, the physician calculated the total person-years for the 200 patients and then the incidence density. Figure 10.6 shows the departure information and calculations. The incidence density (ID) was 16 cases/194.25 person-years = 0.0824 or 8.24%. Because the number that left was small, the ID is about the same as the CI in this example. If new hypothyroid patients had joined the clinic during the year, he would have added them by counting the months they were at the clinic.

Figure 10.6—Calculation of Annual Incidence Density for Suspected Medication-Related Hyperthyroidism Cases for the Clinic

Total population at the start of the year was 200

No new patients were admitted, but 10 patients left during the year:

5 left at 3 months (0.25 year) = 5 persons x 0.25 years = 1.25 person-years

3 left at 6 months (0.5 year) = 3 persons x 0.5 years = 1.5 person-years

2 left at 9 months (0.75 years) = 2 persons x 0.75 years = 1.5 person-years

TOTAL person-years for patients leaving the clinic: 4.25 person-years

190 stay all 12 months (1 year) = 190 persons x 1 year = 190 person-years

Incidence Density is 16/(4.25+190) = 8.24%

Types of Epidemiology Study Designs

To answer the five questions posed in the previous section, one needs to know the types of epidemiological study designs that are used. Questions such as how big, how many people, timing, and location can be measured with frequency data and then studied with descriptive epidemiology. Questions about why the disease occurs (i.e., causation) can be answered with analytic epidemiology. Intervention epidemiology study designs can be used to explore the impact of removing risk factors or adding protective measures in a community on the development of disease. All of the epidemiology study designs employ comparisons as part of their methods. Where the various study designs will differ is in terms of whether the researcher controls or just observes the exposure and whether data are collected before or after the disease develops.

Most of the study designs encountered in epidemiology are **observational** because they follow and record the natural course of exposure and subsequent disease development. In an observational design, the researcher or field investigator does not control the exposure. Instead, the researcher identifies those who have been exposed to the risk factor of interest through their usual course of daily living. Observational designs tend to be used early in the investigation of disease cause and effect. The other general class of epidemiological study designs are **experimental** designs, which means the researcher *does* control the exposure variables. Such designs do not purposely expose subjects to disease-causing risk factors. Rather, these studies investigate whether removing a risk factor or adding a protective factor will reduce disease in a given population. Experimental design is used only in intervention epidemiology.

Descriptive epidemiology

Descriptive epidemiology consists of several study designs that use observational methods to begin identifying and linking exposures to the risk of developing a disease and identifying populations with increased risk of disease. Three types of study designs are used in descriptive epidemiology; they are case reports or case series, cross-sectional surveys, and correlational studies. Results from these studies are often used to determine where resources for care are needed and to develop subsequent studies that will test whether certain exposures cause disease.[6]

Correlational Study

This type of descriptive study uses population level disease information to compare frequencies of disease in different populations or in the same population, at different points in time, to discern whether differences exist. These comparisons can provide clues about disease risk factors. By comparing other characteristics of the populations, such as age, race, lifestyle, or country, patterns may emerge that show a possible association between the presence of specific characteristics and the presence of disease. For example, in populations over 60 years old, the prevalence of type 2 diabetes is 23.1% compared to the prevalence rate for the whole population at 8.7%. Age appears to be a risk factor for type 2 diabetes. To determine whether it is the only risk factor and the extent to which it influences the development of type 2 diabetes, additional study with other epidemiological methods will be needed. Another example is in 2002–03, the incidence rates for types 1 and 2 diabetes in youth 2–12 were 19 per 100,000 and 5.3 per 100,000, respectively. This research seems to indicate that children are at greater risk of developing type 1 diabetes, which is the opposite of adults. A third example using 2004–05 data from the Indian Health Service (IHS) shows that prevalence varies in its patient populations with rates as low as 6% in Alaskan Natives and as high as 29.3% in adult American Indians in Arizona.[13]

The biggest drawback of the correlational studies is their lack of detail about individuals. Because the data are at the population level, it is not possible to make a connection between exposures and the development of disease in individuals. It is also not possible to determine if the exposure occurred prior to the development of the disease. In the third example given above, it is not possible to tell if the increased rate of diabetes in Native Americans in Arizona is due to their location, local customs or diets, or genetic makeup since they are being compared to Alaskan Natives who live in Alaska.

Cross-Sectional Survey

Cross-sectional surveys collect information about exposures and disease directly from the individuals. Unlike the correlational studies, this approach has the advantage of gathering information at the level of the individual so links between exposure and disease can be made. Unfortunately, because the information about exposure and the development of disease is collected at the same time, it is not always possible to determine whether the exposure occurred prior to the disease. In spite of this potential limitation, information gathered through this type of study can be used to better understand possible risk factors and to formulate a research question that can be tested with an analytic epidemiology method.

Case Reports and Case Series

The third category of descriptive epidemiology designs are case reports and case series. These methods provide detailed information about the individual, the exposure, and course of the disease. A case report contains information about a single person, while a case series may include several similar cases. The advantage of case reports and case series is their ability to help establish a clearer cause-effect timeline for exposure and disease development. The disadvantage is that a case report does not indicate the magnitude of the problem in the population.

Case reports and series can provide guidance for defining the populations studied in correlation studies or the type of information about exposures gathered in cross-sectional surveys. Case reports and series usually describe the appearance of a common disease in an unusual population (e.g., pneumocystic pneumonia in apparently healthy young gay men) or a new uncommon disease (e.g., SARS or severe acute respiratory syndrome). Like the other descriptive studies, the results of case reports and series often form the basis for additional research that will test the effect of exposures on the development of disease.

> Descriptive epidemiology study designs can be used to identify populations that need resources and may indicate potential associations between exposure and disease that merit further study. Correlation studies use population level data so they cannot link exposures to disease. Cross-sectional studies gather individual information about exposures and disease, but lack a timeline. Case reports or series collect individual data on exposures and disease, including the timeline.

CASE STUDY 1 *(continued)*

How HC's medication error would be studied with descriptive epidemiology

A correlation study would compare hypothyroid patients at the clinic to see if potential associations exist between various factors and the presence of medication-induced hyperthyroidism symptoms. For this study, the physician might use his medical database to pull all patients with the ICD-9 CM code for hypothyroidism of all causes (244.9). Once identified, he would be able to identify their primary physician, recent lab values, recent appointments at the clinic, and any diagnoses of hyperthyroidism due to medication. Using that information, he could compare his patient population to previous years to see if the occurrence of medication-related hyperthyroidism to this past year was typical or a dramatic increase. The results might look something like the information in Table 10.1 where patients with hypothyroidism during the previous 12 months have been identified and studied. No dramatic increase appears in the number of cases this year.

Table 10.1

Population Level Data for Clinic Patients with Medication-Related Hyperthyroidism for Current Year (n=16) and the Previous Year

Characteristics	This Year (% or mean)	Last Year
Total hypothyroid patient population	200	195
Subset of population with hyperthyroidism due to medication	16	4
Gender (%)	4 (25%) male 12 (75%) female	1 (25%) male 3 (75%) female
Age, years (mean ± std dev)	46 (± 14)	44 (± 12)
Years since diagnosis (mean ± std dev)	15 (± 22)	14 (± 24)
ICD-9-CM code 244.9 (%)	16 (100%)	4 (100%)
Average L-thyroxine dose (mean ± std dev)	38 mcg (± 10 mcg)	45 mcg (± 18 mcg)
Months on current dose (mean ± std dev)	15 (± 56)	14 (± 53)
Months since most recent symptoms appeared (mean ± std dev)	1.5 (± 0.04)	3 (± 4.5)

A cross-sectional survey of the patients who experienced medication-induced hyperthyroidism can be used to collect additional information, which is not contained in the medical database. Based on literature describing causes of medication errors, questions related to the prescription and how the patient took the medication were added to the survey. The results obtained from the cross-sectional survey indicate that a correlation exists between the pharmacy and the brand of tablet dispensed for the Rx Corner and GenX brand (r = 0.855) and ClinicPharmacy and Synthroid (r = 0.644). Table 10.2 shows the descriptive results of the cross-sectional survey.

Table 10.2

Results of Cross-Sectional Survey of Clinic Patients with Medication-Related Hyperthyroidism for 1 Year (n=16)

Characteristics	Total
Gender (%)	4 (25%) male 12 (75%) female
Age, years (mean ± std dev)	46 (±14)
Years since diagnosis (mean ± std dev)	18 (± 29)
Average L-thyroxine dose (mean ± std dev)	32 mcg (± 16 mcg)
Months on current dose (mean ± std dev)	18 (± 64)
Months since most recent symptoms appeared (mean ± std dev)	1 (± 0.34)
Pharmacies used during past year (can list more than one)	Rx corner 12 (75%) Chain Scripts 4 (25%) Clinic pharmacy 8 (50%) VA mail order 1 (7%)
Brand name of medication	Synthroid® 4 (25%) Levothroid® 4 (25%) Levo-thyroxine (GenX brand) 8 (50%)
Usual number of days in prescription (mean ± std dev)	30 (± 2)
Self-reported compliance (mean days/month took dose ± std dev)	28 (± 3)
Medical lab where T4 /TSH analyzed	MML 16 (100%)

The medical lab was removed as a potential source of the error when it was discovered that the high level of use was independent of whether a patient experienced medication-related hyperthyroidism. Apparently, the clinic changed its contract to a new medical lab about 9 months ago and all T4 and TSH levels were now done at the new lab, MML. New information about a potential role of a specific pharmacy and brand of medication requires further exploration.

Case series could be used in this investigation to gather individual level information that has a timeline. These in-depth reports will follow events through time to help the investigator better understand what happened before the medication-induced hyperthyroidism appeared. Table 10.3 summarizes the information gathered about potential risk factors and when they happened relative to when the medication-induced hyperthyroidism episode occurred.

Table 10.3

Sample of Case Report Data for Five of the 16 Clinic Patients with Medication-Related Hyperthyroidsim

Characteristics	CF	LA	CW	HT	HC
Gender	F	F	M	F	M
Age	62	23	43	13	37
Date of diagnosis	02/1988	04/08	11/1997	05/04	02/09
Current L-thyroxine dose	25 mcg	25 mcg	50 mcg	25 mcg	25 mcg
Pharmacy filling last prescription	Rx Corner	Rx Corner	Rx Corner	Rx Corner	Rx Corner
Brand of L-thyroxine last dispensed	GenX	GenX	GenX	GenX	GenX
Date last prescription filled prior to onset of hyperthyroidism symptoms	Jan 29	Feb 1	Jan 24	Jan 29	Jan 25
Date hyperthyroidism symptoms appeared	Feb 2	Feb 5	Jan 29	Feb 4	Jan 30

Based on the results of the case series, a link appears to exist among dose prescribed, pharmacy, date of fill, and the brand of the product used. The outbreak of medication-related hyperthyroidism appears to be clustered around a 2-week time period. Although these results look promising, they do not establish causation. Additional study using comparison groups is needed to make that interpretation.

Analytic epidemiology

Once descriptive studies have identified potential associations between exposures and disease, further investigation is needed. This is the role of analytic epidemiology. Study designs in this group may employ either observational or experimental methods, and they may collect data from individuals **prospectively** (e.g., as events unfold and before end results are known) or **retrospectively** (e.g., by going back to old medical records or through patient recall).[12]

Several key concepts in epidemiological studies designed to determine causes of disease need to be kept in mind. First, as Figure 10.7 shows, the exposure to a risk factor or protective factor must occur prior to the development of the disease. In other words, the studies must be able to determine the order of exposure and disease. Second, any one risk factor may be necessary but not sufficient to cause a disease. The study must be able to determine whether other risk factors must be present in order for the disease to manifest. Third, the study must be able to determine whether the risk factor is a direct cause of the disease or an indirect cause whose impact is mediated through another risk factor. Fourth, the study must be able to rule out or control for confounding factors that may lead to a flawed conclusion. Finally, the study must be able to reduce or eliminate any systematic bias introduced by the researcher. These concepts and study issues are addressed by the various study designs used in analytic epidemiology.

Two types of analytic studies that use observational methods are the **cohort** and **case-control** studies. Both approaches are used to study individuals in terms of their exposure status and disease status to explore the strength of the association between exposures and the development of disease. A primary distinction between the two study designs is the point in the exposure-to-disease timeline when study subjects are identified. See Figure 10.7 to see the different points in time.

Figure 10.7—Study Subjects Selected on Basis of Exposure Status (Cohort Study) or Disease Status (Case Control)

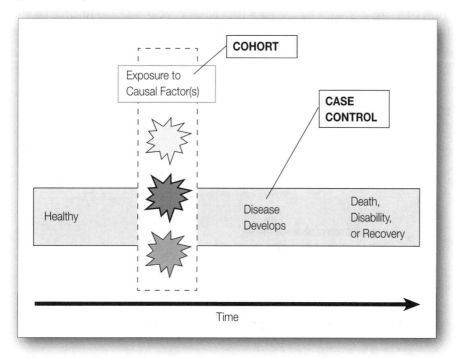

Cohort study design

Subjects in a cohort study are classified into groups on the basis of their exposure history. At the time they are enrolled in the study, the researcher does not know if they will get the disease being studied. The study will seek to answer the question, "Does the exposure change the likelihood that the person will get the disease?" Cohort studies may be either prospective or retrospective. In a prospective study, the subjects who were identified as being either exposed or not exposed are followed forward through time to see if the disease eventually develops. The Framingham Heart Study is a good example of a prospective cohort study that collects lifestyle and health information every 2 years as subjects age and grow older to determine who does and does not get heart disease.[6,12] It is also possible to conduct a retrospective cohort study, too. The subjects are still categorized by their exposure status. The difference is that there is no need to wait to collect their disease status. Once subjects are assigned to their group based on their exposure status, the researcher can look at the existing records to determine if they developed the disease. Large medical databases can be useful in this type of study if they contain the right exposure and disease information. Cohort studies are used most often when exposures are rare and the resulting disease is common. Results from a cohort study are usually reported as relative risks, although odds ratios may also be calculated.

Measure of Association: Relative Risk

One of the more commonly encountered risk estimates is **relative risk**, which is a ratio of cumulative incidence rates that compares the number of people who are at risk of getting a disease after being exposed with the number of people who got the disease but were not exposed. It is a measure of the magnitude of the association between an exposure and disease.

The relative risk (RR) ratio is calculated using numbers from a 2x2 table. As shown in Figure 10.8, the 2x2 table will contain four boxes or cells that describe the possible combinations of exposure status and disease status, and each person in the study population should fit into only one of those boxes.

Figure 10.8—Calculating Relative Risk Using a 2x2 Table

	Disease	No Disease	
Exposed	a	b	a + b
Not Exposed	c	d	c + d

a + c   b + d

Total population equals a + b + c + d
Each person falls into only one category

$$\text{Relative Risk (RR)} = \frac{a/(a + b)}{c/(c + d)}$$

Once the population numbers have been divided into the appropriate cells in the table, the relative risk can be calculated. Figure 10.8 shows the formula shown for calculating relative risk.

After the relative risk is calculated, it must be interpreted. Since relative risk is considering risk of disease based on exposure status, a RR that equals "1" means both the exposed and non-exposed groups have equal likelihood of developing the disease. Said another way, no apparent association exists between the exposure and the development of disease. When RR is greater than 1, then the ratio is interpreted to mean that exposure does increase the likelihood of disease. The larger the RR value gets, the stronger the association between exposure and disease. If an exposure is protective and tends to reduce the formation of disease, the RR value will be less than 1 (the value will be a fraction somewhere between 0 and 1).

When the RR is reported using a 95% confidence interval (95% CI), the key to interpreting the information is whether a "1" is included within the interval. If it is, one would say there is no difference in relative risk. For example, if the RR 95% CI is (0.05, 2.5), the interpretation is no risk; however, if the 95% CI was (1.2, 3.4) or (0.13, 0.35), then there would be a difference in risk based on exposure. The second set of numbers is less than 1, so there appears to be a protective effect.

CASE STUDY 1 *(continued)*

How a cohort study of medication errors might be done

A cohort study would begin by defining the exposure or risk factor that will be used to identify subjects for the exposed and non-exposed (control) arms of the study. For this proposed study, a medication error is broadly defined as any error in the prescribing, dispensing, taking, and monitoring process regardless of whether the error was corrected before it reached the patient. The patients will be ambulatory, and the errors studies will be those that occur in community retail pharmacies. With a cohort study, data collection can be either prospective or retrospective. The researchers will use a prospective method for this study. Data collected at the start of the study is used to place subjects into the appropriate exposure category. During the subsequent months, the dispensed medication, patient compliance, symptoms, lab work, and medications will be monitored and recorded. At the end of 1 year, errors are counted and risk ratios are calculated. The results of the study are shown in Figure 10.9. It appears that the exposure to medication errors at any point in the process is linked to an increased risk of medication-related disease.

Figure 10.9—Relative Risk from the Cohort Study of Medication Errors

	Medication-Related Disease	No Med-Related Disease	
Exposed to Error	40	360	400
Not Exposed to Error	15	585	600
	55	935	

Error is defined as any error related to prescription, dispensing, use, and monitoring regardless of whether it was caught and corrected prior to delivery to the patient. (Adverse drug reactions not due to errors were NOT included.)

Total population is 1,000

$$\text{Relative Risk (RR)} = \frac{a/(a + b)}{c/(c + d)} = \frac{40/400}{15/600} = 4 \text{ or } 4{:}1$$

Case-control study design

This observational design starts at the opposite end of the exposure-disease process and selects subjects on the basis of their disease status. The study then attempts to answer the question, "Were people who have the disease more likely to have been exposed than those without the disease?" The study design can only be conducted retrospectively because this design starts with the end result (e.g., disease status). Once subjects are categorized by whether they have the disease, the researcher will look back in time to determine whether the exposure to the risk factor occurred.[6,12] Results from a case-control study can only be calculated as odds ratios because information about the size of the population that was exposed is not usually known and that information is needed to calculate relative risk. For rare diseases, however, odds ratios can be used as an estimate of the relative risk.

Measure of Association: Odds Ratio

Odds ratios (or relative odds) are used to compare the likelihood that people who have the disease were exposed to those who were not exposed. In considering odds, it is important to distinguish them from probabilities. An odds ratio is a ratio of two probabilities: probability case was exposed (p) over probability case was not exposed (1-p). Suppose 100 people have a disease, and it turns out that 80 were exposed and 20 were not. The probability (p) of exposure is 80/100 or 80%, but the odds of exposure are p / (1-p) or 80 / 20 = 4:1. The odds of a person with the disease having a history of exposure are 4 to 1.

As shown in Figure 10.10, an odds ratio can be calculated from the data in a 2x2 table although the groups are compared in a different manner. Because the odds ratio calculation uses values in opposite corners of the table, it is also called a cross-products ratio. Unlike relative risk, odds ratios can be calculated for either cohort or case-control studies since the calculation does not require numeric information about the total population at risk.

Figure 10.10—Calculating an Odds Ratio (Cross-Products Ratio) Using a 2x2 Table

	Disease	No Disease	
Exposed	a	b	a + b
Not Exposed	c	d	c + d
	a + c	b + d	

Total population equals - a + b + c + d
Each person falls into only one category

$$\text{Odds Ratio} = \frac{a/c}{b/d} = \frac{ad}{bc}$$

Interpretation of the odds ratio is the same as that of relative risk where a value greater than 1 indicates an increased likelihood that the cases were exposed to the causal factor being studied. If the value equals "1," then there are equal odds that the cases were exposed or not exposed. A value less than "1" indicates that the exposure conferred some protective effect against the disease. If a relative risk value for a case-control study is desired then the odds ratio can be considered a reasonable estimate, especially if the disease is rare and the subjects in the comparison groups truly represent their whole populations.[16]

CASE STUDY 1 *(continued)*

How a case-control study of medication errors might be done

If the problem was studied with a case-control study design, the researchers would first identify the patients with a medication-related disease during the past year as well as those who have not had any problems. Once these subjects are categorized into their disease arm of the study, data will be collected retrospectively to determine whether they were exposed to a medication error. The results of this study were calculated as odds ratios and presented in Figure 10.11. The results indicate someone with a medication-related disease or injury probably had experienced a medication error, but the association is not a strong one.

Figure 10.11—Calculating Odds Ratios from the Case-Control Study of Medication Errors

	Medication-Related Disease	No Med-Related Disease	
Exposed to Error	240	200	440
Not Exposed to Error	260	300	560
	500	500	

$$\text{Odds Ratio} = \frac{a/c}{b/d} = \frac{ad}{bc} = \frac{240 \times 300}{200 \times 260} = 1.385{:}1$$

Two types of observational analytic study designs are used to establish causal relationships between exposures and disease or death. Both use comparison groups, but differ in how subjects for the study are identified and when data are collected. Cohort studies select subjects based on their exposure status and use either prospective or retrospective data collection; case-control studies select subjects based on their disease status and use only retrospective data collection. Relative risk, which is used with cohort studies, indicates the likelihood of getting a disease based upon exposure status. An odds ratio, which is used with case-control studies, considers the likelihood that someone who has the disease was exposed to a causal agent.

Experimental study design

Unlike all the previous designs, this aspect of epidemiology uses an experimental design because the researcher will decide who is exposed. The process of assigning subjects to the group to be exposed or not exposed should be a random one. This is done to avoid researcher bias in assigning subjects and to spread the other characteristics of the subjects evenly among both arms of the study.[6] For ethical reasons, this type of study cannot be used to study exposure to risk factors that are thought to cause disease. Instead, this experimental design is used to test whether the removal of a risk factor lowers the incidence of a disease or whether a factor thought to be protective can be added and result in a lower incidence of disease. For example, a study that purposely exposes healthy young adults to tobacco smoke for 20 years to study whether they will develop cancers at a higher rate than a group of non-smokers would clearly be unethical and unacceptable. However, a study that took smokers and used a new intervention to reduce their use of tobacco products and compared it to the effects of current smoking cessation practices would be acceptable.

Intervention studies are analytic epidemiology study designs that use an experimental rather than observational approach. This means each subject is randomly assigned to an exposure arm by the researcher, and data are collected prospectively. These studies are used to analyze how reducing a risk factor or increasing a protective factor will reduce subsequent disease or death.

Another acceptable intervention study may be one that adds vitamins or supplements thought to protect against cancer to the smokers' daily diets. Subsequent reduction in cancer can then be compared between the group with the supplement and the one without it. Data collected in interventional epidemiology may be analyzed with a variety of statistical methods. Choice of statistical analysis methods will depend on the research question and level of measurement of variables.

CASE STUDY 1 (continued)

Effective methods of reducing errors after finding the cause

Further investigation into the cause of the five unusual cases of sudden hyperthyroidism was eventually traced to the pharmacy where all of the patients had filled their prescriptions within the same 10-day period. Although the bottle of GenX brand levo-thyroxine used to fill their prescriptions had been emptied and thrown away, two other bottles were still on the shelf. It became clear very quickly that the labels on the generic product were very similar looking for all the doses, and another unopened bottle of GenX L-thyroxine 0.2mg (200mcg) was sitting on the shelf behind the open bottle of GenX L-thyroxine 0.025mg (25mcg). A complete inventory of the L-thyroxine products revealed that one of the 250mcg dose bottles was missing, and there was an extra, unopened bottle of the 25mcg product. The prescriptions had probably been filled with a product that was 10 times stronger than the dose prescribed. Luckily, none of the patients, including HC, suffered any long-term effects and their symptoms quickly subsided once they resumed lower doses.

The cause of the medication error appeared to have several factors, including poorly written prescriptions that included an unnecessary (and dangerous) terminal zero, look-alike labels on the product bottles, and a dispensing process that did not include sufficient double checks to catch the errors. The pharmacist and physician decided to test methods for reducing errors in their respective parts of the medication-use process.

How an experimental study of HC's medication error might be done

Now that the causal factors for the medication error experienced by HC have been elucidated and causal associations have been explored by observational analytic designs, an experimental study design can be used to test methods for reducing either the errors (i.e., exposures) or protecting the patient from injury or death if an error occurs. The intervention that will be tested by the physician and pharmacy involved in HC's error will be participation in a large, multi-center trial of electronic prescribing. A multi-center study was chosen to ensure that enough subjects would be included in the study and to consider results across a variety of populations.

The researchers will randomly assign the medical clinic and pharmacy to either the intervention arm (i.e., use electronic prescribing) or the control arm (i.e., continue using handwritten prescriptions as usual). Until assignments are made, the physician and pharmacy won't know which group they will be assigned. The researchers will count errors at baseline before the intervention begins and then again at 6-month intervals for 2 years to track changes. They are hypothesizing that the electronic prescribing system with built-in medication names, doses, and instructions will reduce the number of errors related to poor handwriting, improper use of terminal zeroes, dangerous abbreviations, and transcription errors.

Roles for Epidemiology in Public Health

Epidemiology has several important roles in public health. When an outbreak of disease occurs, it can be used to monitor the spread of the disease and guide response efforts. Epidemiological methods can also be used to monitor a population for changes in health status or emergence of a disease, investigate outbreaks, find potential risk factors, and identify exposures that tend to lead to disease. Finally, epidemiological studies can be used to determine whether a public health intervention is producing results (i.e., incidence and prevalence of the target disease is decreasing faster than it would naturally). Epidemiology can also assist with the development of public health policy.[12]

Monitoring health and responding to public health problems

Field investigations of disease outbreak and ongoing surveillance of disease behaviors in populations are key activities of public health. Epidemiology methods (e.g., collecting and comparing descriptors of disease frequency to historical norms) are very useful in monitoring a population for early signs of abnormal disease activity. Should an outbreak of disease occur, such as food or waterborne poisoning, a contaminated medication product, infectious disease, or lifestyle-related injuries or disease, field investigations will be used to determine the source and cause of the outbreak so it can be contained, controlled, and eventually eliminated.

Promoting research to seek effective evidence-based interventions

Understanding the relationships between exposures and disease will allow for the creation of more effective treatments and prevention programs. As the research in the various disciplines of the physical, biological, environmental, and socio-behavioral sciences make advances and discover new knowledge, that information can make epidemiological research more effective. Research is needed to provide the foundation for evidence-based interventions to promote decision making and action based on current understanding of the complex relationships of humans to their environment and one another. Because some of the relationships are so complex, using limited or inaccurate anecdotal information to formulate a response to an outbreak may be merely ineffective or possibly harmful because it delays implementing an effective intervention or actually increases risk.

Determining whether an evidence-based program actually works in a specific community

Evaluators use many of the same methods and study designs as researchers, including epidemiological methods. They differ primarily in the purpose of their work. While research can help to identify approaches and interventions that appear to be superior in their efficacy in a controlled testing environment, that same program or intervention may not necessarily perform at the same level when applied to a specific community or population. Evaluation is used to answer the question about whether the intervention is actually working in a specific community.

Developing public health policies and laws

Epidemiology can provide information that supports the development of new mandates or laws designed to reduce exposures and improve recovery from disease. At the population level, these laws may restrict unsafe behavior (e.g., not alcohol sales to minors), promote protective behaviors (e.g., wear seat belts), or change the environment (e.g., smoking ban in public buildings). Epidemiology helps to identify populations at increased risk so mandates or laws can target the high-risk populations. It also helps to identify relationships between risk factors and disease, so behaviors or environmental factors can be regulated or controlled through laws and policies.

Funding priorities for research and intervention programs

Epidemiological data can guide decisions for setting national and state research priorities. If a problem is shown to be of sufficient magnitude or has great impact, it will be easier to convince lawmakers to provide federal funds for more research into causes and mechanisms of disease development. Likewise, it is easier to convince federal and state funding authorities to provide financial support for the implementation of programs or interventions that have been shown to be efficacious through research or effective through evaluations of programs in other communities. Funding priorities are not limited to just public health interventions; the same data can drive interest and support into research and care programs that focus on individuals.

Epidemiology is used in many aspects of public health, including surveillance of disease behavior in a population; response to disease outbreaks; identification of interventions; evaluation of the effectiveness of the interventions; shaping of public health law, policy, and research agendas; and funding priorities.

How studies of medication errors like HC's have shaped practice

HC's experience is not unique. Luckily, he recovered completely from a mistake that has been fatal in some patients. The problem of injuries and deaths caused by medication errors is sufficiently large to capture the attention of policymakers. Initial efforts to quantify the problem are represented by landmark works such as the Institute of Medicine's 1999 report on medication errors [IOM here] and the data collected by voluntary medication error reporting systems such as the Institute of Safe Medication Practices (ISMP) and U.S. Pharmacopeia's (USP's) Medication Errors Reporting Program (MERP). The Food and Drug Administration (FDA) has expanded its MedWatch program to include reporting of product use errors. Based on the reports received and research into causal factors, recommendations have been made for improving medication ordering, dispensing, administering, and using of systems. Specific recommendations that relate to HC's experience are the appropriate use of zeros in numeric information, avoidance of abbreviations that can be misread, and use of multiple checks in the dispensing process. Additional recommendations and access to the voluntary medication error reporting systems are available at both web sites. The ISMP also offers a free error-risk assessment for a pharmacy.

Funding for research into methods for improving care and reducing errors related to poor writing and transcription has appeared since the IOM report. Recent efforts have focused on the use of technology, such as computerized physician order entry (CPOE), electronic prescribing, and use of infrared scanners and bar coding to match products and patients. Educational efforts to increase patient awareness of potential problems and ways to identify potential problems with medications before they are taken have been provided by numerous professional and lay groups. Clinical pharmacy services that cater to patients with increased risk of medication errors and other drug-related problems due to their use of multiple medications have been implemented through Medication Therapy Management (MTM) among others.

For HC, the error in dispensing has resulted in the pharmacy reviewing and revising its dispensing procedures. All labels are now double checked against the prescription at two separate points in the process. In addition, the pharmacist has begun to show patients the tablets in the manufacturer's bottle so they know what their medication should look like then they compare it to the contents of the dispensed prescription. The manufacturer has redesigned its label and added color to the tablets to make the different doses easier to identify visually. Finally, the physician has begun neatly printing his prescription information, stopped using terminal zeroes and abbreviations, and added the indication to the prescriptions.

Chapter 10 Summary

This chapter focused on epidemiology and its roles in public health. Several key concepts and terms related to the description of disease in a population, such as prevalence, incidence, and epidemic, were presented. Epidemiology uses a variety of study designs to describe how a disease behaves in a population, provides information about diseases relative to other populations or points in time, identifies potential relationships between risk and protective factor exposures and disease development, and investigates whether these are causal relationships. Observational study designs are the primary method used in epidemiology, although some experimental designs are used when it is important to test whether removing a risk factor will reduce disease.

Results from epidemiological studies are used in field investigations into public health problems to guide response and contain the problem. The results can also provide a foundation for the development of public health policies and laws as well as determine where and how to spend public funds on services and research. Evaluation of public health interventions also use epidemiology to determine whether the evidence-based approach that was most promising in research is also effective when applied to a specific community or population. The case in this chapter focused on medication-related disease related to a medication error to explore how epidemiology is used in public health issues closely tied to pharmacy.

References

1. Hepler CD, Strand LM. Opportunities and responsibilities in pharmaceutical care. *Am J Health Syst Pharm.* 1990; 47:533–43.

2. Committee on Identifying and Preventing Medication Errors. *Preventing Medication Errors: Quality Chasm Series.* Aspden P, Wolcott J, Bootman JL, et al., eds. National Academies Press; 2007.

3. Committee on Quality of Health Care in America, Institute of Medicine. *To Err is Human: Building a Safer Health System.* Kohn LT, Corrigan JM, Donaldson MS, eds. Washington, DC: National Academy Press; 2000.

4. Phillips J, Beam S, Brinker A, et al. Retrospective analysis of mortalities associated with medication errors. *Am J Health Syst Pharm.* 2001; 58(19):1824–9.

5. National Coordinating Council for Medication Error Reporting and Prevention (NCCMERP). About Medication Errors web page. Available at: http://www.nccmerp.org/aboutMedErrors.html. Accessed March 3, 2009.

6. Hennekens CH, Buring JE. *Epidemiology in Medicine.* Boston, MA: Little, Brown and Co.; 1987.

7. International Epidemiological Association. *A Dictionary of Epidemiology,* 4th ed. Last JM, Thuriaux MC, Spasoff RA, et al., eds. New York, NY: Oxford University Press; 2000.

8. Vandenbroucke JP, Eelkman Rooda HM, Beukers H. Who made John Snow a hero? *Am J Epidemiol.* 1991; 133(10): 967–73.

9. Doll R, Hill AB. Lung cancer and other causes of death in relation to smoking: a second report on the mortality of British doctors. *Br Med J.* 1956; 2(5001):1071–81.

10. The Framingham Heart Study. Available at: http://www.framinghamheartstudy.org/about/background. html. Accessed March 27, 2009.

11. World Health Organization. *Introduction to Drug Utilization Research.* WHO International Working Group for Drug Statistics Methodology; WHO Collaborating Centre for Drug Statistic Methodology; WHO Collaborating Centre for Drug Utilization Research and Clinical Pharmacological Services. Oslo, Norway: WHO; 2003.

12. Centers for Disease Control and Prevention. *Principles of Epidemiology in Public Health Practice: An Introduction to Applied Epidemiology and Biostatistics,* 3rd ed. Self-study course SS1000. Atlanta, GA: DHHS/CDC/Office of Workforce and Career Development; 2006.

13. National Institute of Diabetes and Digestive and Kidney Diseases. *National Diabetes Statistics, 2007 Fact Sheet.* Bethesda, MD: U.S. Department of Health and Human Services, National Institutes of Health; 2008.

14. *SEER Cancer Statistics Review, 1975–2005.* Ries LAG, Melbert D, Krapcho M, et al., eds. National Cancer Institute. Bethesda, MD. Available at: http://www.seer.cancer.gov/csr/1975_2005/, based on November 2007 SEER data submission, posted to the SEER web site, 2008. Accessed March 31, 2009.

15. Pneumonia and Influenza (P&I) Mortality Surveillance. *Pneumonia and Influenza Mortality for 122 U.S. Cities: Week Ending 02/21/2009.* Epidemiology and Prevention Branch, Influenza Division of the Centers for Disease Control and Prevention. Updated information available at http://www.cdc.gov/flu/weekly/. Accessed March 31, 2009.

16. Gordis L. *Epidemiology,* 3rd ed. Philadelphia, PA: Elsevier Saunders; 2004.

Suggested Readings

Centers for Disease Control and Prevention. *Principles of Epidemiology in Public Health Practice: An Introduction to Applied Epidemiology and Biostatistics,* **3rd ed. Self-study course SS1000. Atlanta, GA: DHHS/CDC/Office of Workforce and Career Development; 2006.**

The Framingham Heart Study. Available at: http://www.framinghamheartstudy.org/about/background.html. Accessed March 27, 2009.

Committee on Identifying and Preventing Medication Errors. *Preventing Medication Errors: Quality Chasm Series.* **Aspden P, Wolcott J, Bootman JL, et al., eds. National Academies Press; 2007.**

Chapter 10 Review Questions

1. Using the data in the 2 x 2 table, calculate and interpret the relative risk.

	Disease	No Disease
Exposure	50	300
No exposure	10	400

Relative risk is (50 / 350) ÷ (10/410) = 0.142857 / 0.02439 = 5.857

Because the RR is greater than 1, it implies that risk of disease increases if a person is exposed to the risk factor being studied.

2. Using the data in the 2 x 2 table, calculate the odds ratios.

	Disease	No Disease
Exposure	50	300
No exposure	10	400

Odds ratio is (50 x 400) ÷ (10 x 300) = (20,000 / 3,000) = 6.667

Because the OR is greater than 1, it implies an increased likelihood that someone with the disease had been exposed to the risk factor being studied.

3. Describe what pharmacoepidemiology is and when it might be used.

Pharmacoepidemiology is the application of epidemiological methods to investigations and research focused on clinically used medications and their effects on the population. Pharmacoepidemiology has applications in phase IV post-marketing studies, investigations into medication errors, and sources of contaminated or counterfeit medications.

4. List the types of descriptive epidemiology study designs and describe their strengths and weaknesses.

The three types of descriptive studies are correlational, cross-sectional surveys, and case reports or case series. Strengths and weaknesses are summarized in the table below.

	Correlational	Cross-Sectional	Case Reports
Individual level data	No	Yes	Yes
Timelines for exposure and disease	No	No	Yes
Compare to other populations	Yes	No	No

5. List the two types of observational analytic epidemiology study designs and describe how they are alike and how they are different.

The two types of observational analytic epidemiology study designs are cohort studies and case-control studies.

	Cohort Study	Case-Control Study
Identification of subjects	Exposure status	Disease status
Outcome being measured	Development of disease	Prior exposure to risk factor
When is data collected	Prospectively or retrospectively	Retrospectively only
Calculations of risk	Relative risk Odds ratio	Odds ratio only (may estimate RR from OR)
When used	Use when exposures are rare	Use when disease is rare

Applying Your Knowledge

1. Study the Tuskegee Syphilis Study in Negro males, an example of an observational study that should have stopped when penicillin became available. It has important ethical issues related to the use of human subjects in the study of disease. Discuss a current disease with no known cure such as HIV/AIDS, and describe how you would study it with epidemiological study designs.

2. Identify a recently recalled medication product and track the process of identifying a problem and determining causation. Determine all the epidemiological studies and methods used during the process.

3. Find a case report or series of unusual reactions that could be potentially linked to medications. Discuss how that link or association could be studied.

Describing Populations

Learning Outcomes

1. Identify examples of demographic data and source(s) for the data.
2. Identify examples of health status data and source(s) for the data.
3. Interpret data in a population pyramid by comparing it to the population pyramid for the United States.
4. Interpret demographic and health status data by comparing it to the data for the general population of the United States.
5. Identify demographic and community factors that are risk factors for vulnerability to poor health status.

Introduction

Public health is aimed at improving health and preventing illness for an entire population group. To identify appropriate public health interventions, you need to know the demographic and health status characteristics of the target population. In this chapter, demographic data and health status data are discussed that can be used to describe the target population. This discussion includes demographic, social, and economic characteristics. Included is a discussion of how to interpret the data using corresponding data for the general U.S. population. Population pyramids also are described. The discussion of health status data includes incidence or prevalence of selected diseases as well as mortality rates for common causes of death. Moreover, the use of health services data also is described. The final section of the chapter includes a discussion of vulnerable populations and the factors associated with them.

The different types of data are presented and interpreted in the context of a fictitious case study. In this study, a pharmacist has relocated from his hometown in the Midwest to a small town in the Southwest. The pharmacist feels that he isn't knowledgeable about the characteristics of the community's residents and that he doesn't understand their health issues. To become better informed about his community, the pharmacist retrieves demographic data and health status data on the population. The case study describes the process of retrieving and interpreting such data.

Population or Community Level Data

Types of data available

When pharmacists work with individual patients to address their health issues, particularly those related to the use of medications, they need to know some basic information about them (e.g., sex, weight, age, hypertension or diabetes status). Patient data typically is obtained through patient interviews, lab tests, and clinical procedures (e.g., blood levels for cholesterol, blood pressure readings). In a similar manner, if pharmacists want to collaborate with communities or populations to address a public health issue, they should have some basic information about the population, such as **demographic** and **health status information**.

Sources of data

Community or population level data typically must be obtained from an agency or organization that collects population data. Sources of population level data are shown in Table 11.1. As the table shows, most data is available from some type of governmental agency at the local, state, or national level. Multiple sources of data likely will be needed to obtain relevant statistics on different aspects of the population. The **census bureau** provides demographic data, which can be accessed for zip codes, community, state, or national levels.[1] Health status data may be available through the **National Center for Health Statistics**[2] or through state health departments. The type of data provided by a state health department tends to vary among states, with some states providing a great deal of locale-specific data and others providing very little. Clinics, hospitals, and phar-

Table 11.1
Sources of Population Level Data

Source	Type of Data
State Health Departments	Often provide county level data for selected statistics; varies somewhat from state to state; some state health departments provide health profiles of communities
Centers for Disease Control and Prevention, National Center for Health Statistics	Offer wide range of national and state level data
Census Bureau	Offer data (basic demographic data) from the local to the national level
County Health Departments	Often provide data on specific issues (e.g., the number of cases of flu), but may provide only limited population level data
Community Web Sites	Generally provide demographic, economic, and geographic data on the community
State Department of Commerce	May provide community-specific data, particularly economic data
Clinic, Hospital, or Pharmacy Data	Offer data, but it is generally limited to patients who are seen in the clinic

macies also have data on the populations they serve, although it is limited because it usually includes only the patients seen at a clinic or those who are patrons of the pharmacy. For more general cultural and economic data, community web sites can be useful sources or the state department of commerce.

CASE STUDY 1

Zach relocates to a new community

Zach's new community

Zach is a 33-year-old pharmacist who graduated from pharmacy school in the Midwest; he has practiced for about 8 years in his hometown. Zach works as a clinical pharmacist in the pharmacy of a **community health center** located in a small, western town. (Community health centers receive federal funds to provide services to low-income persons without health insurance.) Zach and his family hope to make this town their home. The location of the town is spectacular; it sits high on a mesa overlooking a lake and the surrounding area, which is covered with sagebrush, the silvery shrubby bush that grows in dry areas of the high western plains. The sage is so ubiquitous and characteristic of the area that the town is called Sage (a fictitious name). Zach and his family are looking forward to spending their free time on the lake fishing, swimming, and boating as well as hiking or bicycling in the surrounding mountains or on the plains.

Getting to know the community

Zach has enjoyed meeting the town residents because they are friendly and welcoming. However, he wishes that he had a better understanding of who the pharmacy is serving and how activities in the pharmacy relate to improving the health of the community. Zach begins to look for information on the town. One day, he talks to a nurse from the county public health department who suggests that he look at statistics from the state health department on health-related issues. (The county health department is located over 100 miles away in the county seat, but public health nurses visit this community.) The data is available online. When Zach gets online, he discovers that census data for the community also is available so he decides to check it too.

Demographic Description of a Population

Types of demographic data

A demographic description of a population provides basic statistical information on the age, race, sex, socioeconomic status, education, family size, and language spoken at home for a specified population. In the United States, this type of information is collected on the decennial census; it is public information and is available through either paper publications or from the Census Bureau web site. Demographic data are typically presented as a number and a percentage. As shown in the box, the number indicates the absolute number of persons who belong to that demographic category; the percentage indicates what proportion the persons of that demographic category represent of the entire population. Percentages allow comparisons across the populations of different communities, cities, states, or countries.

Comparison to the general U.S. population

When working with population groups within the United States, you will notice that demographic data typically is compared to the general U.S. population. The comparison indicates whether the local population group is similar to or different from the general population. For example, the percent of persons over the age of 80 might be 9% in one community while it is about 5% for the general population, indicating that one could expect more residents of the community to be over the age of 80 than for the general population. A comparison of other demographic characteristics to the general population of the United States gives an idea of whether the community is demographically similar to or different from the general population. To the extent that the population is demographically different, the needs of the residents and the services provided will be different than those required for the general population.

Use of demographic data

Knowledge of the general demographic characteristics of the community can provide a general impression of the types of health issues that residents may have[3] and the types of health services that may be needed, including pharmacy. For example, a substantial proportion of older, mostly retired adults in one community have implications for pharmacy services. Older adults are more likely to have chronic diseases like hypertension, heart disease, diabetes, and COPD (chronic obstructive pulmonary disease), so older adults will require medications and services to meet those needs. In contrast, a community with many young families may require services suitable for young families, for example, services related to pregnancy and child care. For the pharmacist, young families will require medications related to birth control, treatment of the common infectious diseases of childhood, and pain medications.

Presentation of data for populations

Census data and other data for populations are usually reported as both a number and a percentage.

- The number provides specific information relative to the community; for example, a population of 20 school-age children is very different than a population of 2000 school-age children.

- The percentage allows comparisons across communities or to the general population; for example, the 20 children in a very small community could represent 30% of the population, while 2000 children in an urban area could represent 0.1% of the population.

Population pyramid for the United States

Age and sex data also can be displayed in a **population pyramid**, which is a type of graph that visually presents the relative proportion of males or females and the relative proportion in each age group. The population pyramid for the general U.S. population is shown in Figure 11.1. In the general population, the largest proportion of the population is in the 35 to 55 age group with a lower proportion in the younger and older age groups. The bulge in the middle of the pyramid is attributed to **baby boomers**, adults who were born in the generation after World War II. In general, the proportion of males and

Figure 11.1—Population Pyramid for the United States

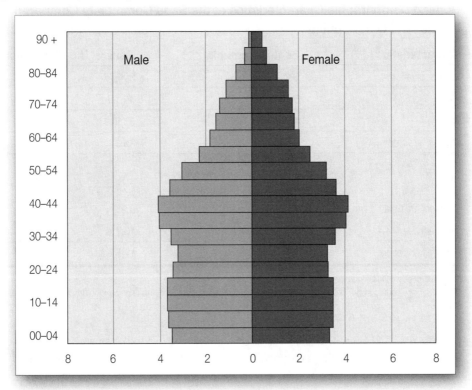

females is approximately equal until about age 70 when females outnumber males. By drawing a line at the age 20 row and the age 65 row, the proportion of the population that is between the two lines is considered self-supporting. The population above and below the lines is considered non-self-supporting, that is, not in the work force because of either youth or old age.

CASE STUDY 1 *(continued)*

Demographic characteristics of Sage

The general demographic characteristics of the Sage community are presented in Table 11.2. The first item provided in this table is the total population of the community; at 6809, it is a small community. The second item is the percent of the population that is male and female; the Sage community is slightly different than the overall U.S. population because it has a few more males than females (by 0.2%), whereas the overall population has more females (by 2.8%).

The second item describes the age of the population. The median age of the community is 32.4, while the median age of the general population is 35.3. The younger age of the community also is evident in the percentage of the population in each age group. A greater percentage of the community is under 5 years of age and a smaller percentage is age 65 or older, again illustrating that the population is younger.

Table 11.2

General Demographic Characteristics of the Sage Community Compared to the General U.S. Population[a]

Characteristic	Sage Community	General U.S. Population
Total population	6809	305,724,504[b]
Male	50.2%	49.1%
Female	49.8%	50.9%
Median age (years)	32.4	35.3
Race		
White	67.3%	75.1%
American Indian	26.7%	0.9%
Other race	3.1%	13.7%
Hispanic or Latino	4.7%	12.5%

[a]This type of data can be obtained from the census web site.
[b]The U.S. population number is continuously updated on the census web site; this is population as of November 23, 2008.

The race and ethnicity of the community population differs too. A smaller percentage of the population is White and a larger percentage is American Indian, which is different than the general population that tends to be primarily White with more other races and a higher percentage of Hispanics.

Population pyramid for Sage

The population pyramid for the Sage community is shown in Figure 11.2; its shape is somewhat different than for the general U.S. population. A substantial proportion of the population is below age 20, and a substantial proportion is between the ages of 35 and 50. Few adults are over age 65, either male or female, compared to the general population. The relatively low proportion of the population between ages 20 and 35 is characteristic of small rural towns where many young adults have left the community to attend college or begin careers. Based on the proportion of the population below age 20, one would assume that there is substantial demand for services aimed at children and teens and less demand for services geared toward older adults.

Social and economic characteristics of Sage

The social characteristics shown in Table 11.3 also indicate that the Sage community differs from the general U.S. population. Adults in the community appear to be slightly better educated than the general population, and fewer of them are foreign born. The family size is only slightly larger. However, over 20% of the community speaks a language other than English at home.

The economic characteristics of the Sage community are shown in Table 11.4. The unemployment rate for the community is low: 5.1% compared to 7.6% for the general population. However, the per capita income is lower than for the general population. A greater percentage of families in the community also are below the poverty level, indicating that salaries may be somewhat lower than for the general U.S. population even though most people are employed.

Figure 11.2—Population Pyramid for the Sage Community

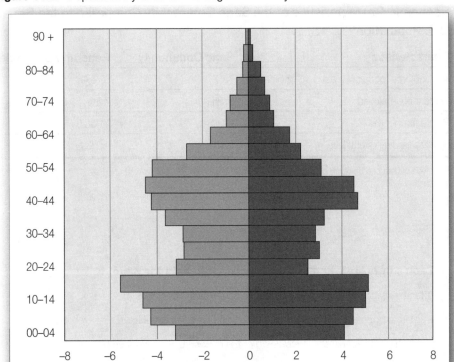

Table 11.3

Social Characteristics of the Sage Community Compared to the General U.S. Population[a]

Characteristic	Sage Community	General U.S. Population
Population, 25 years or older	4011	195,899,193[b]
Education (adults 25 or older)		
Without high school diploma	12.3%	16.4%
High school graduate or higher	87.7%	80.4%
Bachelor's degree or higher	19.4%	24.4%
Average family size	3.3	3.1
Foreign born	1.0%	11.1%
Speak language other than English at home (population 5 years and over)	22.1%	17.9%

[a]This type of data can be obtained from the census web site.
[b]Population, 21 years or older.

Table 11.4

Economic Characteristics of the Sage Community Compared to the General U.S. Population[a]

Characteristic	Sage Community	General U.S. Population
In labor force (population aged 16 or older)	72.7%	63.9%
Percent unemployed	5.1%	7.6%
Per capita income ($)	18,691	21,587
Families below poverty level	12.8%	9.2%

[a]This type of data can be obtained from the census web site.

■ ■ ■

Zach's interpretation of the demographic data for Sage

After reviewing the demographic data for Sage, Zach concludes that:

- With a population of less than 10,000, Sage is truly a small town.

- The population is not a microcosm of the general U.S. population because it is:

  ◆ Younger, with fewer older adults residing in the community;

  ◆ Better educated, with a lower unemployment rate; and

  ◆ Characterized by a substantial American Indian population, but with few other minority groups represented and a substantial proportion of the population speaking a language other than English at home.

The two largest employers in the community are the electric power generating plant, where a substantial portion of men are employed, and the hospitality industry that serves the 3 million visitors to the area every year. For women, the primary employer is the school system but a substantial number also work in the hospitality industry.

Zach interpreted the data by comparing figures for the community to data for the general U.S. population. Zach was surprised to learn that the community residents appeared to be younger than he expected. Zach came from the Midwest where small rural towns are known for the large number of residents who are very old, often with substantial numbers above the age of 80. Zach also was surprised that the educational level of adults was higher than average. Zach didn't remember being told about the language issue at his practice site, and decided to ask about the need for language interpreters. Zach was glad he had taken the time to get to know community residents better by understanding their demographic characteristics; however, he intended to verify his conclusions from the data by checking with community members.

Health Status Description of a Population

Sources of health status data

Several types of data are available related to the health status of communities; the state health department provides statistics on the most common causes of death. For example, **mortality rates** could be reported for total mortality, suicides, cancer, and diabetes. Additionally, the state health department may provide community **health profiles** that can be used to identify the health issues related to a specific community. Types of data include birth statistics such as the birth rate, and the proportion of low birth weight babies. Immunization rates and tooth decay may be reported because they are important factors in the health of children. Hospitalization rates for chronic diseases can indicate what diseases may be a problem in the community. County departments of health also may provide some data on health status but it is usually very limited, particularly for counties with relatively small populations. Health status statistics typically are reported as rates; rates allow comparisons with the general U.S. population or comparisons with other population groups.

■ ■ ■

Presentation of health status data

Data related to health status such as deaths related to cardiovascular disease are usually reported as rates. Death rates are typically per 100,000 population. Birth statistics often are presented per 1000.

Rates allow comparisons across populations; for example, overall mortality for a specific community can be compared to the general U.S. population.

Health services data

Data on health services also are useful; one such example is the number of hospitals, clinics, and health care personnel serving a specific population. State health departments may collect data on health services and on health personnel. Health services data in the United States usually includes statistics on health insurance, the proportion of the population without insurance, and the proportion with particular types of insurance (e.g., Medicare, Medicaid). **Medicare** is a federal insurance program for older adults, aged 65 or older,[4] and **Medicaid** is a combined federal–state program for health insurance to very low-income individuals, including persons with disabilities who are not able to work.[5]

Interpretation of health status and health services data

Health status data can be interpreted by comparing it to the general U.S. population; this comparison can indicate if the rates for certain diseases or for overall mortality are higher than expected or lower than expected. High rates can indicate that residents are at high risk for specific diseases, for example, leukemia and other types of cancer. If the risk is high, then the community can take steps to identify the source of the increased risk and take action to reduce it.

Health status data also can be interpreted by referring to **Healthy People 2010**, a document developed by the Centers for Disease Control and Prevention (CDC) that specifies population health objectives for the nation.[6] States can use the target objectives developed by the CDC or they can develop their own target objectives related to specific health issues. For example, the Healthy People 2010 objective for the proportion of adults at a healthy weight is 60%.[7] A specific community can compare their rate to the 2010 objective; if the proportion of adults at a healthy weight is less than 60%, the community would conclude that excess obesity or overweight is a problem in their locality.

 CASE STUDY 1 (*continued*)

Health status data for Sage

Several health status characteristics of the Sage community compared to the general U.S. population are shown in Table 11.5. The measures related to birth show that the birth rate is higher; a greater proportion of births occur in teens; most pregnancies are paid for by Medicaid or the **Indian Health Service (IHS)**; and a greater proportion of births are to unwed mothers. However, the percent of low birth weight babies is less, and the immunization rate is higher than the national rates. With respect to children's health, 68% of children 6–8 years of age have untreated tooth decay compared to 29% nationally.

Table 11.5
Health Status Characteristics of the Sage Community Compared to the General U.S. Population[a]

Characteristic	Sage Community	General U.S. Population
Birth measures		
Birth rate per 1000 females aged 10–19 years	32.9	20.3
Births paid by Medicaid or IHS[b]	72.5%	52.2%
Births to unwed mothers	56.4%	41.2%
Low birth weight babies[c]	4.7%	7.1%[d]
Immunization rate for 2 year olds	>90%	80.3%
Untreated tooth decay (children 6–8 years old)	68.0%	29.0%
Average age at death	67.1	72.2[c]
Hospitalization rates[e]		
Asthma	937.1	197.4
Diabetes	881.1	205.3
Heart attack	363.6	374.1
Stroke	167.8	332.2

[a]This type of data can be obtained from the state health department web site.
[b]IHS = Indian Health Service.
[c]Low birth weight is defined as babies weighing less than 2500 grams.
[d]For the state population; data not available for general U.S. population.
[e]Rates are per 100,000 population.

In examining adult health, the average age at death (67.1) is less than the state average (72.2). Hospitalization rates are much higher in Sage than the national rates for asthma and diabetes, but are less for heart attack and stroke.

Examination of the data for infectious disease reported by the state health department indicates no new cases were reported of hepatitis A, HIV/AIDS, or tuberculosis in Sage in the past year. Very few (only two) cases of vaccine-preventable disease (e.g., measles, mumps) and food borne diseases (only three) were reported; however, there were more sexually trans-mitted diseases (37).

Data on cause-specific mortality for the Sage community are shown in Table 11.6. The total death rate is somewhat higher for the community. The rates are lower for deaths second-ary to cancer, cardiovascular disease, and homicide. The rates are higher for motor vehicle-related deaths, suicide, and diabetes.

Table 11.6

Mortality for the Sage Community Compared to the General U.S. Population[a]

Type of Mortality	Sage Community	General U.S. Population
Total deaths	957.0[b]	872.0
Motor vehicle-related deaths	26.3[c]	15.7
Suicide rate	36.3	10.6
Homicide rate	4.8	6.1
Cardiovascular diseases	288.5	339.9
Cancer	190.4	201.0
Diabetes	31.7	25.2

[a]This type of data might be available from the state health department web site.
[b]Total deaths are reported per 100,000 age-adjusted population.
[c]The rates are reported per 100,000 population.

Insurance data and health service data also can provide insight into the health issues of the community. For Sage, 9.8% of the population has Medicare insurance compared to 11.1% for the state; 26.5% of the population has Medicaid insurance compared to 18% for the state. So Sage appears to have fewer Medicare recipients than would be expected for the state, which is consistent with the census data that indicated fewer persons greater than age 65 live in Sage. A greater portion of the population has Medicaid insurance than for the gen-eral state population, again consistent with the census data that indicates a greater portion of the Sage population is below the poverty level (12.8% vs. 9.2%).

Health personnel data indicate there are no mental health providers in the community, 33 primary providers (including physicians, nurse practitioners, and physician assistants), and eight dentists. Three pharmacies are located in the town; one independent pharmacy, one pharmacy in the hospital (it is the only hospital and has 25 beds; the next closest hospital is 49 miles away), and one pharmacy at the community health center. There are no school-based clinics. Therefore, the limited health services available in the community might dispro-portionately affect low-income persons.

Interpretation of data

Zach's conclusions related to the health issues in Sage are shown in the box. As Zach did for the demographic data, he interpreted the statistics by comparing the data points for Sage to the general U.S. population. If the rates were higher, then Zach concluded that Sage might have a health issue. However, Zach considered this a preliminary analysis and decided that he would check out his conclusions with some of the other health professionals in the community. Zach felt like he understood the health issues in Sage; for example, he looked at what types of information the pharmacy provides on dental hygiene, particularly for children. Zach also wanted to check out what type of **disease management services** were being offered to persons with diabetes or asthma.

The state in which the Sage community is located has selected a number of goals from Health People 2010 and monitors the progress of each county toward those objectives. For the county in which Sage is located, the deaths from unintentional injuries is very high (68.1 compared to the 2010 target of 17.5); for diabetes, it is 68.4 with a target of 45.0; and, for cirrhosis deaths, it is 13.3 compared to the target of 6.7. The county death rates for cancer and heart disease are already below the 2010 targets.

Zach also located data on the population served by the community health center. The patients seen at the center are about 60% White, 30% American Indian, and 10% another race. About 50% of patients are indigent, and 3% of the prenatal patients have gestational diabetes. Over 160 patients are in the diabetes disease management program offered through the community health center. Of the patients in the diabetes program, 67% are female, 70% are American Indian, and about 60% require both oral drug treatment and insulin to control their diabetes.

Zach's conclusions related to health issues in Sage

- Care related to pregnancy and childbirth may be an issue because of the high birth rates, particularly for teens.

- Dental services for children appear inadequate as the prevalence of untreated tooth decay is very high.

- Mental health services appear to be an issue because no mental health providers are located in the community.

- Given the lower per capita income and the lack of sliding fee scale clinics in the community, the working poor may have inadequate access to health services.

- Accidental injury and motor vehicle-related deaths may be an issue.

- Diabetes and asthma management appear to be a problem.

Characteristics of Vulnerable Populations

Within the context of health, **vulnerable populations** are those groups with a higher than average risk of having poor health.[8,9] Vulnerability can result from demographic characteristics that decrease individuals' ability to care or otherwise provide for themselves, for example, disability that prevents a person from earning a living. Vulnerability also is increased by selected community factors such as inaccessible services, including health care. Factors that increase the vulnerability of a population group to poor health[4] are shown in Table 11.7.

Table 11.7

Factors Associated with Increased Vulnerability to Poor Health

Population Characteristic	Examples
Demographic Characteristics	
Age and household characteristics	Race/ethinicity, age (either young or old but not able to be employed), large family, one-parent family, adult dependent(s) in household
Health status	Disability, chronic illness (self or member of household)
Poverty	Unemployment, underemployment, low paying jobs, jobs without benefits (e.g., health insurance or vacation)
Education	Unskilled or low skills; limited literacy
Community Characteristics	
Lack of affordable housing	Lack of permanent address needed for many services or to obtain employment; stress of homelessness
Deprived environment	Exposure to crime, violence; inability to obtain services (e.g., heating in winter, no accessible employment); no health clinics
Inadequate public transportation	Dependent on others for transportation or on public transportation

Source: Adapted from Mullen K, Curtice L. The disadvantaged—their health needs and public health initiatives. In: Detels R, Holland WW, McEwen J, et al. *Oxford Textbook of Public Health*, 3rd ed. New York, NY: Oxford University Press; 1997.

Demographic characteristics

Age and Household Characteristics

Demographic characteristics can increase a group's vulnerability to poor health; for example, infants and the very old are at higher risk for poor health because of their respective ages. The elderly population is at risk because many cannot work and are living on fixed incomes that barely cover the costs of food and shelter. The costs of prescriptions and health care become a much lower priority. Figure 11.3 shows a way in which the elderly can find inexpensive or free health care by attending school health fairs or screenings. The elderly are often times also dependent on someone else for support and thus more likely to live in poverty. Other demographic characteristics that can increase vulnerability to poor health are one-parent families, large families, or adult dependents in the household. These factors may increase vulnerability due to their effects on the economic status of the family, but they also may produce increased stress associated with poor health.[9]

Figure 11.3—An Elderly Couple Seeks Inexpensive Health Care by Attending a Pharmacy School Health Fair

Source: Used with permission of The University of Montana IPHARM program.

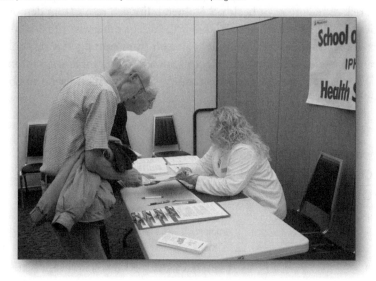

Health

Illness and disability can increase vulnerability because the person may not be able to engage in activities, for example, going to the grocery store, required to maintain health. Additionally, if the person cannot work, then he or she will lack monetary resources. Illness or disability is particularly problematic when health insurance is dependent on employment. If a person is too ill to work or has disabilities that preclude employment, then he or she will be at increased risk of additional illness or for an illness increasing in severity.

Education

Low levels of education affect vulnerability through one's inability to obtain a well paying job but also through an inability to identify and use resources that promote health. For example, if a mother cannot read and understand information about care during her pregnancy, she may not understand that her prenatal vitamins are covered as part of prenatal care or that vitamin supplements are important for her and her child's health.

Lack of education and limited literacy probably increases the effect of any one of the other vulnerability factors. Education and literacy are needed to obtain services for which one is eligible; for example, transportation. Even using public transportation requires the ability to read the bus schedule and identify the bus stops. To use specialized transportation requires even more effort on the part of the user; users have to know about the service and, if they are eligible, then they must be able to request the service and provide directions if necessary.

Poverty

Poverty, in this context, is defined as the lack of resources required to maintain an average level of health. Poverty could result from being unemployed or having a low-paying job without access to health insurance. Poverty also could result from other characteristics such as age, poor health, including disabilities, and lack of education.

Community characteristics

Lack of Affordable Housing

Lack of affordable housing can create homelessness, a factor that increases vulnerability to poor health. Persons who are homeless cannot protect themselves from the weather or keep their possessions safe; they are forced to move constantly, and they lack the ability to obtain adequate food or to take other actions to protect their health. Additionally, homeless persons cannot obtain adequate health care or the medications needed to treat even minor conditions.

Deprived Environment

Residence in a deprived neighborhood implies that many services are not readily available or are deficient. Living in a house without heat in the winter is a major health hazard for infants and elderly persons. Residents of remote rural areas may lack services because of their remote location; they may not have electricity, indoor plumbing, or telephone service. (Cell phones often do not work in remote areas.)

Inadequate Public Transportation

Lack of private transportation may seem unrelated to health, but in most U.S. communities private transportation is required for employment and necessities (e.g., shopping for groceries, going to the doctor). Even if public transportation is available, it is often unreliable because of restricted routes and difficulties for persons with disabilities or small children. Hence, lack of private transportation can result in failure to obtain preventive care or medication. It also could result in one's purchase of food items with poor nutritional content at the local convenience store instead of better quality options at a grocery store.

CASE STUDY 1 (*continued*)

Zach's conclusions about vulnerable populations in Sage

Based on this information, Zach can review the data he has collected on the Sage community to identify vulnerable population groups. Two groups may be vulnerable based on their demographic characteristics: teen mothers and children. Two groups could be vulnerable based on the fact that they already have a chronic disease: persons with mental health problems and persons with diabetes or asthma. Zach knew that some pharmacy patrons lived in areas remote from the community, but he wasn't sure if they also were more vulnerable to poor health. Zach felt like he had been alerted to possible issues with these population groups; however, he also felt he needed more information and planned to consult with other health professionals in the community.

Chapter 11 Summary

In this chapter, statistics were explained relevant to the demographic and health status characteristics of a specific community. Data on the age, sex, educational level, employment status, and ethnicity of a community are available from the decennial census. The data were presented as absolute numbers and as percentages; percentages allow comparison of community characteristics with the characteristics of the general U.S. population. The age and sex structure of a specific population can be compared to the general U.S. population using population pyramids. The relative proportions of different population groups are readily discernable from the population pyramid. Through the National Center for Health Statistics, state health departments, or county health departments, health status data for communities are available. Example health status data include birth measures, immunization rates, untreated tooth decay, and hospitalization rates as well as total mortality rate and cause-specific mortality.

Most of the health status data were presented as rates to allow comparison with the general U.S. population. The chapter ends with a discussion of the factors that increase the vulnerability of specific population groups to poor health. Demographic factors include age and household characteristics, health status, and education. Community characteristics that increase vulnerability include the lack of public transportation, lack of adequate housing, and residence in deprived neighborhoods or in remote rural areas.

References

1. Census Bureau Home Page. Home page available at: http://www.census.gov/. Accessed December 3, 2008.

2. Centers for Disease Control and Prevention. National Center for Health Statistics. Available at: http://www.cdc.gov/nchs/. Accessed December 3, 2008.

3. Anderson ET, McFarlane J. *Community as Partner*, 4th ed. Philadelphia, PA: Lippincott Williams & Wilkins; 2004.

4. Medicare. Overview. Available at: http://www.medicare.gov/. Accessed December 3, 2008.

5. Medicaid. Program Overview. Available at: http://www.cms.hhs.gov/MedicaidGenInfo/. Accessed December 3, 2008.

6. National Center for Health Statistics. NCHS—Healthy People 2010—About Healthy People 2010. Available at: http://www.cdc.gov/nchs/about/otheract/hpdata2010/abouthp.htm. Accessed December 3, 2008.

7. National Center for Health Statistics. NCHS—Healthy People 2010—About Healthy People 2010. Available at: http://www.healthypeople.gov/data/midcourse/html/focusareas/FA19Objectives.htm. Accessed December 3, 2008.

8. Sebastian JG. Definitions and theory underlying vulnerability. In: Sebastian JG, Bushy A, eds. *Special Populations in the Community: Advances in Reducing Health Disparities*. Gaithersburg, MD: Aspen Publishers; 1999:3–9.

9. Mullen K, Curtice L. The disadvantaged—their health needs and public health initiatives. In: Detels R, Holland WW, McEwen J, et al. *Oxford Textbook of Public Health*, 3rd ed. New York, NY: Oxford University Press; 1997.

Suggested Readings

Healthy People 2010. Read the section *About Healthy People 2010* **and the section** *Healthy People 2010 Midcourse Review.* **These sections give an overview of the current health issues for Americans and the progress, or lack thereof, toward the 2010 goals.**

Chapter 11 Review Questions

1. Identify two examples of demographic data and source(s) for the data.

Any two of the following demographic characteristics would be acceptable: total population, gender, median age, race, Hispanic or Latino ethnicity. Social characteristics also would be acceptable, for example, education, average family size, foreign born, or language. This data is available from the Census Bureau. Census data may be available from other sources such as community web sites, but the data originates from the Census Bureau.

2. Identify two examples of health status data and source(s) for the data.

Any two of the following health status data would be acceptable:

- Mortality available from state health department, Centers for Disease Control, National Center for Health Statistics;

- Incidence or prevalence of diseases such as obesity, diabetes, cardiovascular disease available from state health departments, Centers for Disease Control, or the National Center for Health Statistics; and

- Incidence of flu in a particular county or city that is available from county or city health departments.

3. Compare the demographic characteristics of Birmingham, Alabama, to the general U.S. population by referring to the data provided in Table 11.8.

The ratio of males to females in Birmingham (0.90) is slightly less than for the general U.S. population (0.96). Based on the median age, the population of Birmingham appears slightly younger. The race and ethnic characteristics of Birmingham are very different than for the general U.S. population; the largest population group is Black or African American (74.6%), while the largest group is White (73.9%) for the general U.S. population. In addition, proportionately fewer Hispanics live in Birmingham (3.7%) than for the general U.S. population (14.8%).

Table 11.8

General Demographic Characteristics of Birmingham, Alabama, Compared to the General U.S. Population[a]

Characteristic	Birmingham, AL	General U.S. Population
Total population	217,131	305,724,504
Male	47.4%	49.1%
Female	52.6%	50.9%
Median age (years)	35.5	36.4
Race		
White	22.3%	73.9%
Black or African American	74.6%	12.4%
Other race	3.1%	13.7%
Hispanic or Latino	3.7%	14.8%

[a]This type of data can be obtained from the census web site.

4. **Compare the population pyramid in Figure 11.4 for Smith County, Kansas, to the population pyramid for the United States to answer the following questions:**
   (a) Does the population of Smith County appear older or younger than the U.S. population? Explain your answer.

   The population of Smith County appears older than the general U.S. population because the largest single population group is adults over age 74 (about 16% of the population).

   (b) Do certain age groups have more males than females, and vice versa?

   Females over age 74 appear to substantially outnumber males—about 10% of the population is composed of females over age 74, while only about 6% are males. Other age groups appear about equal until age 55 and then women begin to outnumber men.

   (c) Do certain age groups appear unusually small?

   The smallest age group is the 20–24 age group; the next smallest age groups are young adults aged 25–29 and 30–34. The small proportion of young adults is reflected in the relatively small number of children under age 5 because young adults would be expected to have babies and small children.

Figure 11.4—Example Population Pyramid for Smith County, Kansas, a Rural County with a Total Population of 5549 in 2000

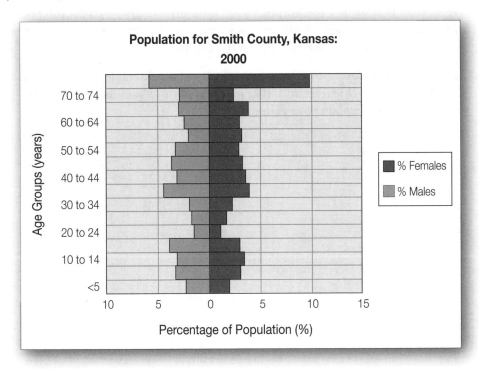

5. **Identify two demographic factors and one community factor that are risk factors for vulnerability to poor health status.**
   Any two of the following would be acceptable responses for demographic factors: age; household characteristics such as race/ethnicity, large family, one-parent family, or adult dependents; and poor health status such as disability or chronic illness, poverty, and limited education.

   Any of the following would be acceptable responses for a community factor: lack of affordable housing, deprived environment, and inadequate public transportation.

Applying Your Knowledge

1. Go to the census web site at: http://www.census.gov/ and find the current population of the United States. How much did the population increase from the 305,724,504 number used for this book?

2. At the census web site, look up the community profile for your home state or for the state where you attend pharmacy school. Compare it to the profile for the general U.S. population. The profile is available at http://www.census.gov/Press-Release/www/2001/demoprofile.html or the home page for the census web site; locate Census 2000 Data Release, then Demographic Profiles.

3. Go to the web site for Healthy People 2010, Guide to Clinical Preventive Services at http://www.ahrq.gov/clinic/cps3dix.htm, and identify two clinical preventive services that involve medications and could involve pharmacists. Interview a pharmacist to determine if pharmacists currently offer these services or if they would be interested in offering them in the future.

4. Refer to the table describing the characteristics of a vulnerable population and identify one of the characteristics that might apply to a population group in your community. Explain your rationale.

Community Health

Learning Outcomes

1. Recognize the characteristics of community health.
2. Describe a systems framework for identifying data on health determinants in a community.
3. Describe the SOAPE framework for developing a health intervention for a community.
4. Describe task roles that can be used to facilitate group work.
5. Identify the types of activities that occur during each management phase of community group work.

Introduction

The community in which an individual resides constitutes his or her immediate external environment; it is characterized by living conditions that may affect health. Efforts to modify the environment for improving the health of community residents are known as community health. In this chapter, the case study is about a pharmacist who moves from the Midwest to a fictitious rural town in the southwest to practice in a community pharmacy. As a pharmacist who wants the best health possible for his patients and community residents, he becomes involved in community health.

The purpose of this chapter is to provide pharmacists with the basic concepts of community health and to provide tools for participating in community health activities. The chapter begins by providing a model to guide data collection that will enable health issues in the community to be identified. The next section describes the SOAPE framework for guiding the process of identifying, implementing, and evaluating a community health intervention. Because community health involves working with other professionals and community residents, the final section discusses issues related to working with community groups and managing group activities.

Health in the Context of a Rural Community

Rural defined

Sparse population or low population density is the central component of the definition for rural. Rural areas represent geographic areas (1) in which relatively small numbers of people reside and (2) in which the density of the population is relatively low and distances to services or between services are large. In other words, rural residents may have difficulty accessing services because of the distances involved and because road conditions may exacerbate difficulties in access.[1,2] The small population also has implications for practitioners' ability to provide services. The number of people who would patronize a pharmacy might be too small to offset the costs of doing business so that many medical services may not be available without traveling long distances to larger towns or urban areas.

Implications for the health of rural residents

The reduced access to services has implications for the health of rural residents, particularly related to preventive services. Rural residents are more likely to report untreated tooth decay, and older adults are more likely to have lost their teeth. Poor dental health is partly attributable to the lack of fluoridated water for drinking in rural areas because many residents live outside of areas with centrally treated water supplies. Rural residents also tend to have less education in general so their need for health education is greater. This education is more difficult to provide when residents must travel long distances to attend classes or meet with providers. Obtaining care is exacerbated by poverty; household income tends to be lower in rural areas, and residents are more likely to be underemployed or unemployed. They often lack health insurance, which means that rural residents have less ability to obtain preventive care.[1]

CASE STUDY 1

A pharmacist participates in community health

Zach reviews health status data

Zach is a 33-year-old pharmacist working in a community pharmacy who has recently moved to Sage, a rural community in the southwest bordered by the Sierra Blanca Indian Reservation. In his hometown, Zach participated in community activities such as health fairs but he knew very little about similar activities in Sage. At the suggestion of the Sage public health nurse, Zach had been collecting demographic and health status data for the community from census and state health department web sites. From the data, it appeared to Zach that type 2 diabetes was an issue. The pharmacy where Zach worked had a disease management program for diabetes and Zach participated in it; however, it seemed that the ideal approach would be to prevent diabetes as well as assure that it was managed as effectively as possible.

Disease prevention and effective disease management

Effective disease prevention and management involve both nutrition and exercise. Zach knew that he could provide information in the pharmacy on nutrition and exercise, but nutrition seemed like a bigger issue than handing out information at the pharmacy. If residents were going to eat healthy foods, they needed access to affordable, high-quality foods; knowledge about the foods with the most nutrition per unit cost; and information about the nutritional needs of specific groups, for example, children and persons with diabetes. Additionally, food programs were already present in the community such as school lunch programs; Meals on Wheels, which delivers meals to homebound residents; and the food bank, which provided emergency food supplies to persons who needed it. Zach also had heard something about a program called WIC, but he didn't know much about it. Thus, Zach wasn't sure what to do since trying to address an issue like nutrition on his own didn't seem very workable.

Zach discovers community health

The public health nurse who had recommended that Zach retrieve demographic and health status data came into the pharmacy again to ask about services for a homebound elderly resident and asked Zach if he had managed to find any data about the community. Zach told her what he had discovered and then shared his concern that he didn't know how to act on the information he had acquired except in a minor way. The public health nurse told him that she had talked to the social worker at the hospital, and a group was forming to address several health issues in the community; she recommended that Zach call the social worker and find out about the group. The public health nurse also told Zach that it sounded like he was interested in community health and suggested he check the CDC web site to learn more about it.

Definition of Community Health

Characteristics of community health

The characteristics of community health[3] are delineated in the box. Community health is based on the belief that the community creates an environment in which its residents have the ability to be healthy.

Collaboration and community health

Collaboration is a key feature of community health; residents must collaborate to identify the primary health issues in the community and then develop and implement plans to address them. Some health issues may be addressed entirely by the community, but often collaboration and access to outside resources is required to effectively improve the local environment. Outside collaborations can involve health departments, economic development groups, legislators, and universities. Ideally, the outside collaboration will increase the capacity of the community to address health issues rather than make the community more dependent on outside resources.

Community health is characterized by:

- A focus on the health of the population;

- Collaboration among community residents and others interested in health;

- Health promotion and disease prevention;

- A healthy physical, social, and economic environment;

- Concern that all residents have the ability to be healthy; and

- Concern that limited resources are used as effectively as possible to improve health status.

Focus of community health

The focus of community health is the local population and subgroups within the population that might be at risk for poor health. A population cannot be considered healthy if a significant number of people have a higher than average risk of health problems. Groups within the population that traditionally are at risk for poor health include dependent populations such as children and older adults or disadvantaged groups such as the economically or educationally challenged.

Community health is primarily concerned with health promotion and disease prevention rather than the treatment of disease. A group formed to address a community health issue would be expected to focus on preventing the disease rather than developing new treatments for persons who already have the disease. For example, community health is concerned with the prevention of obesity through nutrition and exercise interventions rather than the treatment of persons who are already obese or have diseases resulting from obesity and sedentary lifestyles.

Community as Partner Model to Guide Data Collection

Community as partner model

Because community health is focused on changing the local environment to improve residents' health, data is needed not only to identify specific health issues of residents but to obtain information on aspects of the community that are determinants of health and on the resources available to address the issues. The assessment wheel from Community as Partner, a model for community health from nursing, provides a systematic approach to the collection of relevant data.[3]

The community core: community residents

As shown in Figure 12.1, residents are considered the core of the community; therefore, data must be collected to describe its residents. One such example in describing a community's residents is to consider whether a community has become a retirement destination with a substantial number of older adults who may not have other family members living near them. Data should be collected not only on the demographic characteristics of the community but also on the health status of the residents (e.g., prevalence of cardiovascular disease, incidence of gastrointestinal disease).

Systems and subsystems of the community

The assessment wheel[3] (shown in Figure 12.1) provides a model for systematically collecting data by dividing the community into eight subsystems in which the residents, the core of the community, live and work. The subsystems identify the parts of the community where informa-

Two guiding frameworks are described for community health activities:

- The Community as Partner model, which guides collection of data on community determinants of health; and

- The SOAPE framework, which guides the process of collecting and analyzing data, identifying a priority health issue, and evaluating the intervention.

Figure 12.1—Assessment Wheel (Community as a System) Consisting of Eight Subsystems

Reprinted with permission from Anderson ET, McFarlane J. *Community as Partner*. Philadelphia, PA: Lippincott Williams & Wilkins; 2008.

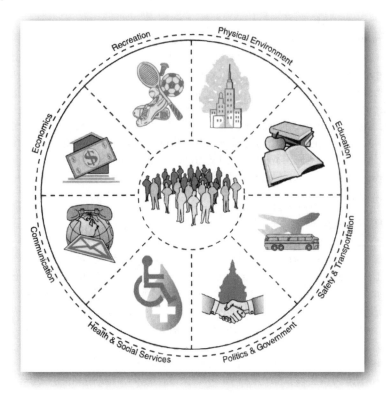

tion related to determinants of health can be located. For example, the health and social services subsystem indicates where data can be obtained about access to primary care and social support. Safety and transportation includes not only data on the types of transportation accessible to residents of the community but also data on food supplies, water, and sanitation. Housing is included in the physical environment subsystem, while education has its own subsystem. The economics subsystem enables data to be obtained on employment and the economic base of the community. A communication subsystem is also available.

Systematic collection of data on the community subsystems provides information on both the resources available in the community as well as on factors that might be contributing to health problems. For example, if the community lacks effective mass media channels for educating residents, then an educational campaign that requires some type of mass media could not be implemented. However, if most community members attend Wednesday evening bible classes, then asking class leaders to distribute information might be an effective method of communication.

SOAPE Framework (Subjective, Objective, Assessment, Planning, Evaluation)

A shared framework

A shared framework for community health work is essential to the success of community health activities. A framework provides a logical process for collecting data, interpreting the data, identifying the primary health issues, planning and implementing the agreed-upon intervention to address the problem, and evaluating the outcomes of the intervention. Without a shared framework, individual community members or groups may just "do something" without consideration of whether it meets the needs of the target group or whether it may result in additional problems. Fortunately, most health professionals, including pharmacists, who provide individual care have learned a framework, SOAP, to guide the provision of care. The SOAP framework can be readily adapted for use with community health.

The SOAPE framework

The SOAP framework to guide individual care and the SOAPE framework for community health are contrasted in Table 12.1. The components of each framework are very similar. Subjective and objective data are used for both individuals and communities. For individuals, subjective data refers to their feelings and beliefs about their health problem. For the community, subjective data refers to the community members' opinions about the health issues of their area and what causes them. Objective data for an individual refers to measurements on particular factors, for example, age or BMI; for the community, the analogous data would be percent of the population aged 65 or older or percent of the population with a BMI greater than 30. While assessment for the individual provides a

Table 12.1
SOAPE for Community Health versus SOAP for Individual Care

SOAP Component	Individual Care	Community Health
S—Subjective	Patient's feelings and beliefs (e.g., feeling fatigued caused by excessive stress)	Residents' opinion of community health problems and causes
O—Objective	Patient data (e.g., age, BMI, blood sugar level, blood pressure)	Statistics on demographics and health status (e.g., % of population 65 or older, % with BMI >30)
A—Assessment	Identified problems (e.g., type 2 diabetes associated with poor diet and sedentary lifestyle)	Above average incidence of diabetes; lack of health clubs, lack of walking or cycling paths; only grocery store nearby is a convenience store
P—Plan	Begin metformin; refer to nutritionist and trainer	Organize a farmer's market
E—Evaluation	Blood sugar level, calories consumed, minutes of exercise	Number of residents purchasing food at the market; residents' opinion of market

diagnosis of an individual health problem, the assessment for a community provides a diagnosis of a community health problem. Both diagnoses may include information on probable causes, which may be either individual (e.g., lifestyle) or community (e.g., lack of exercise facilities). The plan for the individual versus the community seem quite different because medication, exercise, and diet therapy appear directly related to health, while organizing a farmer's market seems to have little to do with health and a lot to do with business. An E for an evaluation component has been added to the SOAP framework for community health to emphasize the need for collection and analysis of data related to the outcomes of the intervention.

Timeline for community health

The community health timeline differs from individual care in that it can be much longer because community health involves a group of people. The typical clinical encounter involves a single professional, for example, the pharmacist and an individual patient. The SOAP process describes how the professional obtains data, prioritizes issues, and implements a plan. Because organizing a group and conducting meetings take time, the community health process probably requires, at a minimum, several months. Several years may be required if a wide variety of data must be collected and analyzed before the group can identify the priority community health issues and implement a plan, including the intervention and the evaluation.

Subjective data

Key Informants

Subjective data or opinions should be obtained from community leaders, key informants, residents, or anyone who could be considered a stakeholder.[4] The opinions of community leaders, official and unofficial, are important because they may have a particular perspective or may be critical to implementing an intervention to address a specific problem. Key informants include a variety of residents with an interest in the community's health or the health of a particular population group.[5] Health professionals, including pharmacists, may have knowledge concerning health issues. Others with a knowledgeable perspective could include, for example, the owner of a used clothing store who may have information about the issues of economically disadvantaged residents or the manager of a senior citizens' home who knows about the needs of older adults.

Opinion Survey

Collection of subjective data on the community can begin by using the opinion survey[4] shown in Figure 12.2. The opinion survey can be used as a tool to guide the interview and obtain information from community leaders, key informants, and lay residents. The survey contains general questions concerning health issues in the community; if data is being collected on an issue, specific questions can be added to the survey. If students will be conducting the interviews, it is usually a good idea for two students to go to each interview. One student can assume primary responsibility for asking questions and the other for taking notes (Figure 12.3).

The number of interviews conducted will depend upon the size of the community and the resources available. For a group of students working in community health for one semester, each student can expect to interview at least two to six key informants related to the issue. Persons representing community leaders, key informants, and lay residents from each of the subsystems will need to be interviewed.

Figure 12.2—Example Opinion Survey for Collecting Subjective Data about the Community

Questions for Community Opinion Survey[4]

1. What are the main health problems in your community?

2. What are the causes of these health problems?

3. How can these problems be reduced or eliminated in your community?

4. Which one of these problems is the most important one?

5. Can you suggest three other people with whom I might talk about the health problems in your community?

Thank you for your help. Right now I do not have any more questions, but I may contact you in the future.

Informant Demographics

(Collect demographic data on separate sheet of paper; informant demographics should not be associated with data.)

6. Sex: ___ Female ___ Male

7. Ethnicity: ___ White ___ Black ___ Hispanic ___ American Indian ___ Asian ___ Other

8. Affiliation: _____

9. Number of years at agency/organization: ____ years

10. Number of years lived in community: ____ years

11. Commutes from outside the community: ___ Yes ___ No

Figure 12.3—Pharmacist Conducting an Interview

Photo credit: M.A. Hartshorn, Biomedical Communications, University of Arizona.

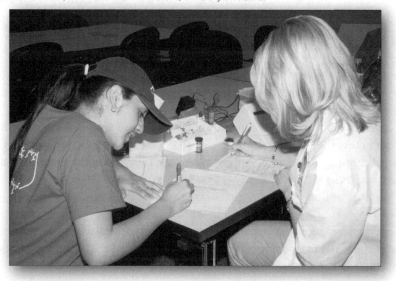

Zach uses the SOAPE framework

Zach liked the idea of using a framework like SOAPE to learn about community health. Community health was a new experience for him so the tool seemed like something that would guide his study and activities. Additionally, collecting data about community health issues seemed like a good place to start. Pharmacist friends had told Zach about an experience that they had developing a cardiovascular disease management program for an employer. Zach's friends had worked hard on the program. When they were ready to implement it, they discovered that only three people at the work site had cardiovascular disease!

Zach volunteered to interview two community residents about health. The first interview was with his neighbor who worked as a waitress in one of the three restaurants patronized primarily by Sage residents. When the topic of health came up, the neighbor volunteered her opinions about the diet of Sage residents; she thought most residents tried to avoid vegetables, and fruit was consumed only occasionally. Few vegetables or fruit were offered on the menu at the restaurant where she worked; diners could have fruit juice for breakfast, and they could order a dinner salad or get it from the salad bar on Sundays.

The second interview was with the fire chief to obtain information on emergency services. This interview surprised Zach because he had not realized that the fire chief would have so much information about health issues in the community. The fire chief told him that a large portion of emergency calls were to visitors participating in outdoor recreational activities who were involved in some kind of accident. These calls were problematic as they involved traveling long distances and working under difficult conditions. As for local residents, most calls were for either accidents (especially for children) or for residents with chronic disease, including diabetes and heart disease. The fire chief was very interested in the community health group and offered to help in any way. The fire chief also recommended that Zach or someone from the group be sure to interview the practitioner of traditional Indian medicine from the Indian reservation to get his perspective on the health issues associated with that population.

Objective data

Observational Data

Observational data is obtained by visual examination of the community; it is the information that one could obtain by driving through the community and looking for the schools, the city offices, hospitals, clinics, and playgrounds. Included in observational data is information about groups using the playground, for example, toddlers or older children. A systematic visual examination of the community can provide a useful orientation to the community.

General Community Survey

A general survey, also known as a windshield survey, is one way to collect data from visual examination of the community and, for most American communities, can be obtained by driving through the community. Using a guide such as the one illustrated in Figure 12.4, one could drive through the community and obtain basic information on the subsystems of the assessment wheel, for example, on the number of grocery stores in the community and number of convenience stores.[3] The observations should include observed activities of the residents, for example, the number of mothers out with their preschool children, the number of children using playgrounds, the numbers of people running or cycling for exercise, and the traffic on the streets.

Figure 12.4—Tool for Guiding the Collection of General Observational Data Describing the Community

Reprinted with permission from Revised "Learning about the community on foot," which incorporates all aspects of the assessment wheel from Anderson ET, McFarlane JM. *Community as Partner: Theory and Practice in Nursing*, 5th ed. Philadelphia, PA: J.B. Lippincott; 2008:172–4.

General Observations about the Community: Windshield Survey[3]

I. Community Core	Observations
1. History—What can you glean by looking (e.g., old, established neighborhoods; new subdivision)?	
2. Demographics—What sorts of people do you see? Young? Old? Homeless? Alone? Families? What races do you see? Is the population homogeneous?	
3. Ethnicity—Do you note indicators of different ethnic groups (e.g., restaurants, festivals)? What signs do you see of different cultural groups?	
4. Values and Beliefs—Are there churches, mosques, temples? Does it appear homogeneous? Are the lawns cared for? With flowers? Gardens? Signs of art? Culture? Heritage? Historical markers?	

II. Subsystems

1. Physical Environment—How does the community look? What do you notice about air quality, flora, housing, zoning, space, green areas, animals, people, human-made structures, natural beauty, water, climate? Can you find or develop a map of the area? What is the size (e.g., square miles, blocks)?	
2. Health & Social Services—Evidence of acute or chronic conditions? Shelters? "Traditional" healers (e.g., curanderos, herbalists)? Are there clinics, hospitals, practitioners' offices, public health services, home health agencies, emergency centers, nursing homes, social services facilities, mental health services?	
3. Economy—Is it a "thriving" community or does it feel "seedy?" Are there industries, stores, places for employment? Where do people shop? Are there signs that food stamps are used/accepted? What is the unemployment rate?	
4. Transportation and Safety—How do people get around? What type of private and public transportation is available? Do you see buses, bicycles, taxis? Are there sidewalks, bike trails? Is getting around in the community possible for persons with disabilities? What types of protective services are there (e.g., fire, police, sanitation)?	

Continued

Figure 12.4—*Continued*

5. Politics and Government—Are there signs of political activity (e.g., posters, meetings)? What party affiliation predominates? What is the government jurisdiction of the community (e.g., elected mayor, city council with single member districts)? Are people involved in decision making in their local governmental unit?	
6. Communication—Are there "common areas" where people gather? What newspapers do you see in the stands? Do people have TVs and radios? What do they watch/listen to? What are the formal and informal means of communications?	
7. Education—Are there schools in the area? How do they look? Are there libraries? Is there a local board of education? How does it function? What is the reputation of the school(s)? What are major educational issues? What are the dropout rates? Are there extracurricular activities available? Are they used? Is there a school health service? A school nurse?	
8. Recreation—Where do children play? What are the major forms of recreation? Who participates? What facilities for recreation do you see?	

III. Perceptions

1. The residents—How do people feel about the community? What do they identify as its strengths? Problems? Ask several people from different groups (e.g., old, young, field worker, factory worker, professional, minister, housewife) and keep track of who gives what answer.	
2. Your perceptions—General statements about the "health" of this community. What are its strengths? What problems or potential problems can you identify?	

Secondary Data

Objective data includes secondary or statistical data on demographics, health status characteristics, and other characteristics (e.g., economics), which are usually retrieved from local, state, and national governmental agencies that collect the relevant data. Typically, a community health assessment would include statistical data related to each of the subsystems in the assessment wheel. For example, assessment of the economic subsystem requires data on the median income or per capita income, the unemployment rate, and the major employers in the community. The education subsystem requires data on the number of children in school; the number of schools; and the availability of adult education, including both post-secondary education and classes for English as a second language or GED classes.

> ■ ■ ■
>
> **Data provides the evidence for community health interventions or evidence that:**
>
> - A health issue exists in a specific community; and
>
> - An intervention actually had an effect on health or on the determinants of health.

CASE STUDY 1 (continued)

Objective data for Sage

When Zach called the social worker at the hospital, she was very pleased that he was interested in the health of the community and welcomed him into the group. The social worker also offered to give Zach a tour of the community; she thought that a general orientation to the community would help him understand the unique location of the town and its special characteristics. When the social worker came by the pharmacy one afternoon, they went on a tour.

The social worker told Zach that Sage was a relatively new town. It was not founded until the 1960s so there were no "old" sections to the town, with buildings dating from the late 1800s. The town also was quite isolated; it was over 50 miles to the next town of comparable size and over 200 miles to a city. The town was located on a high mesa where there were few trees and no fields of corn or wheat that one would see in the Midwest. Perhaps because the town was new, the lack of suburbs or outlying residential areas made the town seem self-contained—like a ship on the ocean. A few miles outside of Sage, one entered a sparsely settled Indian reservation.

The few people on the streets seemed to be children, some riding bicycles, or mothers pushing strollers along the edge of the streets because sidewalks were scarce. Everyone else seemed to be driving. Zach already knew about "Church Row," the street where 12 different churches were located. Houses seemed to be set in large yards with well kept lawns, and many had lots of flowers. Few apartment buildings of any size existed, and the social worker told Zach that low-income rental housing was a problem. The most prosperous area of the town was the area near the motels that served the tourists; small shops sold souvenirs, apparel, and equipment for the recreation associated with outdoor activities such as hiking, camping, and fishing. Several convenience stores were located in the tourist area; the one grocery store was in the central part of the town.

The social worker took Zach to the city hall and introduced him to the mayor. The city hall was next to the fire station, which was bigger than city hall. Outside city hall was a large glass-encased bulletin board; the social worker told Zach that information in the community was communicated via bulletin boards since there was no local paper or even local TV stations. The social worker drove past the two elementary schools (Zach's children attended one) and past the campus shared by the middle school and the high school. Recreational activities for children seemed to be centered on the facilities associated with the schools such as the playgrounds and gymnasium. The social worker's perception was that two groups lived in the community: (1) those who participated in outdoor activities and who were prone to accidents and (2) those who did not participate, had a sedentary lifestyle, and often were obese with some type of chronic disease. That was a new perspective for Zach; he thanked the social worker for taking him on the tour and told her that he looked forward to working with the community health group.

Assessment

Data Analysis: Interview Data

Because the data obtained will be from multiple individuals, it must be analyzed and summarized. This process usually is not required to provide care to individuals. A simple analysis guide[2] is provided in Figure 12.5. Using this guide, the 10 top health problems as perceived by community members can be identified. A similar analysis can be conducted for causes of each problem and for what the respondents believe can be done to address the problems.

Ranking Community Health Issues

Selection of priority health issues involves reviewing the collected data by checking one source against the other so that the critical issue is not identified based only on one type or one piece of data. An example framework for ranking health issues is shown in Table 12.2. Subjective data obtained from the opinion survey is listed in the first column, then related objective data. Issues identified though the analysis of the objective data that are not included in the subjective data should be added to the list. The health status and demographic data corresponding to each issue are listed in the second column. The third column lists comments that offer an additional perspective on the issue.

Data Interpretation: Identifying a Priority Health Issue

Using the framework shown in Table 12.2, the health issue that the group wants to work on can be identified after all the data related to it has been analyzed. Selection of the priority issue is likely to involve a number of factors, some of which seem to have little to do with health. If the group is from an agency or organization, the issue selected will need to be compatible with the services they provide. Similarly, a volunteer group would need to select an issue that was appropriate for a volunteer group to address and for which members of the group have skills to address. Additionally, the group would want to consider whether the issue seems important to the health of residents and whether their interventions are likely to have an impact.

Figure 12.5—Template for Analyzing Data Obtained through the Opinion Survey

---

Summary of Opinion Survey Data[4]

Date data collected: From _____ to _____

Total number of people interviewed: _____   Number of interviewers: _____

Rank	Health Issue	Number of Persons Identifying Issue	Percentage of Persons Identifying Issue
1.			
2.			
3.			
4.			
5.			
6.			
7.			
8.			
9.			
10.			

Table 12.2

Selecting a Priority Health Issue

Subjective Data	Objective Data	Comments
Nutrition: Most persons (90%) interviewed mentioned healthy eating as an issue and believed obesity was a problem.	*Observational:* Only 1 grocery store in community; 10 convenience stores. *Health status:* Death from diabetes is 52% higher than 2010 goal; hospitalization rate for diabetes is 4x that for general U.S. population. *Demographic data:* About 28% of population is American Indian at high risk for diabetes.	More data on obesity and other factors directly related to nutrition would be helpful. Nutrition affects entire community.

A priority health issue in Sage

In the example from the Sage community, nutrition was identified as the priority issue through the opinion survey. But no data was examined directly related to nutrition. However, one of the health status issues identified was diabetes; given the relationship between diabetes and nutrition, the high rates for diabetes supported the opinion that nutrition for community residents is an issue. In the comment column, a remark is included identifying the need for more data relevant to the specific issue (i.e., nutrition). The need for more data at this stage of the analysis is typical because the original collection process was not designed to obtain all, or even most, of the data required to address a specific issue. For example, the group may decide that they would want specific figures on the prevalence of obesity in school-aged children or they want to know the prevalence of obesity among patients seen at the medical clinic. The example data in Table 12.2 represents the nutrition data considered by the Sage community.

The group in Sage decided to address the nutrition issue. One reason was that it was clearly an issue for the community, and the second reason was that improvement in nutrition would benefit the entire community. The community group also felt that they had the level of expertise needed to address the issue and that nutrition issues could be divided into smaller subsets for ease of resolving them and increasing their likelihood of success. The group recognized that they had little experience in community health interventions so they needed to begin with smaller interventions. Thus, a number of factors ultimately led the community health group to select the one issue for which they would devote their time and energies.

Planning and implementation of an intervention

Planning

Once the priority problem has been identified, a plan is developed to address the issue. Additional data may be required specifically related to resources in the community, for example, the availability of nutrition information from the clinic, the hospital, or through the school system. Planning may be relatively straightforward and simple, or it may involve extensive planning of complex activities. Even with simple activities, explicit efforts are needed to identify the resources required, both monetary and personnel, and to plan ways the activity will be evaluated.

Implementation

Implementation involves actions that will lead to accomplishment of the goal. Implementation typically requires substantial coordination and collaboration. Members of the community group need to decide tasks and responsibilities, locate resources, arrange for any facilities required, organize the team, and arrange for cleanup or closure. Finally, implementation involves collecting evaluation data to determine the effect that the activities had on accomplishing their goal.

CASE STUDY 1 (*continued*)

Planning the intervention in Sage

The community groups had several ideas about addressing nutrition issues in their community. One idea was to conduct a weekly farmer's market; another idea, given the lack of knowledge by many residents about nutrition, was an educational campaign. A third suggestion was to collect more data on food programs to determine if they were adequate and if the food offered through the programs was nutritious. After considerable discussion, the groups decided to implement all three components. They felt that they might have more impact on residents' nutritional status with the three-part plan.

Some members of the group, including Zach, said that they would work on the educational campaign. Zach agreed to distribute literature on nutrition through the pharmacy as well as to identify other venues for distribution, including the clinics and the grocery stores. The second part of the plan, establishing a farmer's market, was selected by other members of the group. They planned to contact hobby farmers from 20 miles downriver about bringing their produce 1 day a week. They also discussed ways to promote the market to the community. The third part, collecting data on other food programs in the community included the food bank, the WIC program (providing food to pregnant women and young children), and the school lunch program. Zach decided that he also would serve in this group as it would give him an opportunity to become better acquainted with community resources. Zach was sure that he could use this information in his pharmacy practice when patients asked questions about local services or if he was working with a patient who had problems obtaining adequate nutritious food.

Evaluation: measuring outcomes and evaluating progress

Process Measures

Evaluation is an important component of a community health program. Because evaluation is not closely tied to the subjective and objective data used to develop the intervention, it is easy to omit. Measures are needed to describe the process as well as to evaluate the impact of the intervention. If the intervention is education, using brochures or fliers, a process measure could be the number and type of sites where brochures were distributed; an outcome measure could be the number of brochures distributed or a short survey on satisfaction with the information in the brochure. Process measures can indicate which part of an intervention was most effective, for example, whether it was more effective to distribute brochures through the pharmacy or through the churches.

Outcome Measures

Outcome measures indicate impact, for example, the total number of people who received a brochure or the number of people who now exercise regularly. For interventions related to health, the ideal outcome measure would be a health status indicator such as the proportion of residents who are obese. However, an extended period of time may be required before an effect can be discerned in health status. Therefore, for many small interventions, interim outcomes are measured such as the number of people who now exercise regularly.

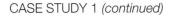

CASE STUDY 1 *(continued)*

Outcome measures in Sage

The Sage community health group wanted some way of assessing their progress toward better nutrition in the town. Outcomes such as reduced prevalence of obesity or diabetes probably would not be detectable for several years, and the group felt that they needed data on more immediate outcomes. Therefore, the group identified several types of data that would be relatively easy to collect over the next year, including:

- Number of nutrition brochures distributed over the next year for the informational component;
- Progress toward a farmer's market made within the next 6 months (i.e., number of vendors identified, location identified, manager/coordinator of the market identified) and at the end of the year, the number of markets held, number of vendors, and satisfaction of vendors and residents with the farmer's market; and
- Types of data collected on the three food programs and progress toward addressing these issues.

Collaboration and Management of a Community Group

Collaboration

Productive Collaboration

Fundamental to community health is collaboration among residents and others interested in the health of the community. Collaboration implies that residents will be working together to collect data, analyze the data, identify the priority health issues, and agree on how to address the issues. Typically, this type of collaboration requires the formation of a group of interested residents[4] and participants' skill in interacting with others to address an issue.

Interaction within the context of a group whose purpose is to address a health issue is somewhat different than the social interactions with which most individuals are familiar. Productive collaboration requires a structure, usually consisting of leadership and working groups, composed of persons who are focused on the issue. Collaboration and appropriate behavior in a task group are facilitated if training is provided to members on the types of skills required for group work. In this section, examples are provided of task roles that individuals can assume to facilitate group work. Also provided are the management phases of the group process that are required to address a community health issue.

Task Roles

Task roles that facilitate group work[6] are described in Table 12.3. Because groups typically schedule meetings to discuss issues, the task roles are related to the discussion of a topic with example statements that would facilitate the discussion. As shown in the figure, overall task roles relate to conducting a collaborative meeting. The gate keeping and expediting roles are related to focusing the meeting on the issue at hand and not getting distracted by side issues or other interests. Attention to time allows one to conduct an efficient meeting that does not waste attendees' time and facilitates being able to address the relevant issues. Evaluation is related to assessing the group process and possibly discussing how the next meeting should be conducted. If, for example, having a handout was helpful to the group, then asking other presenters to provide a handout would facilitate future meetings.

Procedures for Group Meetings

A collaborative group meeting typically requires that participants proceed through the discussion in a logical sequence.[6] As shown in the table, initiating the discussion is the first step. While a formal group meeting for the dissemination of information may rely on a designated group leader, anyone can initiate the discussion in a collaborative group. The first part of the discussion of a particular topic typically involves a short presentation or report on the topic that solicits comments by other group members. Questions need to be asked and information provided until the group feels that they understand the issue and a majority of the members participate. Group members can participate by giving and asking for reactions from other group members and by restating or giving examples. Throughout the discussion process, group members need to be sure that misinformation is not being presented; if they have doubts, then a group member needs to verify the source of the information and its reliability. As the discussion proceeds, the primary task role is to clarify, synthesize, and summarize in preparation for identifying actions and the individuals who will execute them.

Table 12.3

Task Roles[6] Required for Effective Collaboration

Task Role	Statements Appropriate for Task Role
Overall Task Roles	
1. Gate keeping and expediting	T. has expressed a concern about ____; when would be a good time to discuss this issue?
2. Timekeeping	We have only 10 minutes before we need to ____; I am wondering if we should continue this discussion at our next meeting.
3. Evaluating group process	We have addressed a number of issues today, which seemed to take longer than we anticipated. Does our next meeting need to be longer?
Sequence of Task Roles Specific to Discussion of a Topic	
1. Initiating	OK, what do we need to discuss today?
2. Giving and asking for information	I think several of you have participated in similar activities; can you describe what you did?
3. Giving and asking for reactions	We haven't heard from J.; J., can you share your perspective?
4. Restating and giving examples	If I understand correctly, you are saying that...
5. Confronting and reality testing	That is an interesting perspective. Are there any studies examining the issue?
6. Clarifying, synthesizing, and summarizing	We've talked about several issues. It sounds like the group wants to ....
7. Identifying actions and actors	It sounds like we need more information about...; Z., is it possible for you to...?

Management phases of community group work

The Five Management Phases

Management of a collaborative group can be an issue if group members have not identified a leadership group or if leaders have misconceptions about how a collaborative group operates. Failure to recognize the need for management can result in members not having the requisite skills to participate or in not having an organizational structure that will facilitate work. However, management tasks will need to be adjusted according to the phase of the group's activities.

The five phases of a single effort by a community health group and the appropriate management tasks are delineated in Table 12.4. The phases correspond to sequence of the group's activities. As the group is getting organized, management tasks are related to organization; as the group's work proceeds, management tasks are related to facilitating the work and assuring the group has resources and is structured appropriately for the task. For example, in Phase III, the group is making a decision on what they will do to address a health issue. Because collaborative groups work by consensus and most group members have had little experience with consensus meth-

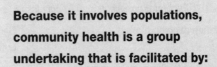

Because it involves populations, community health is a group undertaking that is facilitated by:

- A shared view of the problem or goal;

- A shared understanding of effective procedures for group work; and

- Group members assuming roles that result in collaboration.

Table 12.4

Phases in the Activities of a Collaborative Group[6] and Associated Management Tasks

Management Phase and Tasks	Comments
Phase I: Organizational Phase	
Identify community members interested in participating	Group should contain a mix of professional and lay community members
Develop the organizational structure required for a functioning group	Typical structure consists of a leadership group, working groups, and the entire group
Assess level of experience to identify novice groups	Novice groups typically require much more time to organize and learn collaborative skills
Assure that group members have requisite knowledge and skills for collaboration	Few people have been trained to collaborate; review basic information on collaboration; an outside consultant might be helpful
Assure that group has a basic understanding of community health	Provide information on community health
Identify support that the committee needs to function effectively	Office support will be needed for efficient and effective group function; identify and provide

Continued

Table 12.4 *Continued*

Management Phase and Tasks	Comments
Phase II: Working Together to Collect Data	
Review committee structure (e.g., is the number of working groups appropriate?)	Reorganize and adjust responsibilities and working groups as needed; meet with working groups as needed to facilitate progress
Review participation; right people assuming responsibility for each task	Adjust group membership to best utilize members' skills
Monitor need for additional knowledge and skill development	Review group norms and rules; conduct additional training as needed
Phase III: Facilitate the Selection of Priority Issues and Planning	
Facilitate decision making	Determine if consensus procedures are needed and obtain outside expertise if necessary
Phase IV: Monitor Implementation	
Monitor for problems with implementation; need to recruit members with requisite skills	Provide support; meet with persons primarily responsible for implementation to assure success
Phase V: Evaluation and Dissolution	
Facilitate evaluation of the intervention; evaluate the function of the committee	Assure that intervention is evaluated; obtain feedback on group function; arrange for records storage, etc.

ods, training may be needed. In a collaborative community health group, implementation probably will depend to a large extent on activities of the group members. Often the leadership group will want to meet with the groups doing the work to assure that they are moving forward and have the resources they need. When the group completes their work on a particular issue, then management activities are focused on facilitating evaluation and turning over the activity to an appropriate person or agency. If the group will be dissolved, then management tasks are related to ending the group and assuring that records are stored in a safe place.

The Organizational Phase Is Critical

The organizational phase is critical to the development of a functional community-based group. Participating volunteer community leaders, professionals, and lay members may have little experience working in collaborative groups and may have little knowledge of community health. Therefore, organizing a new group can require a substantial amount of time as the group members learn about the issues, develop skills (e.g., how to identify and retrieve data, analyze the data), and use consensus procedures to prioritize issues. Additional time will be required if members are diverse and have differing levels of education, cultural backgrounds, and possibly languages.

Community group work at Sage

At the first meeting, the social worker who had organized the group suggested that the members decide how they were going to work together. She then posted a procedure and asked the group to modify it to suit their needs. The suggested procedure for conducting meetings included an opening, a review of what happened at the last meeting, and a brief discussion of what they wanted to accomplish at this meeting. Other suggestions included reports from subgroups that had collected data or obtained relevant information, discussion of the information, and then identification of actions and actors for activities. The social worker also handed out a list of task roles that group members could assume during the meeting, which was something new to Zach. Zach found the suggested roles (see Table 12.3) to be very helpful. For the first time, Zach knew it was allowable to ask a silent member of the group for his or her perspective; by restating what someone else had said, he could clarify what the group was discussing.

The procedure and the roles described made the meetings much more productive. Any of the group members was willing to initiate the meeting by saying something like "OK, we're here to hear reports from Jane and Olivia, so I think we need to get started." Several group members, Zach included, would restate what they thought someone else had said or give an example and ask if that was what they meant. One member, who was always on time, served as their timekeeper and would frequently say "We need to hear from Harry and Zach yet, so how do you want to handle the discussion of transportation—put it on the agenda for the next meeting or do you think we can finish the discussion now?" After several meetings, Zach became quite adept at clarifying, synthesizing, and summarizing as well as suggesting what action the group could take next. These roles seemed to facilitate the group work, and Zach frequently complimented the group on being easy to work with.

Overall, Zach felt like the group had spent a lot of time getting organized and collecting data, but it all seemed worthwhile in the end. Once the group identified what they wanted to do, it seemed like things happened quickly. The brochures were obtained and distributed and then the farmer's market was organized. The group was in the process of collecting the additional data they wanted on the programs in the community. Zach was sure that once the group decided what they needed to do, it would happen quickly. On the whole, it was a positive experience and Zach was sure that he would participate in other community health activities.

Chapter 12 Summary

This chapter introduced the concepts of community health and collaboration. Community health consists of health-related activities for the purpose of improving the health status of the community. Similar to providing care to individuals, community health requires a systematic process for work. An adaptation of the SOAP process, SOAPE includes both subjective and objective collection of data. The data is analyzed, and the priority health issues in the community are identified. An intervention is planned and operationalized and then the outcomes of the intervention are evaluated. The Community as Partner model was presented to provide a systematic guide for obtaining and interpreting data about the community. Because community health involves local residents as well as health care professionals, most of the work in community health is conducted through groups. The management phases and management tasks associated with a group that was formed to address a community health issue were delineated. The task roles required for successful group work, for example, gate keeping and giving and asking for reactions, also were provided.

References

1. Stamm BH, ed. *Rural Behavioral Health Care.* Washington, DC: American Psychological Association; 2003.
2. Glasglow N, Morton LW, Johnson NE. *Critical Issues in Rural Health.* Ames, IA: Blackwell Publishing; 2004.
3. Anderson ET, McFarlane J. *Community as Partner.* Philadelphia, PA: Lippincott Williams & Wilkins; 2008.
4. U.S. Department of Health and Human Services. Planned Approach to Community Health: Guide for the Local Coordinator. Atlanta, GA: U.S. Department of Health and Human Services, Department of Health and Human Services, Centers for Disease Control and Prevention National Center for Chronic Disease Prevention and Health Promotion. Available online at: http://wonder.cdc.gov/wonder/prevguid/p0000064/p0000064.asp. Accessed December 16, 2008.
5. Murray SA, Tapson J, Turnbull L, et al. Listening to local voices: adapting rapid appraisal to assess health and social needs in general practice. *BMJ.* 1994; 308:698–700.
6. Rabow J, Charness MA, Kipperman J, et al. *William Fawcett Hill's Learning through Discussion*, 3rd ed. Thousand Oaks, CA: Sage Publications; 1994.

Suggested Readings

Durch JS, Bailey LA, Stoto MA, eds. *Improving Health in the Community: A Role for Performance Monitoring.* Washington, DC: National Academy Press; 1997.

The Community Health Improvement Process (CHIP) developed by the Institute of Medicine is described. CHIP uses a problem identification and prioritization cycle to identify critical health issues that are addressed in the analysis and implementation cycle. The book provides a good, although advanced, discussion of assessing the outcomes of community health interventions.

Anderson ET, McFarlane J. *Community as Partner,* 4th ed. Philadelphia, PA: Lippincott Williams & Wilkins; 2004.

The Community as Partner assessment is described and then an extensive case study that includes a wide variety of statistical data is provided. Additional short examples, illustrating the application of the model to a variety of settings, also are described.

Rabow J, Charness MA, Kipperman J, et al. *William Fawcett Hill's Learning through Discussion,* 3rd ed. Thousand Oaks, CA: Sage Publications; 1994.

This book provides instruction for group learning. Although a small, easily read book, it provides multiple examples of the concepts involved in group learning. The description of the criteria for effective groups and group members' roles and skills is the best that I have ever encountered. The authors do not assume that the reader has any knowledge of group work and so they delineate the basics—for example, that group members need to arrive on time if the group is going to function well.

1. **List two characteristics of community health.**

   Any two of the following are acceptable responses:
   (1) Focus on health or health promotion and disease prevention as opposed to the treatment of disease; (2) focus on a population rather than on an individual patient; (3) be concerned with creating an environment in which a resident can be healthy; (4) be concerned with the economical use of limited resources; and (5) collaborate among community residents, both lay and professional.

2. **The Community as Partner model could be considered to represent an ecological approach to health.** _____ **True** _____ **False**

   True.

3. **Fit the items listed below into the SOAPE framework by indicating whether the item is an example of (a) subjective data, (b) objective data, (c) assessment, (d) planning, or (e) evaluation.**

   _____ The volunteers took a total of 20 patients shopping at the grocery store. (e)

   _____ The community health group decided to provide assistance shopping for healthy foods by having a volunteer accompany patients to the grocery store. (d)

   _____ There are 10 hospitals in the city; one is a county hospital, one is a Veterans hospital, two are non-profit hospitals, and the remaining six are for-profit hospitals. (b)

   _____ The director of the food bank believes that that most health professionals do not know when to refer a patient to the food bank. (a)

   _____ The community health group concluded that the accident rate for children was very high. (c)

4. **The statement "If I understand correctly, you are saying that your organization could bring the tables and chairs and set them up for the meeting" is an example of which task role related to collaborative group work?**
   (a) Initiating

   (b) Giving and asking for reactions

   (c) Clarifying, synthesizing, and summarizing

   (d) Confronting and reality testing

   The correct response is (c).

5. **The development of a common understanding of the problem occurs during which phase?**

   (a) Phase I: Organizing

   (b) Phase II: Working together to collect data

   (c) Phase IV: Monitoring implementation

   (d) Phase V: Evaluating and dissolving of the group

   The correct response is (a).

Applying Your Knowledge

1. **Consider the Case of Mr. Smith (quoted from Smith RE, Olin BR, Madsen JW. Spitting into the wind: the irony of treating chronic disease. *J Am Ph A.* 2006; 46:397–400).**

   "...let's examine an actual 64-year-old white man who we will call John Smith. He is 5′7″ tall and weighs 225 pounds (body mass index [BMI], 35 kg/m^2). He does not exercise and eats enough to maintain his current weight. He has been diagnosed with hypertension, diabetes mellitus, hyperlipidemia, osteoarthritis, fluid retention related to possible congestive heart failure, sleep apnea, slight memory loss, and depression, all of which can be related to his sedentary lifestyle. If he could...bring himself close to ideal body weight,...many of his chronic problems would improve or be resolved."

   "Mr. Smith's pharmacist continues to provide him with his medications and perhaps even counsels him on the importance of taking them correctly. However, the importance of each medication is simply to keep him alive so he can continue to be obese and live a sedentary life."

   Assuming that Mr. Smith is typical of many patients seen in a community pharmacy, would you say that this might represent a community health problem? Why or why not? Assume that you work at the pharmacy where Mr. Smith obtains his prescriptions. What might you do to determine if Mr. Smith's problems are characteristic of the residents of the community? What might you do at the community level to help address the problem of patients such as Mr. Smith?

2. **Related to the Mr. Smith case described in question #1, identify the role that pharmacists might have related to:**

   Medications;

   Assuring conditions for effective medication use; and

   Assuring healthy living conditions.

3. A friend of yours is in the leadership group of a community health committee. Your friend has no experience in community health nor do other members of the committee. What two things would you suggest to your friend related to management of the entire committee?

4. Referring to the situation described in question #3, could you recommend readings or references that your friend might use that would help him or her learn about working in groups to improve community health?

PART three

Pharmacist-Run Public Health Programs

This section of the book is dedicated to providing detailed examples of pharmacists' involvement in public health activities. As such, the models are based on either a single program or created by combining information from several programs. Details about the planning, implementation, intervention, and outcomes are used in each chapter to provide examples of program evaluation as well as interventions. The chapters are ordered specifically to move the reader from familiar ground to activities that have not traditionally involved pharmacists. Chapter 13 begins with a tobacco cessation program followed by chapters on pharmacy-based influenza service, a community-based obesity prevention program, and a campus-based tuberculosis screening and monitoring service. The last two chapters on emergency response and domestic violence were designed to push the limits of the readers' vision of what pharmacists can do in public health.

These chapters provide detailed models by using a case study format. The models use the concepts and tools presented in earlier chapters; the reader should be able to identify examples of their use in the case study employed to present the models. After completing the chapters in this section, the reader should have a basic understanding of what is involved in identifying, operating, and evaluating public health services or interventions.

CHAPTER 13

Tobacco Control Programs

Learning Outcomes

1. Give one example each of subjective data and objective data that may be used to determine whether a tobacco cessation program is needed in the community and describe where that data might be found.
2. List three health risk factors associated with tobacco use.
3. Describe how a needs assessment can be used to start building support for a new program.
4. Explain the role of program evaluation and why objective and subjective data can be useful in the analysis.
5. Prepare an argument to support the involvement of pharmacists in tobacco control efforts.

Introduction

Tobacco use can increase the risk of illness and premature death. Because it is a preventable cause of morbidity and early mortality, tobacco use is a target area for public health interventions. These interventions focus on either preventing members of the population from beginning to use tobacco or helping those who currently use it to quit, or both. This chapter will first look at the scope of the tobacco use problem in the United States and the health risks associated with it. It will then look at the various cessation programs that have been studied before focusing on two fictitious model tobacco cessation programs proposed by a staff pharmacist. One of the programs is designed for employees at a local hospital, while the other targets patients who use tobacco. Hospitalization often interrupts the use of tobacco, so it can be a good time for an intervention aimed at reducing use or quitting.

This chapter will emphasize the importance of gaining support from stakeholders early in the needs assessment and planning process. Once a need for programs is established, the chapter will follow the planning and implementation of the two programs. Initial results of these programs will be examined through a formative evaluation process. At the end of the chapter, a discussion will focus on (1) ways new programs can garner support, (2) implications of voluntary or mandatory programs to change behavior, and (3) the need to change the environment as well as personal behaviors when trying to reduce health risks.

Public Health Issue: Tobacco Use

Tobacco use is a source of preventable disease and death, so it is no surprise that reducing tobacco use and exposure to second-hand tobacco smoke is one of the 10 leading health indicators for Health People 2010 (HP 2010). According to the midterm report for HP2010, progress is being made in a number of areas related to tobacco use because a concerted effort has been made across many levels of society.[1] Although tobacco use has been reduced, the objectives have not yet been fully met; additional, ongoing effort is needed.

Epidemiology of tobacco use and its associated health risks

The midterm report for HP 2010 indicates that the teen-to-young adult population appears to be increasing its interest in and use of tobacco, which makes this group ideal to target.[1] Statistics for the state of Arkansas, where the model program is located, indicate that the smoking rates have fallen from 43% in 1997 to 21% in 2007.[2] This trend is contrary to national trends and indicates that current interventions are having an effect. However, the adult population in Arkansas appears to need the most effort because it has maintained the same level (77%) of smokers for the past 10 years.[2]

According to the HP 2010 midcourse review, tobacco use in the United States directly causes over 400,000 deaths each year. Indirect (or second-hand) smoke exposure increases the death rate by 10% or almost 40,000 people. For every person who dies, the report estimates there are 20 people who suffer illnesses caused by or exacerbated by exposure to tobacco smoke.[1] Cancer, heart disease, and stroke are the leading causes of death in the United States and all occur more frequently in smokers. Lung cancer occurs in men who smoke more than 23 times its rate in non-smoking men.[3] Cigarette smokers are 2 to 4 times more likely to develop heart disease than nonsmokers, and smoking doubles the risk of stroke.[3] The risk of dying from chronic obstructive lung disease is 10 times higher in smokers, and 90% of all deaths from such disease are related to cigarette smoking.[3]

Master Settlement Agreement of 1998

The historic **1998 Master Settlement Agreement (MSA)**, better known as the tobacco settlement between states and tobacco companies, has resulted in an infusion of funds to state budgets. The purpose of the funds is to promote health, including bolstering tobacco control efforts. Each state is free to decide how to best use these funds.[4] A recent American Lung Association report card on tobacco-control efforts by state gave Arkansas an "A," which means it was spending at least 90% of the amount recommended by the CDC for control and prevention activities. Arkansas is one of only four states that achieved a grade of A.[5]

Model Program

Two Tobacco Cessation Programs: Hospital Patients and Employees

This model program will focus on cessation programs in two different populations, those who are patients in a local hospital and those who are employees. Other interventions that would form part of a comprehensive tobacco control effort in a community (e.g., prevention awareness campaigns, restrictions on where tobacco may be sold or used) will be presented only as they pertain to the model. While reading about the programs, note the steps in planning and implementation that are missed and consider how they probably contributed to the initial results or lack thereof produced by the interventions.

Background

Bob Gordon, R.Ph., recently lost his beloved mother. She smoked two packs of cigarettes a day for 40 years when she died from lung cancer. The experience of watching her suffer and eventually die from a preventable disease was the catalyst for his interest in helping other smokers to quit and reduce their health risks. Bob works in the local hospital pharmacy where he has limited contact with patients. However, he does have a lot of contact with other health care providers; almost a third of them are cigarette smokers. Bob is very involved in his state pharmacy association, and was recently appointed to his local county health board. Bob is interested in developing a tobacco cessation program for patients as well as getting involved in awareness and prevention activities in the community. Bob's wife is a supervisor at the local manufacturing firm where she is required to be present in the manufacturing areas at least 4 hours a day. At his wife's company, smoking in the staff lounge and within the building is currently allowed.

Objective Data

Community characteristics

The fictitious community of Midville, Arkansas, where Bob lives and works has a population of around 300,000. The major industries for the town are manufacturing, telecommunications, tourism, and higher education. The community is also a regional hub for agriculture and air travel. The community has a robust economy with an unemployment rate of less than 3%. The larger employers (i.e., more than 50 employees) offer fairly comprehensive forms of health insurance, but the smaller employers and service-sector employers are not able to afford complete coverage for their employees; 28% of the population is under- or uninsured. Of those, 16% are children under 18 years of age. The college students receive health care through the university health center located on the campus. The number of health insurance plans that pay for tobacco cessation programs is not known.

Population demographics

The population of Midville is estimated at 280,000 year-round with an influx of 20,000 college students during the school year. Table 13.1 shows the general characteristics of the town in terms of age groups, gender, and race. A number of the older, retired residents are former employees of the local manufacturing firm, Mysterious Substances, Inc.

Tobacco use statistics

Tobacco use statistics for the community of Midville do not exist, so Bob has opted to use county, state, and national data. He also talked to the campus student health service and local manufacturing firms to see if they collect data on tobacco use in college students and employees, respectively. Bob did not collect data from the local high schools or elementary schools. Based on his research, Bob estimated the smoking habit in Midville at 23% of males and 20% of females in the total population. By age, the smoking percentages are highest in the over 65 category (28%) and young adults between 18–30 years (33%). Many of the younger smokers are enrolled at the local college. The Mysterious Substances, Inc. employees have the highest rate of tobacco use in the community, with 41% of the personnel reporting they smoke at least ½ packs per day (ppd). Based on observation, Bob estimated tobacco use at 20% at his hospital. The smokers were primarily older nursing staff on evening and graveyard shifts and the support staff. The majority of the tobacco users smoke (85%), but a small subset of users prefers smokeless chewing tobacco. Bob also found a published study that indicated around 70% of smokers want to quit.

Table 13.1

Demographic Characteristics of Midville (2005)

Characteristic	Midville
Total Population	300,000
Under 12 years	45,000
13–21 years	80,000
22–50 years	110,000
51–75 years	50,000
Over 75 years	15,000
Male	140,000
Female	160,000
Caucasian	180,000
Hispanic	30,000
African American	62,000
Asian/Pacific Islander	1,600
American Indian/Alaska Native	1,600
Other	400

In addition to tobacco use data, Bob sought information about the incidence and prevalence of diseases associated with tobacco use because he had a feeling it would tie directly to hospital patients and reasons for their admission. Tobacco use is tied to higher rates of cancer, heart disease, and stroke, which are all diagnoses that tend to result in hospital admissions. In his hospital, Bob estimated that the 2,200 patients admitted each year smoked regularly and could be potential participants in a cessation program. Because smoke from tobacco products has been shown to put non-smokers at risk through second-hand smoke, the scope of the problem with tobacco use is often much bigger than statistics indicate. These people would be helped indirectly if their family member stopped smoking.

Current interventions and tobacco control measures in the community

At this time, smoking is not allowed in the hospital where Bob works. Smokers must go outside to have their cigarette; patients who smoke either stop "cold turkey" or are given nicotine replacement treatment (NRT) to reduce their cravings or withdrawal symptoms. On rare occasions, patients talk their nurses into letting them sneak a smoke by going into a corner of the courtyard. Aside from the no-smoking policy, no protocol is in place for treating nicotine withdrawal and promoting smoking cessation after discharge. Other public buildings in town also forbid smoking inside, so the courthouse, library, and city hall are now smoke free. A group of residents have begun a campaign to extend this ban on smoking to business establishments such as restaurants and bars.

At home, Bob has begun asking visitors to refrain from smoking inside to reduce his exposure to second-hand smoke. Most visitors respect his wishes and step outside when they need a cigarette. A couple of friends and two of his in-laws were offended and now refuse to visit him.

The local medical clinics and two retail pharmacies offer smoking cessation courses for adults. These programs vary widely in what is covered and the methods used to inspire a change in behavior. Bob decided to explore the evidence-based cessation methods described in the literature before approaching these groups to discuss their programs.

The state health department has been using funds from the tobacco lawsuit (MSA), which settled with each state to prepare and run an awareness campaign on smoking dangers via television and billboards. The funds are also made available to local health departments to support smoking cessation classes for medically underserved populations as well as prevention campaigns targeted at the general population. In Midville, professional students' organizations in pharmacy have become actively involved in smoking prevention education and awareness activities within the local high schools and college.

State law prohibits selling tobacco products to minors (anyone under 18 years old), but a recent sting operation by local police indicated that only 55% of the retailers were complying with the law. Most of the clerks who were ignoring the law were under 25 years old and many smoked or used chewing tobacco themselves.

Literature on tobacco cessation programs

First, Bob sought information about cessation program effectiveness. He found the most effective methods for reducing tobacco use appear to be those that offer a multi-prong approach to changing personal behaviors and opinions.[1] These comprehensive programs include interventions such as increasing the price of tobacco while reducing costs of smoking cessation services; increasing support systems for quitting such as free phone "quitlines" and clinician counseling; raising awareness of risks and options; and creating smoke-free workplaces and public areas. Both the CDC and USPHS have free, online-accessible community and clinical guidelines for comprehensive tobacco control programs.[6-8] Examples of pharmacy-based tobacco control programs can be found in the literature, so this is not a new area of activity.[9-11]

Bob also sought information about the impact of smoker behavior on productivity and health care costs for employers. He figured hospital administrators might be convinced to let him create an employee tobacco cessation program. Studies show smoking employees are less productive due to smoke breaks, have an increased number of sick days, and cost more for health benefits.[12,13]

Subjective Data

Community culture

The historical ties that the town has to the tobacco industry are apparent when one looks at names on grade schools, the college, and the hospital where Bob works. Although somewhat obscured by the passage of time, the link appears to be associated with the childhood home of a founder's spouse of one of the more successful cigarette manufacturers. This has created a tradition and acceptance of smoking in public places and homes that persists to this day. Many businesses that support other public health initiatives will not help with "anti-tobacco" programs.

Workplace interest

Bob informally polled his coworkers and local residents about tobacco use and illness they have observed. Because Bob works in a hospital, he figured his coworkers would observe the worst cases and have a high-end estimate of illness due to tobacco use. To balance his information, he intentionally sought input from people who work with healthy teens and adults. The results of this informal poll of Midville residents indicated that they knew of people who smoked who also had lung cancer, emphysema, heart disease, diabetes, and stroke. Many of these people also currently or previously worked at the local manufacturing firm, Mysterious Substances, Inc. (MSI). Some noted that most of the cancer cases seemed to come from the northeast side of town, which is downwind and downstream from the MSI factory.

Key stakeholders

Bob's final step was to poll the hospital pharmacy director and two members of the hospital executive board to determine whether they would be interested in tobacco cessation programs for patients and employees. Using his objective data on smoking trends and cost effectiveness of cessation programs, Bob received an enthusiastic response from his boss, the pharmacy director, who promised some release time at work to pursue planning and implementation. The hospital administrators said they would work with the Chief Financial Officer (CFO) to ensure that materials and medications could be provided free-of-charge to employees as well as with supervisors to enable employees to attend tobacco cessation education sessions. Bob was asked to submit a budget for each proposed program, including ideas for reimbursement. This led to his feasibility estimates for a couple of interventions.

Assessment

Data analysis

Findings from the Informal Polls

Within the hospital where Bob works, his colleagues indicated an interest in a tobacco cessation program for employees as long as it was free, voluntary, and effective. The Chief Executive Officer (CEO) and CFO would support the program as long as it "paid for itself" through savings in health insurance. For the patient program, both the clinicians and administrators agreed that cessation efforts should be initiated at discharge.

Findings from the Literature Search

From the literature, Bob determined that the most effective tobacco cessation programs address the problem at several levels of influence—from personal to work to whole community to national levels. For example, an effective program might focus on changing personal behaviors, restricting where a person can smoke, setting a minimum age for purchasing tobacco products, and regulating how the products are advertised to the various age groups. Tobacco users interested in quitting need support for themselves as well as support in the community that makes tobacco use more difficult.

Feasibility of Proposed Programs

For the patient tobacco cessation program, the costs would include training of cessation counselors ($800/trainer including travel costs); release time for personnel during their shifts to provide the counseling (no additional cost); materials for a packet for patients ($2/packet), including samples and non-medication products; and administration costs for tracking and followup phone calls. For the first year, Bob estimated they would need six trained counselors and enough packets for 1,000 patients. Based on these estimates, Bob calculated a cost of $6,800 for the first year with about $2,000 for each year thereafter. The sessions would occur in the patient room, so no costs would be incurred for meeting rooms.

To help with the costs of the program while patients were in the hospital, Bob found sources of reimbursement, including Medicare, which would cover physician interventions for smoking cessation as long as it was not the reason for the hospital admission. Some private insurers and **Medicaid** had limited coverage for post-discharge, outpatient tobacco cessation treatments. It was not clear if the insurers would pay for pharmacy-based services for outpatients, but studies showed smokers may be willing to cover costs that their insurers do not pay.

For the employee program, the hospital would have to pay extra for the additional 4 hours of sessions (mean $20/hr/employee) for each smoker as well as the cost of materials and medications not covered by the health insurance. Bob assumed 70% of the smokers who account for 20% (100/500) of the workforce would participate. Of those who participated, he estimated about 30% would require some medications ($50/person) and half of them would not have the costs covered by their insurance.

Both programs would be conducted by the counselors who were trained to provide the patient cessation services. The materials in the employee packet would cost about the same ($2/packet). Based on this information, Bob estimated salary and program costs at around $6,600 for employees with some of those expenses covered by insurance. Subsequent years would cost less because fewer employees would be smokers. The sessions would be conducted in conference rooms within the hospital during shift changes, so no costs were associated with meeting rooms. The CFO said both programs could easily be integrated into the budget. The savings due to reduced sick leave pay, lost productivity, and health insurance benefit costs would easily provide a positive return on the program costs.

Data interpretation

Assessment Summary

Bob determined that the existing interventions in the community tended to focus on adults who were already smoking, although the health department and local college *did* have some prevention activities for their clientele. The areas for improvement included expanding the no-smoking ordinances to include restaurants and bars, increasing prevention activities geared towards young smokers (teens and college students), reducing access to tobacco products at local retailers, and ensuring that tobacco cessation programs were based on evidence of effective methods. Bob determined roles for both patient and employee tobacco cessation programs; the administration at the hospital would support both programs because they anticipated a positive return on their investment. The proposed plans appear to be financially feasible and should be revenue neutral. The inpatient program may actually generate revenue if health insurers are willing to pay for the service. The administration and clinicians appear to support both programs, which should facilitate implementation.

Planning

Inpatient smoking cessation program

Results have been mixed with tobacco cessation programs that are started in the hospital.[14] The keys to success appear to be using staff trained in tobacco cessation, devoting time for in-depth counseling while in the hospital, and calling up to 6 months after discharge since abstinence behaviors are most likely to be dropped between 3–5 months after discharge and initial counseling. Furthermore, the overall rate of abstinence is better for a smoking patient who has more interaction with a smoking cessation trained counselor.

Based on this information, Bob is planning to create a program that begins while the patient is in the hospital and extends 6 months post-discharge. He planned to become a counselor, so he needed five other individuals (one pharmacist, two nurses, one hospital-employed physician, and one social worker) who would also be willing to be trained as cessation counselors. He was excited about being able to assemble a multi-disciplinary team. Bob delayed preparing packets and other materials until after the counselors were trained since they were likely to get ideas about materials to include during the training process.

Counselor Training

Bob found a training program for health care providers being offered in a nearby state within the next 4 months. The names of the volunteer trainers and the program information were submitted to the central administration for approval and registration.

Upon their return from the training program, the newly minted counselors were excited to meet and get the program organized. They began with chart stickers alerting them that a patient was a smoker and indicating the level of interest he or she had in quitting (ready or not ready). They identified materials for the packet and prepared a list of items to cover in the initial meeting with patients. They also planned a series of inservice presentations for their colleagues because they would need their help in identifying patients and scheduling initial encounters. The social worker volunteered to conduct the monthly followup phone calls with help from student interns. The pharmacy **APPE** students were also asked to help with the followup calls. Due to restrictions on reimbursement for the initial encounters, only the trained counselors were allowed to provide sessions. Standing orders for the smoking cessation program were created, and all physicians were encouraged to initiate them for their patients.

The trained counselors developed a protocol for the inpatient smoking cessation service. It focused on the adult patients (18–75 years old) who had a history of smoking and had smoked within the past week before being admitted. To ensure post-discharge continuation of the program, the service was offered only to those patients who live in Midville where community pharmacies and medical clinics agreed to participate.

Intervention

The intervention would begin with a smoking cessation trainer while the patient was still in the hospital. (See Figure 13.1 for intervention steps.) During the initial session, patients would be assessed for readiness to quit, nicotine withdrawal symptoms, and willingness to change their lifestyles. They would be matched with a community resource for monthly followup sessions; a permanent phone number would be determined for contact calls after discharge. Patients would be followed for 6 months after discharge. The plan for each patient would be individualized and could include medications in addition to the counseling sessions.

The post-discharge sessions were dependent on the site where the patients chose to receive the care. Sites included retail pharmacies, medical clinics, and the health department. Insurance coverage of the outpatient care service also varied by site, provider, and insurance. Bob designed a protocol for the community pharmacists and medical clinics to use. He also created a template for a collaborative practice agreement for the pharmacies. Furthermore, he worked with the local and state health departments and state pharmacy and medical associations to find options for using some of the state's tobacco money to reimburse patients whose insurance did not cover the service.

Employee smoking cessation program

As with the patient program, Bob postponed most planning until the counselors returned from training. The team of counselors designed the employee program as a combination of individual initial sessions followed by group meetings to build peer support. All sessions were scheduled in mornings or mid-afternoon to ensure employees on all three shifts would have access to counselors (i.e., morning sessions for graveyard and day shift workers and mid-afternoon for day and evening workers). The group support meetings would be monthly, and employees will be compensated for up to 6 months. Beyond that time, employees could still attend meetings, but they would not be compensated for their time.

Voluntary, Not Mandatory

The group was uncomfortable with a mandatory program for employees, although it had strong support within the administrative team. The voluntary program would allow smokers to refer themselves to the program (i.e., self-refer). The goal of the team was to

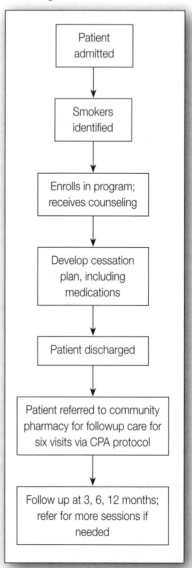

Figure 13.1—Flowchart of Inpatient Tobacco Cessation Program

Patient admitted

Smokers identified

Enrolls in program; receives counseling

Develop cessation plan, including medications

Patient discharged

Patient referred to community pharmacy for followup care for six visits via CPA protocol

Follow up at 3, 6, 12 months; refer for more sessions if needed meet with smokers who signed up for the program within 1 week of enrolling. In addition, the team decided to promote the program and cessation awareness through posters, human resources memos, and inservice presentations to staff in all areas of the hospital.

The team also decided to start holding monthly meetings on Wednesdays and Thursdays during the second week of each month as soon as they started getting employees enrolled. They reserved one centrally located meeting room through the end of the year.

Employees who enrolled in the program were asked to obtain a written referral order from their primary care physician to ensure that they were physically able to participate. Once referred, the employees' cessation treatment was guided by a protocol that was similar to the inpatient protocol. The administrative team started negotiating with its health care benefits manager to get the service covered.

Implementation

Both programs were implemented with a publicity push that included inservice presentations to hospital employees; letters to physicians with privileges at the hospital, local medical clinics, and pharmacies; and posters in the hospital hallways, lounges, and areas identified as smoker hangouts.

Inpatient smoking cessation program

The inpatient program began with the identification of patients who were smokers. Self-adhesive labels were applied to the charts as patients were admitted to the various units in the hospital. The presence of the label indicated the patient was a regular user of tobacco, but the interest in cessation services had to be indicated by checking the appropriate box. Figure 13.2 shows the label. The designation was the responsibility of the nurse, pharmacist, or physician completing the intake medical history. At the same time, Bob or another trained counselor made a round of the units in the morning to identify which patients were interested in the cessation program so they could schedule the initial consult.

Consults were shared unevenly among the counselors due to different demands on their time and availability. The physician had the hardest time participating due to other existing duties. The pharmacists and nurses were best able to provide the initial sessions because of more flexibility in their schedules.

Figure 13.2—Label for Patient Chart

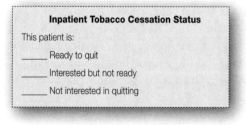

Follow-up phone calls began roughly 6 weeks after the first inpatient encounter. The social worker quickly suggested obtaining preferred calling times in addition to phone numbers to reduce the number of unanswered calls.

Employee smoking cessation program

The first group meeting was held on a Wednesday during the second week of the same month that the inpatient program began. This initial meeting was designed to enroll employees in the program; subsequent monthly meetings would focus on behavior change and support activities. Packets were handed out, and initial reactions were gathered. The trained counselors prepared a 6-month schedule to ensure all the sessions were covered.

Evaluation

Because these programs are new, the administrators asked Bob and the team of counselors to conduct formative assessments during the first year to fine tune the process and catch problems early. They agreed that a 6-month interim assessment of outcomes would provide information that could be used to modify the program process, if needed. The primary outcome would be number of days smokers were tobacco-free. A secondary outcome would look at cost-per-person smoke-free days.

Inpatient smoking cessation program

Objective Data

During the first 6 months of the program, 320 patients were identified as smokers and 155 of them were enrolled in the cessation program. Followup calls showed that 75 of the 155 were still abstinent at 2 months. Of the 60 who were contacted 6 months post-discharge, 12 were still abstinent. A majority of them (7/12) were patrons of a specific pharmacy on the east side of town. A review of 30 charts showed that one in three smokers did not have a sticker on his or her chart, and 27% of the stickers did not have a preference checked. The surgical and ICU units had the best record of applying stickers and checking preferences. The medical units were less likely to use the stickers. The cost for 6 months for 155 patients was $3,150. Reimbursement for providing the service was still zero, although the pharmacy had submitted paperwork for 96 patients with health insurance with tobacco cessation benefits.

The counseling team also discovered almost 6% of patients with stickers, indicating interest in smoking cessation, were never referred to or identified by the counselors as interested in the program. The communication breakdown was further explored, and it was discovered that these patients (and their charts) were often off the unit at radiology or other departments at the same time that the team made its rounds to find patients.

Subjective Data

Physicians and nurses were informally polled about the new program. One in three said they had not heard about the program. Of those that knew about the program, all said they used the stickers. Several physicians said they had seen their patients after discharge, and the program was well received. Even their patients who had not been able to sustain their abstinence status were positive about the program and interested in trying again. The counseling team members checked the ease of finding stickers on the units several times during the first 6 months. They found some units had stickers prominently displayed near the chart storage area, while others had them in drawers in the medication room or a private desk. Two of the units that had used the stickers heavily at the start of the program ran out and did not request more. Even the posters, reminding personnel to use the new system, were not always visible.

Analysis and Interpretation

The initial results from the formative assessment indicate adjustments to the program are needed. Additional education and reminders are needed to ensure that all units are identifying patients who smoke and that the sticker system is used. Prominent and consistent locations for stickers on each unit need to be found. A unit liaison person needed to be identified so there was someone responsible for reordering stickers and maintaining communication with the counselors to ensure all patients interested in the cessation program received the service. Additional inquiry into the post-discharge activities is needed, but the voluntary nature of the community participation would make it difficult to reinforce follow through. The initial costs were high per patient because of the cost of training and paying for the counselors.

Employee smoking cessation program

Objective Data

At the initial meeting, no one except the counselor showed up. This necessitated an immediate assessment of how the program was announced. Subsequent months had an average attendance of six with a range of two to nine employees per session. The enrollment in the cessation program was 12 at the 6-month mark. None of the employees had completed the series of cessation group meetings at the 6-month formative assessment mark. Of the 12 enrollees, however, five appeared to be on track to complete the program within the next 2 months. Of the 16 units and departments in the hospital, five had at least one employee enroll. The oncology unit and the housekeeping department had the greatest number of employee participants. The medical ICU reported that none of its employees smoked, so they would not be participating.

Subjective Data

Among the employees participating in the program, a consensus was reached that the sessions *did* help them change their behavior and maintain abstinence. They also said that they felt better overall, once they got through the initial withdrawal phase. They were concerned about what would happen in the long term due to cravings. Several said they were having a hard time maintaining their abstinence because they could see smoking or smell smoke on co-workers. Four employees said they had a family member interested in the program, and they wanted to invite them to attend the sessions.

For employees who admitted to smoking but did not participate in the program, the biggest barriers to participation were the timing of the sessions and lack of incentives. They did not want to give up their smoke breaks ("It's the only time I get to sit down for three minutes"), and some were offended that no one asked their opinion about the whole thing ("Just another example of administrators telling us what to do"). At least three out of five smoking employees who responded to Bob's inquiries said they would have to make the program mandatory before they would quit smoking. A subset said that if it happened, they would rather quit working at the hospital. Other counselors said they had heard grumbling and negative comments about the employee program. Ironically, many of the people who were not happy about the employee program were very diligent about helping the team identify patients interested in quitting.

Analysis and Interpretation

The current employee program is falling short of its goal, and appears that it may have inadvertently created a hostile environment. Bob and his team of counselors were advised to create several **focus groups** with smokers from all the units and departments to explore the barriers and identify an approach that would work for those interested in quitting. To ensure employees would be honest in their opinions, the administrative team paid an external evaluator to meet with the focus groups initially. After the initial meeting, Bob and the counseling team joined the focus groups to discuss methods for revising the program.

Discussion

Using a needs assessment to build support for a new program

This case illustrates the importance of identifying all key **stakeholders** during the initial planning process to ensure program success. Early involvement of stakeholders often achieves (1) increased support for the program when it is finally implemented, (2) early notification of the program, and (3) better acceptance of the program because all points of view were considered in its creation. In his excitement, Bob got permission and buy-in from his bosses and feedback from a few of his friends, but he neglected the target population—smoking employees. Although the initial misstep may require time to overcome resistance, the use of focus groups may provide some damage control. It is probably a lucky thing that the program was voluntary. Imagine the mess and hard feelings if a mandatory smoking cessation program had been implemented!

Using focus groups for the patient smoking cessation program prior to initiating the program may have been more difficult; however, Bob could consider convening a group of patients who represent smokers who completed the program, began it but dropped out, or never tried along with community health care providers to discuss barriers and successes to date.

Changing behaviors and the environment to reduce health risks

When working to change behaviors that put health at risk, a multi-faceted approach is most effective. Even the most dedicated individual will have a hard time sustaining efforts to not use tobacco if it is readily available and being used in many places in the community. Behavior change programs should be part of a larger effort that also changes the environment to make it easier avoiding unwanted risky behavior. For smoking, the number of communities banning smoking in public buildings and enforcement of laws restricting the sale of tobacco products to minors has been increasing. Controls on how tobacco products are advertised is another example of how an intervention at the state and national level can support behavior change. All of these interventions need to be sustained for a long period of time to ensure behaviors are maintained. It is very likely that the unwanted, unhealthy behavior will return again if programs end, ordinances or laws are removed, or tobacco advertising resumes targeting potential smokers.

Using voluntary versus mandatory behavior change programs

One of the key decisions made in the model program was whether to make the employee program mandatory or voluntary. Arguments exist both for and against these approaches. Proponents of mandatory programs support requiring all smokers to participate in cessation programs and to quit smoking or be fired. Of course, a mandatory approach can only affect employees while they are at work, so it may not impact smoking behavior at home or elsewhere. It is also difficult to determine if a person is a tobacco user unless he or she is observed smoking or chewing while at work. Examples of other mandatory programs designed to protect the health of workers include the use of safety goggles or gloves. Some companies may even enforce sick leave policies and send workers home who are contagious.

In contrast, a voluntary cessation program is based on the smoker's own desire to quit. It is assumed that this will carry over into all aspects of the person's life, making it a more effective deterrent of smoking-related health risks. A voluntary program does not require identification of smokers; instead, it allows those who use tobacco products to self-identify when they enroll in the cessation program. As a voluntary program, the tobacco cessation program may be seen as a benefit of employment rather than another mandated behavior. Since smoking is not the only health risk of employees, a voluntary cessation program also avoids issues of targeting certain behaviors while ignoring others (e.g., drinking, overeating, sedentary lifestyle).

Chapter 13 Summary

This chapter focused on two types of smoking cessation programs, which are part of a more comprehensive community tobacco control effort that also includes prevention activities (e.g., awareness and education programs, restricted access to tobacco, no-smoking bans in building). The smoking cessation programs were based in a hospital setting, and initial results fell short due to a failure to include key stakeholders early in the planning process and lack of assigned oversight responsibilities. Luckily, the strong administrative support allowed the hospital to revise the programs and continue working with employees and patients who smoke to increase their success in tobacco abstinence efforts. Although initial results in the 6-month formative evaluation were not great, they *did* provide information about programmatic strengths and weaknesses and guide further refinement of the programs.

References

1. Chapter 27: Tobacco Use. Healthy People 2010 Midcourse Review web page. Available at: http://www.healthypeople.gov/data/midcourse/pdf/fa27.pdf. Accessed December 27, 2007.
2. Centers for Disease Control and Prevention, Tobacco Activities Tracking and Evaluation (STATE) System: Detailed Report – Cigarette Use (Adults) – BRFSS. Smoking & Tobacco Use web page. Available at: http://apps.nccd.cdc.gov/statesystem/. Accessed October 28, 2008.
3. Centers for Disease Control and Prevention, Fact Sheet: Health Effects of Cigarette Smoking (updated January 2008). Smoking & Tobacco Use web page. Available at: http://www.cdc.gov/tobacco/data_statistics/fact_sheets/index.htm Accessed October 28, 2008.
4. National Association of Attorneys General. Tobacco Master Settlement Agreement Summary. Available at: http://ag.ca.gov/tobacco/resources/msasumm.php. Accessed February 11, 2008.
5. Traynor K. U.S. fails to make grade on tobacco control in health-system pharmacy news on American Society of Health-System Pharmacists web site. Available at: http://www.ashp.org/s_ashp/article_news.asp?CID=167&DID=2-24&id=9396. Accessed February 4, 2008.
6. Centers for Disease Control and Prevention. *Best Practices for Comprehensive Tobacco Control Programs—2007*. Atlanta, GA: U.S. Department of Health and Human Services, Centers for Disease Control and Prevention, National Center for Chronic Disease Prevention and Health Promotion, Office on Smoking and Health; October 2007.
7. Tobacco Use and Dependence Clinical Practice Guideline Panel. A clinical practice guideline for treating tobacco use and dependence. *JAMA*. 2000; 283:3244–54.
8. Centers for Disease Control and Prevention. The Guide to Community Preventive Services: Tobacco Use Prevention and Control. Smoking & Tobacco Use. Available at: http://www.cdc.gov/tobacco/tobacco_control_programs/stateandcommunity/comguide.htm. Accessed February 11, 2008.
9. Kennedy DT, Giles JT, Chang ZG, et al. Results of a smoking cessation clinic in community pharmacy practice. *JAPhA*. 2002; 42(1):51–6.
10. Maguire TA, McElnay JC, Drummond A. A randomized controlled trial of a smoking cessation intervention based in community pharmacies. *Addiction*. 2001; 96:325–31.

11. Stack NM, Zillich AJ. Implementation of inpatient and outpatient tobacco-cessation programs. *Am J Health-Syst Pharm.* 2007; 64:2074–9.

12. Anderson DR, Whitmer RW, Goetzel RZ, et al. The relationship between modifiable health risks and group level healthcare expenditures. Health Enhancement Research Organizations (HERO) Research Committee. *Am J Health Promot.* 2000; 15:45–52.

13. Tsai SP, Wen CP, Hu SC, et al. Workplace smoking related absenteeism and productivity costs in Taiwan. *Tobacco Control.* 2005; 14(suppl):i33–i37.

14. Hennrikus DJ, Lando HA, McCarty MC, et al. The TEAM project: the effectiveness of smoking cessation intervention with hospital patients. *Prev Med.* 2005; 40:249–58.

Suggested Readings

Anderson JE, Jorenby DE, Scott WJ, et al. Treating tobacco use and dependence: an evidence-based clinical practice guideline for tobacco cessation. *Chest.* 2002; 121:932–41.

Kennedy DT, Small RE. Development and implementation of a smoking cessation clinic in community pharmacy practice. *JAPhA.* 2002; 42(1):83–92.

Chapter 13 Review Questions

1. **Based on the model programs described, list one example each of subjective data and objective data that may be used to determine whether a tobacco cessation program is needed in the community and describe where that data could be found.**

   Objective data (source):

   (a) Number of smokers/tobacco users in the community (extrapolate from state or national statistics)

   (b) Number of tobacco cessation programs already in the community (directly from agencies or stores, via the local health department)

   (c) Demographics of tobacco users (local, state, or federal statistics at CDC)

   (d) Prevalence of tobacco-related morbidity or mortality (CDC stats)

   (e) Effectiveness of cessation programs and medications (review of scientific literature)

   (f) Cost effectiveness of cessation programs (review of economic literature)

   Subjective data (source):

   (a) Interest in a tobacco cessation program (smokers, sponsors)

   (b) Impact of smoking or tobacco use on quality of life (smokers, personal contacts of smokers)

   (c) Willingness to pay for service if not reimbursable (smokers, employers of smokers)

2. **List three health risk factors associated with tobacco use.**

Any three of the four risk factors listed would be correct: premature death, cancer, heart disease, and stroke.

3. **Describe how a needs assessment can be used to start building support for a new program.**

By asking key stakeholders for their input on a potential program early in the assessment and planning stages, they have helped to design a program they would like and are aware of the efforts underway to bring it into existence. They may be more inclined to provide support and champion the program early in the process, which may increase support across other individuals or groups.

4. **Explain the role of program evaluation and why objective and subjective data can be useful in the analysis.**

Program evaluation is used to determine whether a program is actually meeting its goals or making an impact. The use of objective measures can be helpful for quantifying results in a manner that allows easy statistical analysis and comparison to other programs with similar goals. If objective data describes what happened, subjective data can often explain why. Input from individuals involved in a program, including patients, personnel, supporters, and sponsors, can often reveal how a program is viewed, its acceptability, and reasons why some approaches work better than others. By combining information obtained from objective and subjective data, a more complete picture of the program is attained. Program evaluation should occur during and after a program is completed to allow for changes while the program is still in use and a summary of its overall effectiveness once it is done, respectively.

5. **Prepare an argument to support the involvement of pharmacists in tobacco control efforts.**

Although not emphasized in the model program, several medications commonly used during tobacco cessation require close supervision by a health care professional. Pharmacists, especially those who work in retail settings, are ideally placed to interact with patients who consider quitting, those who are looking at non-prescription quit aids, and those who are taking prescription medications to quit. Pharmacists who do not want to offer a tobacco cessation service at their pharmacy can always provide information about quitting and refer patients to other cessation programs in the community. At the very least, the pharmacist can remove tobacco products from the store shelves and no longer sell such items.

Applying Your Knowledge

1. Discuss how you would determine whether your pharmacy should initiate a tobacco cessation service in your community.

2. How are the MSA funds ("tobacco money") being used to promote health in your state?

3. Discuss how a smoke-free campus or community could be created.

A Community Pharmacy Influenza Vaccination Service

Learning Outcomes

1. Describe types of data to collect for determining whether an immunization service should be established in the community and where to find such data.
2. Discuss steps to take during the planning and implementation phases to ensure acceptance of a new immunization service.
3. Explain the role of program evaluation and why objective and subjective data can be useful in the analysis.
4. Compare the example used in this chapter with other immunization services, identifying pros and cons of each service model.
5. Prepare an argument to support the role of pharmacists in immunization efforts.

Introduction

One of the basic tenets of public health is finding ways to avoid preventable injury, disease, and premature death. Vaccination against infectious disease is an excellent example of how that public health philosophy is put into action at a primary prevention level. A vaccinated person will have antibodies that help him or her avoid developing disease after being exposed to a causative organism. In spite of the apparent advantages of vaccination, the actual rates remain low so pharmacists are helping to fill the gap by becoming vaccinators.

This chapter will first look at influenza as a specific example of the public health issue of vaccine-preventable diseases; then it will describe a model vaccination program located in a community retail pharmacy. The steps and processes used by pharmacists to identify the type of service needed in the community and plan the services will be explored. Initial results from the first year of the new service will follow a presentation of the implementation steps. At the end of the chapter, the discussion will explore variations on the type of service that can be provided in a retail pharmacy, the role of pharmacy students and interns, and physical space considerations.

Public Health Issue: Vaccine Preventable Disease

Mortality and morbidity of influenza and pneumonia

It is difficult to say exactly how many deaths each year are due to influenza because: (1) most deaths occur from complications or secondary pneumonias and (2) the practice of combining pneumonia and influenza (P+I) death counts into a single measure. The combined P+I rate was 59,644 in 2004, making it one of the top 10 leading causes of death in the United States.[1] While the debate about actual numbers continues, it is generally accepted that the most vulnerable members of the population are the elderly and very young. The P+I death rate is estimated from the excess number of deaths from all causes during the winter months.[2] However, death is not the only indicator of health impact. Hospitalizations due to influenza and its associated illnesses have been estimated at 200,000 each year, with more in years when A(H3N2) viruses predominate and less when A(H1N1) and type B viruses are most prevalent.[2,3] The death rate has remained constant or slightly increased over the past decade. The reasons for this are not clear.

Vaccination rates for influenza

The influenza vaccine is unique in that a new shot is needed each year. This is not a **booster** shot; a new shot is needed because variants (or mutations) of the viruses emerge each year, and the vaccine has to be re-formulated to cover the latest variants. The vaccine is a trivalent product that contains two A type and one B type influenza virus. Annual shots are given because the influenza season, which is the winter months (November to March) in the United States, occurs once a year. The vaccine is very effective and can provide some cross-over protection for influenza viruses that are similar to those whose antigens are in the vaccine.

Rates for **vaccination** against influenza vary by age group, with around 72% of older Americans ($\geq$65 years) receiving flu shots compared to only 23% of healthy adults under 50 years during the 2006–07 flu season.[4] For children under 2 years old, another high-risk group for influenza complications and death, the 2005 vaccination rates were about 33%.[5] Health care personnel (HCP) with a rate of 42% in 2007 are a subpopulation considered at high risk for influenza morbidity, mortality, or spread of the disease.[6]

HP2010 goal: increase vaccination rates

One of the 10 main goals of the **Healthy People 2010** initiative is to increase rates of **immunization** for vaccine-preventable disease, including influenza. Although the efforts of health departments and medical and nursing practitioners have increased vaccination rates, those rates are still below the goal level. For example, adult immunization rates for influenza and pneumococcal disease are now in the mid 50 to low 70% range, but the goal for each is 90%.[7] Reaching the goal has been hampered by difficulties in identifying which at-risk populations are not getting immunized and finding ways to reach them. Because health care workers can spread influenza or pneumococcal disease to their vulnerable patients, HP 2010 has a goal of getting 60% of all health care workers vaccinated for influenza by 2010.

Need for more immunization programs

One potential solution is to enlist the help of other health care workers in the vaccination process, especially those who have access to different populations than those already being served by medical clinics or hospitals. Because pharmacists are often the only health care providers in small, rural communities and they are often accessible during evening and weekend hours, they are in a position to interact with otherwise healthy adults or those who are not scheduled to see their physicians until after the flu season is over. Recent studies have found pharmacy-based vaccination programs to be effective and well received by patients and other health care providers.[8-10] As of March 2008, the scope of practice laws for pharmacists in 96% (48/50) of the states included administration of influenza vaccines to adults.[11] Methods for incorporating the activity into the workflow to further enable and encourage the activity have also been published.[12]

Model Program

Retail Pharmacy Immunization Service

Background

Tracy J. is the owner and pharmacist-in-charge of an independent pharmacy in Roseville, a fictitious town in central Montana. This is a rural community of 26,000 with another 4,200 residents living nearby on ranches, farms, and small towns. There is a critical access hospital, two medical clinics, and three pharmacies. Two of the pharmacies are independently owned, and one is part of a chain of stores. After noticing the attention that pharmacy-based immunizations were receiving at state and national pharmacy meetings, Tracy began exploring options for providing a vaccination service in her pharmacy.

The assessments needed for Tracy to determine the type and scope of immunization service included an analysis of the population's immunization needs, laws governing pharmacy practice with regard to administering vaccines, and feasibility of implementing a new service with current resources. The assessment process required data collection and analysis. The sources of data reflected the groups in the community that would have an interest in immunization: patients, physicians, employers, and the health department.

Tracy plans to collect both objective and subjective data. The objective data will include demographic information (e.g., age, gender) about the populations in the community, influenza and pneumonia activity, and vaccination rates. In contrast, subjective data will include opinions and ideas about vaccination and pharmacy immunization services from a variety of perspectives. Both are important pieces of information for assessing any service or program that will affect people.

Objective Data

Population characteristics

Like many rural communities, the average age of the population is increasing. This is due, in part, to the departure of younger adults seeking better working opportunities in larger metropolitan areas and the decrease in the number of children being born in the community. In Roseville and the surrounding service area, 44% of the residents are over 50 years old and 22% are over 65 years. Many are self employed (i.e., ranchers, farmers) and do not have health insurance. They tend to minimize visits to the medical clinic, waiting until they feel sick or are injured to seek care. In general, the adult population is very stoic and independent.

During the school year, many of the ranch and farm children stay in town with other families so their exposure to illness occurs in school as well as at their boarding home. Children are required by state law to be current on their immunizations prior to attending public schools (MCA 20-5-403). These requirements cover the usual childhood illnesses including measles, mumps, rubella, chickenpox, and pertussis. During the summer, an influx of seasonal farm workers increases the population of the area by another 650. Many of these workers do not have health insurance and receive care at a Migrant Health Center located over 100 miles away in a neighboring county. Most of the seasonal workers are Mexican Nationals (71%) and do not speak English as their primary language. Of the 650 migrants, approximately 100 are infants and 200 are between 2 and 16 years old.

There are no statistics for Roseville regarding the actual rate of immunizations. Using state-level statistics, Tracy estimated about 16% of pre-school aged children are missing one or more recommended vaccinations. Tracy also estimated adult vaccination rates for influenza (73%), pneumococcal disease (72%), and tetanus/diphtheria/pertussis (69%) using the same data source. The actual rates did vary by presence of chronic disease, risk factors, institutionalization, and insurance, so Tracy used middle values. Based on these percentages, Tracy estimated the number of children and adults in need of vaccines as shown in Table 14.1.

Table 14.1

Estimated Number of Unvaccinated Residents Based on State-Level Statistics for 2006

Vaccine/Population	A Percent Not Vaccinated (State-Level Data)	B Number (%) of Population in Age Group[a]	A x B Estimated Number Not Vaccinated
Childhood vaccines (0–5 years)	16%	2,777 (9%)	445
Adult, influenza	27%	20,361 (66%)	5,498
Adult, pneumococcal	28%	20,361 (66%)	5,701
Adult, Tdap[b]	31%	20,361 (66%)	6,312

[a]Total population (30,850) includes residents of Roseville and surrounding area plus seasonal workers.
[b]Tdap = tetanus, diphtheria, pertussis vaccine for adults.

Current service options

After Tracy had a better idea of the population and its immunization needs, she explored the current options available to residents of the Roseville area. Data were collected from the schools, clinics, and health department as well as the customers. For infants, the local clinic and health department provided virtually all of the immunizations during their well-baby checks. For young girls and teens, the medical clinics provided required school vaccines (e.g., *Varicella*, MMR) and offered HPV vaccines during the annual physical or well check exam visits. The source and type of vaccines varied more widely for adults. For booster shots of tetanus/diphtheria/pertussis (i.e., Tdap) and Varicella (chicken pox) vaccines, adults went to their medical clinic. They went to the health department for influenza and pneumococcal vaccines, the annual mid-October flu shot clinic day at the senior center, or their physician if they were already scheduled for an appointment. Several physicians felt confident about getting their patients with chronic illnesses vaccinated because they were coming to the clinic for care.

The group of adults that seemed to "fall through the cracks" every year was healthy and not seen at the clinic on a regular basis. According to the customers, some of those adults got their flu shots while visiting Billings, over 140 miles away, for business or holiday shopping, but most did not bother because they were healthy and believed flu shots were just for old or sick people. For travel vaccines, adults were always referred to the health department. The results indicated pharmacy-based vaccination services in the community were nonexistent.

Current status of pharmacist-administered vaccines laws in the state

Another area in need of assessment prior to planning and implementing an immunization service was the status of pharmacist-administered vaccines according to the current Pharmacy Practice Act. Practice acts are state-level legislation that define the scope of practice for a pharmacist and determine the extent of involvement a pharmacist may have in vaccination. Because practice acts vary by state, it is important to determine what is allowed state by state. In Montana, the practice act had been updated in 2001, allowing pharmacists to administer vaccines to anyone 18 years or older. Infants and children were not included in this state because of the concern about how an alternate source of vaccinations might reduce the number of little ones seen in doctors' offices for well-baby and well-child checks where vaccines are routinely administered. In addition, the **Board of Pharmacy** rules and regulations for immunization practice required training and **collaborative practice agreements** for a pharmacy-based vaccination service.

Resources needed and resources available

Tracy also looked at her physical, time, and financial resources to determine the scope and number of vaccination services that she would provide. All of her pharmacists were willing to attend training sessions to become certified providers of vaccines. The cost of the training would be $150 per pharmacist, and it included the required current copy of the "Pink Book" along with knowledge and injection skills training sessions. Tracy agreed to pay the $150 fee if the pharmacists would provide their own transportation to the session and maintain their **CPR** training. The interns and pharmacy students would get certified at their schools where certification is now part of the curriculum.

Tracy had appropriate storage space in the medication refrigerator for the injectable vaccine, and was willing to purchase the freezer for the intranasal product. She could put $600 towards purchase of vaccines. She liked the idea of pre-filled syringes, but the cost for a day-long flu shot clinic would be prohibitive. Therefore, she decided to use multi-dose vials for the clinic and pre-filled syringes for the drop-in shots. The pharmacy has area within the store to accommodate two tables with two vaccinators per table. Tracy already has the tables, but will need to purchase three chairs with arms ($150 each) for patients to sit in.

The forms and patient information sheets can be printed on the photocopier in the store. Based on 3¢ per copy, Tracy figures the pediatric vaccine information and adult vaccination program printing costs will be around $100 for 3,000+ pages. Record keeping will be done within the current prescription software system for no additional cost. The other resource requirement will be to pay for extra pharmacist time on the day of the flu shot clinic. That will cost Tracy about another $300. The total costs of the services will be approximately $600 for training, $600 for vaccines, $450 for chairs, $100 printing, and $300 for staffing for a total of $2,050. To help defray the cost of the program, Tracy would charge for the vaccines. At $15 per vaccination, she would have to administer 137 doses of injectable vaccine just to cover implementation and first year costs.

Subjective Data

Stakeholders and key informants

Tracy informally surveyed 30 customers during the month of March to determine if they or someone in their families had gotten sick that winter and, if they had gotten vaccinated, what they received and where they got it. Tracy also asked customers about their interest in and likelihood of using a pharmacy-based immunization service. The results of this data collection effort are shown in Table 14.2. This data seemed to confirm the extrapolated state-level data with one exception, which was no interest in getting a booster Tdap vaccine.

Table 14.2

Number (%) of Customers Experiencing Illness and Vaccination Histories (n = 30)

Topic	Yes Number	Yes Percent[a]
Someone had influenza last winter	7	23%
Someone had other infectious illness last winter	4	13%
Got flu vaccine last fall (n=17)	17	57%
• At clinic or doctor office	8/17	47%
• At health department	2/17	12%
• At other site (e.g., flu shot clinic)	7/17	41%
Is over 65 years (n = 18) and got pneumococcal vaccine (n=8/18)	8	26%
• At clinic or doctor office	6/8	75%
• At health department	1/8	13%
• At other site	1/8	13%
Got Tdap or Td booster (n=10)	3	10%
• At clinic or doctor office	3/3	100%
• At health department	0	0%
• At other site	0	0%
Would be interested in getting flu shot at the store	25	83%
Would be interested in pneumococcal shot at the store	26	87%
Would be interested in Tdap booster at the store	12	40%

[a]Denominator is 30 unless otherwise specified.

Tracy also sought information from the local schools and medical clinics to double check the numbers that were emerging. The school and medical clinics could only offer summary data because of requirements to keep student and patient information confidential, respectively. This was fine with Tracy, since the goal was to assess the whole population, not individuals. The school nurses and local health care providers were asked if they would support a pharmacy-based vaccination program. The school and medical clinic data are shown in Table 14.3.

Table 14.3

Estimated Annual Vaccination Rates Based on School Enrollment and Medical Clinic Data

Information	Number/ Total	Percent of Total Population
Number of children entering first grade who are missing one or more vaccinations	24/78	31%
Number of grade school children out sick last winter due to vaccine-preventable illness	135/380	36%
Number of adults getting flu shot at the clinic[a]	8,144	40%
Number of adults treated for the flu last winter[a]	9,163	45%
Number of older adults getting pneumococcal vaccine[b]	1,900	28%
Number of adults treated for pneumococcal disease[b]	814	12%
Number of adults receiving Tdap or Td booster[a]	405	2%

[a]Numbers (%) based on an adult population (18 years and older), which is 66% of 30,850 or 20,361.
[b]Numbers (%) based on older adult population (65 years and older), which is 6,787 (22% of 30,850).

Tracy's approach of collecting data on the same subject from two or more sources is referred to as **triangulating data**. The practice helps validate results from any given source as well as create a more complete picture of a population. Tracy was pleasantly surprised to find that the surveys had served as a link to local supporters and potential medical partners for a vaccination service. Three of the local physicians asked when the service would be available so they could refer their patients!

Assessment

Data analysis and interpretation

Tracy decided that some form of a vaccination service for adults would be a welcomed service in the community and would help increase immunization rates in the Roseville area. According to the state's practice act for pharmacists, immunization services are within the scope of practice for Tracy and her professional staff as long as they meet the training and collaborative practice agreement requirements. Tracy also appears to have sufficient resources to implement both the education program and the influenza vaccination service.

Planning

Once Tracy determined which populations had the greatest need for additional immunization services, the external constraints on the type of services a pharmacist can provide, and the feasibility of implementing them, she decided to do two things: (1) create an advocacy and information role in infant and child immunizations and (2) develop a hands-on vaccination program for adults.

Infant and child vaccine pamphlets

After Tracy decided to provide information about pediatric vaccines, she got her pharmacy intern, Nina, involved in the process. Nina was in charge of contacting local medical care providers and the health department to see if they had any specific suggestions for the advocacy and education service. The nurse at the health department recommended offering the information in both English and Spanish to ensure the migrant families could access it. One of the physicians noticed that some of his patients had strong misconceptions about vaccines and asked for a pamphlet that addressed some of these misplaced concerns. Nina also used the CDC web site to locate some ready-to-use information for patients. It took Nina longer to prepare an information sheet on the common misconceptions about vaccines (also found on the CDC web site), because she had to paraphrase and summarize four pages of information into a more succinct format to fit on one piece of paper.[13] As requested, Nina wrote the summary information so it would be readable at the eighth grade reading level and provided definitions of medical terms in case the reader did not understand them.

To complete the setup, Nina cleaned an old three-sided pamphlet holder with six pockets on each side and placed it near the waiting area in the pharmacy. Once she had finished photocopying the selected pamphlets and vaccine schedules, she stocked the pamphlet holder and awaited the first customer. Tracy put her in charge of answering questions, maintaining the supply of pamphlets, and identifying patients who should be referred for vaccinations. Nina was also asked to give an inservice presentation about the pediatric vaccine information pamphlets at the next staff meeting to ensure that the staff would be on the "same page" with their information.

Adult vaccination service

Tracy decided to offer a day-long immunization event on an October Saturday that didn't conflict with the Senior Center's vaccination event or the local high school football games. She also decided to provide on-demand influenza vaccinations using the recommended approach of weaving the vaccination into the prescription fill line-up so it minimized disruption of dispensing service.[5] She would try these two approaches the following year and evaluate them to see how well they worked. Planning and implementing the vaccination services required seven steps.

Step 1: Training Personnel

First, Tracy and her staff had to become certified to give immunizations through a nationally recognized training program. Two such programs are offered by the American Pharmacy Association (APhA) and the Centers for Disease Control and Prevention (CDC). One of the pharmacists on staff had noticed that the state pharmacy association was offering a day-long certification and continuing education program at both its spring and fall meetings, so Tracy had half of the staff sign up for the spring meeting and the rest enroll in the fall meeting. All the pharmacists and interns already had their basic life support training, so Tracy just asked them to maintain their CPR credentials.

Step 2: Preparing Forms and Protocols

In addition to the training needed to become certified, Tracy also prepared written guidelines for safe handling and disposal of used needles and other wastes in accordance with the current **OSHA** standards. She also verified that current liability coverage for the pharmacy would include the new service, and she recommended that employees check their personal liability contracts. Other pharmacists at other stores shared their protocols and collaborative practice agreements with Tracy so she did not have to re-create them from scratch.

Step 3: Obtaining Collaborative Practice Agreements

Another step in preparing to implement was the identification of medical partners in the community who would be willing to participate in a collaborative practice agreement (CPA). Luckily, Tracy found three physicians who agreed—as long as she was willing—to locate some sample documents they could use to draft the agreement. The Board of Pharmacy and the school of pharmacy both had sample CPAs that she could use to draft her own agreement. Because it was a legal document, Tracy asked her attorney to review it prior to signing it. Figure 14.1 shows elements commonly found in a CPA. Among those elements are the protocols used to identify which patients may receive which vaccine, requirements for monitoring, emergency care protocols (should they be needed), and ways information will be reported to the physician. Most states require CPAs to be renewed at a regular interval, which is usually once a year.

Figure 14.1—Elements of a Collaborative Practice Agreement (CPA)

The required elements of a CPA may vary slightly state by state, but tend to contain these items:

- Name of the pharmacist(s) who will administer the vaccines
- Names of interns or students if allowed by law
- Name of the physician(s) participating in the CPA
- The patient population covered by the agreement
- The vaccines covered by the agreement
- Protocol for screening, administering, and monitoring vaccine recipients
- Instructions about when to refer to a physician
- Protocol for recording vaccine information and reporting to physicians
- Protocol for proper storage and supplies
- Protocol for handling medical emergency related to vaccine administration
- List of required supplies and equipment that must be available
- Instructions about when to call "911" or physician
- Required training for participating pharmacists
- Information regarding when the CPA expires

Step 4: Establishing a Record-Keeping System

One of the interns, Nguyen, and one of the pharmacists, Frank, were both computer and software enthusiasts. They worked with Tracy and her forms to create a computerized record-keeping system that would track patients receiving vaccines, vaccine information such as lot numbers, and vaccination dates. Tracy then personally organized the patient records to determine which patients were due for vaccines. She decided to flag their electronic profiles with a notice so the pharmacists could personally remind patients when they were due for a vaccination.

Step 5: Ordering Supplies and Vaccines

Tracy had her purchasing clerk, Dorothea, place orders for the vaccines and related supplies (e.g., syringes, needles, alcohol swabs, gloves). The clerk's job was to maintain an appropriate level of vaccine stock and to ensure it is stored and handled properly. At the time, two companies manufactured the injectable influenza vaccine and one manufactured the intranasal form. Due to prior incidents in which one of the manufacturers had production problems, the clerk split the order between the three sources. Tracy asked Dorothea to order around 250 doses of the injectable influenza vaccine and 25 doses of the intranasal vaccine. The purchasing clerk discovered several options for obtaining vaccines, including the state health department as a source for populations covered by public insurance such as **Medicare** and **Vaccines for Children (VFC)** programs. For customers who were not eligible to use those supplies, the store would have to place an order with a designated vaccine distributor or directly from the manufacturer. Orders have to be placed about 6 months ahead of time so Tracy asked Dorothea to put that task on her calendar of seasonal "things to do."

Step 6: Setting Up the Vaccination Area

The next step in the preparation process involved setting up an appropriate site for the vaccination service within the retail store. Tracy settled on the counseling area, which is semi-private and has room for a table and two chairs. For the all-day flu shot event, she decided to clear a larger space so up to four customers at two tables could be accommodated simultaneously. She would also increase staffing that day and have one pharmacist and one intern dedicated to the flu shot service.

Step 7: Getting the Word Out

Tracy also realized that she would need to advertise the new service if it was going to be a success. She realized that she had forgotten to include advertising costs in her original cost estimates, but she didn't panic. Luckily, Tracy had already placed funds in her budget for advertising the pharmacy and its services. She decided to augment her "word of mouth" approach with two quarter page ads in the local newspaper; flyers that could be posted on walls and windows at the pharmacy and around town; and letters to clinics, employers, schools, and stores. Her intern, Nguyen, who was very handy with the computer, also had a strong artistic eye so he worked on the design of the flyers and newspaper ad. The next step would be to wait for the customers to come to the pharmacy for information or vaccinations.

Implementation

Infant and child vaccine pamphlets

Implementation of this service was relatively simple once the initial set up and preparation of the pamphlets was complete. Tracy decided to unveil the display on the same day as the flu shot event. Once started, interns and APPE students were placed in charge of maintaining the supply of pamphlets and routinely reviewing them to determine if they needed to be updated.

Adult vaccination service

1-Day Flu Shot Event

Tracy decided to kick off the new service with the 1-day flu shot clinic with the idea that all the pharmacists would be able to practice their new skills on many people. The event had to be scheduled the last Saturday in October because the football team, the Roseville Rebels, was in the state play-offs the weekend before, and the Senior Center had already scheduled its flu shot event for the following Saturday. For the inaugural event, Tracy scheduled a pharmacist and intern to run the event and provide coverage for others who wanted to participate for an hour or two. The pharmacy staff received additional help from two certified pharmacy students and their preceptor who were in an advanced pharmacy practice rotation at the local hospital.

The flu shot event was kicked off with an employee vaccination session. After opening the doors of the pharmacy to the public, Tracy and her staff demonstrated their belief in getting flu shots by leading the line. Tracy offered the shots free-of-charge to all employees of the store. She felt if was important to lead by example, especially after discovering that health care workers are one of the populations that tend to have low vaccination rates.

To facilitate the flow of patients through the clinic, the students and intern drew up 30 doses from multi-dose vials prior to opening the doors. Once the clinic opened, one student and one intern greeted customers and began the intake process using a form to collect information about the patients and vaccination as well as to remind them to cover key points and provide a photocopy of the Vaccine Information Statement (VIS) for influenza. When the paperwork was completed, customers were invited to sit at one of four stations where they received an intramuscular shot of influenza vaccine.

As part of the post-injection monitoring program that included keeping vaccine recipients in the pharmacy area for 10–15 minutes after the injection, customers were then sent to a clerk to pay for the vaccine. Tracy set the price at $18, which covered salary, injectable vaccine, and other supply costs with a $3 profit if up to 50 customers were vaccinated. If more people were vaccinated, the margin would increase because costs would be spread across more customers. For the more expensive intranasal form of the vaccine, Tracy set the customer price at $56, which also generated $3 of revenue. For customers with Medicare or private health insurance that covered the flu shot, the clerk charged a co-pay and billed the insurance source.

After the event ended, Tracy asked Nina to prepare letters to doctors to let them know which of their patients had been vaccinated. Throughout the event, Tracy had the pharmacists, interns, clerks, and students gather data so she could evaluate the service.

On-Demand Vaccination Service

After the kick off event, Tracy advertised the new on-demand vaccination service for influenza. This service was offered between November 1 and March 30 or until the influenza vaccine supply ran out. The seasonal nature of influenza outbreaks allowed Tracy to limit the service to the winter months. To ensure vaccine efficacy, Tracy had opted to use the single dose ready-to-use syringes for the on-demand service to reduce costs associated with wasted doses, which might occur with the multi-dose vials. Tracy monitored the number of doses administered each day to determine use patterns.

To minimize interruption to the workflow, Tracy had the pharmacists and interns treat requests for immunization as they would prescription fill requests. The person's request was queued with other prescriptions, and the vaccine was administered when that request was processed.[3] As with the 1-day flu shot event, patients were interviewed to determine risk factors or contraindications; given vaccine information sheets; injected and monitored; and charged for the vaccine. Letters to their physicians were also sent out once a week. The charge for the flu shots with the on-demand service was increased to $20 to cover the additional costs associated with single-use ready-to-use syringes.

Evaluation

Infant and child vaccine pamphlets

Objective Data

To estimate number of pamphlets taken, the interns set up the pamphlet holder with 30 copies of each type of brochure. As they restocked the holder, they tracked numbers of pamphlets needed to bring the quantity back up to 30. They reported that all categories of pamphlets had each been accessed by at least five people by the end of March. The top five topics appeared to be the **Advisory Committee on Immunization Practices (APIC)** *Child Immunization Schedule* (83), *Flu Shots Fax* (57), and the *True or False: Common Misconceptions* (38). A review of the current recommendations for childhood and adult vaccinations indicated that the pamphlets contained the most current information.

Adult vaccination service: 1-day flu shot event

Objective Data

Tracy was delighted to learn that all but two employees had either already had a flu shot or opted to receive one at the inaugural flu shot event at the pharmacy. Three of them said it was the first time they had gotten one. Excluding employees, by the end of the day, 112 flu shots and five intranasal flu vaccines had been administered. Three flu shot doses and one intranasal flu dose were wasted due to equipment malfunction or possible contamination during handling. No one had an adverse reaction that required medical attention, and no one fainted. Insurance covered the cost of the shots for 42 patients. Six people verbally complained about the price, even though three of them had insurance that paid for it. No single staff member worked the clinic for more than 4 hours total, and everyone on staff who was certified got to administer at least five shots apiece.

Subjective Data

The employees who received a shot for the first time said they would probably get a flu shot again next year. Customers were asked what they thought about the service, and most said it was convenient; they didn't know pharmacists could vaccinate; the shots didn't hurt; and the price was fair. They agreed universally that they would use the service again next year unless they happened to get their flu shot at the doctor's office. Several said they did not realize this was being offered today and suggested more advertising for next year. The pharmacists and interns said they felt nervous at the start, but quickly gained confidence as they administered more shots. Some suggested changes in the process to improve flow, such as preparing more pre-filled syringes and setting up more stations. The young female intern and students said a couple of older customers kept calling them "nurses," even though they wore their white coats and nametags.

Analysis and Interpretation

The first day-long event exceeded the expected turnout by about 60 people. No adverse events occurred and everyone on staff had an opportunity to practice their injection skills. The customers generally supported the idea of another clinic next year. There were some comments about the length of time it took to complete the process, so ideas for better flow need to be explored for next year.

Adult vaccination service: on-demand vaccination service

Objective Data

Data collected between November 1 and March 30 indicated that 132 flu shots and eight intranasal flu vaccines were sold. Two intranasal flu doses were wasted due to premature thawing when someone left the syringes on the counter overnight. Two customers complained of mild flu-like symptoms after receiving the intranasal vaccine, but no one experienced a severe adverse reaction. The average waiting time to receive a vaccination was 26 minutes compared to an average prescription fill time of 12 minutes. The intranasal product took longer due to thawing requirements. As part of the evaluation, Tracy had tracked when customers tend to request the flu shots. She found that the busiest times tended to be around 5 p.m. as customers were getting off work and heading home and on Mondays and Thursdays. Saturday mornings also seemed to be a busy time. The supply of injectable influenza vaccine was running low in late November when the news announced rumors of a vaccine shortage secondary to the discovery of contaminated lots of vaccine from one manufacturer. Since Tracy had "clean" vaccine from the other manufacturer, patients from the health department and medical clinics were referred to Tracy's pharmacy. Most of the purchased doses were either used by the pharmacy or sold to the health department and a medical clinical, but Dorothea had to return five unused intranasal and four (5 ml) multidose vials for credit.

Subjective Data

Patients thought the service was very convenient and appreciated having the pharmacist or intern bill their insurance for them, but they did not like the long wait to receive the shot. Waiting made them more nervous. Several suggested having appointments so there would be little or no wait time. Pharmacists and interns said they had a difficult time leaving the dispensing area to set up for a vaccination. They suggested limiting "drop-in" vaccinations to the 2-hour interval between 1 and 3 p.m. when the shifts overlap and more help is available in the pharmacy.

Two physicians had called Tracy to let her know that their patients seemed to like the service. The physicians discovered that they could refer patients for shots and free that time for appointments with other sick patients.

Analysis and Interpretation

Overall, the on-demand service was well received but it needed to be modified to either appointment only or limited hours for drop-in vaccinations or some combination of the two. Given the information about the days and times that people tend to request flu shots, Tracy can limit the on-demand hours to those dates and times and use an appointment method when two pharmacists are on duty.

Discussion

Other types of vaccination services

The scenario described several different approaches that a pharmacist can take to provide immunization services at the pharmacy. It focused on an "on-demand" model where patients can request an influenza or pneumococcal disease vaccine at any time. Variations of this model include the use of limited hours for drop-in shots (e.g., Mondays, Wednesdays, and Fridays from 3 to 5 p.m.). This approach may be needed if all of the pharmacists are not certified or able to give injections. It has some of the flexibility of the on-demand model, which allows drop-in shots but *does* limit hours of access. Another way to adjust staffing to meet needs is through a "by appointment" model. Like the drop-in models, the hours may be completely open or restricted to certain days or times.

An outreach service provides vaccinations at the site where potential recipients reside, such as an assisted living facility or office building. This approach is most effective for immunizations that need annual updates (e.g., influenza). The requirements are the same as the services provided in the store, but will require additional staffing since it is off site. At the site, a central area may be used for those interested in the vaccine to gather, but office-to-office or apartment-to-apartment services may also be used. The key is allowing enough time to watch for any reaction after the injection and to have emergency supplies and a phone on hand, if needed. Two advantages to this approach include (1) employees do not lose as much work time, and (2) the employers or their health insurance may be willing to pay for the shots. Over time, this event could become an annual affair with employers calling the pharmacy to set up the clinic.

Another way immunization services may vary is in the scope of vaccines offered. A restricted formulary of one or two commonly used vaccines will make the service focused and smaller. In this case, Tracy could consider adding pneumonia vaccine for adults. Some pharmacies have successfully implemented vaccine clinics for travelers and provide a wide variety of vaccinations based on the CDC recommendations for travel to certain areas of the globe.

Involving pharmacy students and interns

Involving pharmacy students and interns in any model is another consideration. The requirements for interns and pharmacy student immunization practice vary by state, so students planning to intern in another state may want to check that state's practice laws regarding intern vaccinations and training requirements.

Finding a good location for the service

Another issue is finding space for the vaccination area. At a minimum, the patient should have a sturdy, hard back chair to sit in and the pharmacist should have a clean, clear space to set up the vaccine, information sheets, intake form, and emergency supplies. The area should not be cluttered, and traffic should be minimized to increase privacy. The area should be sufficiently large to allow a fainting patient to be stretched out comfortably on the floor without hitting shelves or other furniture. Some patients need to remove their shirts, so privacy panels would be good. If the pharmacy already has a counseling area with chairs, this may be the place to do immunizations.

Chapter 14 Summary

As the model program shows, pharmacists can be key providers for vaccines in the community and become part of the national effort to increase immunization rates for vaccine-preventable diseases like influenza. The pharmacist who planned the new service looked at the needs in the community, pharmacy practice laws in the state, resources, and interest to determine the type of services to provide. The pharmacy interventions were provision of educational materials about all vaccines, the 1-day flu shot event, and an ongoing on-demand vaccination service. The pharmacist entered into collaborative practice agreements, completed required training, and prepared a vaccination area in the pharmacy as part of the implementation process. Early results from the evaluation indicate that the service was successful and positively viewed by patients and physicians alike. The model program depicted in the chapter is just one of many approaches that a pharmacist could use to become involved in immunization services.

References

1. National Center for Health Statistics, Fastats. Deaths—Leading Causes Available at: http://www.cdc.gov/nchs/fastats/lcod.htm. Accessed on February 7, 2008.
2. Simonsen L, Reichert TA, Viboud C, et al. Impact of influenza vaccination on seasonal mortality in the US elderly population. *Arch Intern Med.* 2005; 165:265–72.
3. Thompson WW, Shay DK, Weintraub E, et al. Influenza-associated hospitalizations in the United States. *JAMA.* 2004; 292:1333–40.
4. Centers for Disease Control and Prevention. State-specific influenza vaccination coverage among adults—United States, 2006–07 influenza season. *MMWR.* Sept 26, 2008; 57(38):1033–9. Available at: http://www.cdc.gov/mmwr/preview/mmwrhtml/mm5738a1.htm. Accessed November 3, 2008.
5. Centers for Disease Control and Prevention. Prevention and control of influenza: recommendations of the Advisory Committee on Immunization Practices (ACIP), 2007. *MMWR.* June 29, 2007; 56(early release):1–54. Available at: http://www.cdc.gov/mmwr/preview/mmwrhtml/rr56e629a1.htm. Accessed November 3, 2008.
6. National Center for Health Statistics, Centers for Disease Control and Prevention. TABLE: Self-reported influenza vaccination coverage trends 1989–2006 among adults by age group, risk group, race/ethnicity, health-care worker status, and pregnancy status, United States, National Health Interview Survey (NHIS). Available at: http://www.cdc.gov/VACCINES/stats-surv/imz-coverage.htm#nhis. Accessed November 3, 2008.
7. Healthy People 2010 Midcourse Review. Chapter 14: Immunization and Infectious Diseases. Available at: http://www.healthypeople.gov/data/midcourse/html/focusareas/FA14ProgressHP.htm. Accessed December 27, 2007.
8. Hogue MD, Grabenstein JD, Foster SL, et al. Pharmacist involvement with immunizations: a decade of professional advancement. *J Am Pharm Assoc.* 2006; 46(2):168–79.

9. Grabenstein JD, Guess HA, Hartzema AG. People vaccinated by pharmacists: descriptive epidemiology. *J Am Pharm Assoc.* 2001; 41(1):46–52.

10. Madhavan SS, Rosenbluth SA, Amonkar M, et al. Pharmacists and immunizations: a national survey. *J Am Pharm Assoc.* 2001; 41(1):32–45.

11. APhA Immunization Resource Center web page. States where pharmacists can immunize. Updated March 2008. Available at: http://www.pharmacist.com/AM/Template.cfm?Section=Public_ Health2&TEMPLATE=/CM/ContentDisplay.cfm&CONTENTID=15864. Accessed November 3, 2008.

12. Hogue MD. Incorporating adult immunization service into community. *Pharmacy Times.* 2007 (July). Available online at: http://www.pharmacytimes.com/article.cfm?menu=1&ID=4868. Accessed November 20, 2007.

13. National Immunization Program of the CDC. Basic and common questions: Some common misconceptions about vaccination and how to respond to them. Available at: http://www.cdc.gov/vaccines/ vac-gen/6mishome.htm. Accessed December 28, 2007.

Suggested Readings

Epidemiology and the Prevention of Vaccine-Preventable Disease (see current edition). Centers for Disease Control and Prevention/National Immunization Program publication. Available online at: http://www.cdc.gov/vaccines/pubs/ pinkbook/pink-chapters.htm. Accessed December 10, 2007.
This resource is free online and includes current adult and pediatric vaccination schedules in its appendix.

Pharmacy-Based Immunization Delivery: A Certificate Program for Pharmacists (American Pharmacy Association program). Available at: http://www.pharmacist. com/Content/NavigationMenu3/ContinuingEducation/CertificateTraining Program/PharmacyBasedImmunizationDelivery/Pharmacy_Based_Immun.htm. Accessed November 20, 2007.

Guidelines for Pharmacy-Based Immunization Advocacy. APhA Immunization Resource Center. Available at: http://www.pharmacist.com/AM/Template. cfm?Section=Public_Health2&CONTENTID=6253&TEMPLATE=/CM/ContentDisplay.cfm. Accessed December 20, 2007.

Health Resources and Services Administration (HRSA) National Vaccine Injury Compensation Program web page. Available at: http://www.hrsa.gov/vaccinecompensation/. Accessed December 28, 2007.

Occupational Safety and Health Administration (OSHA). Safety and Health Topics: Bloodborne Pathogens and Needlestick Prevention web page. Available at: http://www.osha.gov/SLTC/bloodbornepathogens/. Accessed December 28, 2007.

1. **Give one example each of objective data and subjective data collected during the process to determine whether a vaccination service was needed and indicate where that information was found.**

   Objective data (sources) include:

   - Vaccination rates for adults (National Center for Health Statistics; *MMWR*; state or local health departments)
   - Population demographics to identify high-risk groups in the community (demographics from U.S. Census by county; definition of high-risk groups by ACIP)
   - Number of flu shot clinics in the community (interview health department and local clinics)

   Subjective data (sources) include:

   - Interest in a flu shot clinic at the pharmacy (interview or survey patients and physicians)
   - Willingness to pay for flu shots (survey patients)
   - Interest in participating in the flu shot clinic (pharmacists at the store)

2. **Describe the steps taken during the planning and implementation phases to ensure other local health care providers would accept and support the new immunization service.**

   By contacting the physicians and local health department early in the needs assessment process, the pharmacist did two things: (1) made them aware of her interest in creating the new service and (2) allowed them to have input into how the service would be structured.

3. **Describe the results of the evaluation of the vaccine information pamphlet service. Give an example of subjective data that could have been collected to further assess the pamphlet program.**

   The results of the pamphlet service were measured in terms of number of pamphlets taken, but not in terms of how well received the pamphlets were or if they led patients to seek immunization. A good subjective measure would be satisfaction with the pamphlets, whether they were easy to read and understand, or whether the information was relevant.

4. **Comparing the example used in this chapter with immunization services you have seen, identify pros and cons of an on-demand service model with a 1-day event (i.e., flu shot clinic).**

   On Demand

   Pros—allows a patient to easily combine getting the flu shot with other pharmacy visit needs. Does not require additional staffing if it is treated like any other prescription and filled when its turn is up, and spreads the need to stock vaccine over time.

Cons—requires staff pharmacists to all be certified to vaccinate since no one can predict when a patient will ask for the shot; it may be difficult to do on a busy day; and patients may not allow enough time for one.

1-Day Event

Pros—can plan on increased workload and staff accordingly; can use an alternate site if more room is needed; and can order all vaccine for the season at one time.

Cons—may conflict with other community events that decrease attendance; patients may not be able to attend that 1 day or get to the alternate site; and event requires additional staffing.

5. **Prepare an argument to support the role of pharmacists in immunization efforts.** The main reason for getting pharmacists involved in vaccination is the need to increase the vaccination rates for vaccine-preventable diseases. In particular, pharmacists are highly accessible due to their evening and weekend hours and the ability to drop in when needed. With a majority of states now allowing pharmacist-administered vaccinations for adults, there are no longer any regulatory barriers.

Applying Your Knowledge

1. **How would you determine whether your pharmacy should initiate a vaccination service in your community?**

2. **What pharmacy practice laws in your state relate to the role of the pharmacist in administering vaccinations?**

3. **What liability issues may arise from a vaccination service? Include discussion of OSHA regulations and the National Vaccine Injury Compensation Program.**

CHAPTER 15

A Community Health Worker Program for Obesity Prevention in a Minority Population

Learning Outcomes

1. Identify three examples of objective data that would establish the need for a program to prevent obesity.
2. Identify at least three risk factors for obesity.
3. Identify one cultural issue and how it was addressed in the model program.
4. Identify the rationale for pharmacists' participation in a primary prevention program to prevent obesity.
5. Identify two characteristics of community health workers that enable them to work with disadvantaged minority populations.

Introduction

Public health prevention programs, which are designed to promote or improve health, require individuals to change their behavior. Behavior change is particularly relevant to the prevention of a disease such as obesity. However, behavior change for disadvantaged populations, particularly minority populations, requires special attention to the cultural context and the development of a program that is acceptable to the target population. This chapter begins by providing some background on the problem of obesity and then describes a model program. The fictitious model program involves a pharmacist and uses community health workers (CHWs) associated with a community health center to provide prevention services.

Community health centers receive federal funding to provide services to low-income and uninsured patients. The community health center in the model program serves a population that is primarily Hispanic with limited education and economic resources. The description of the model program follows the Committee for Obesity Prevention through the SOAPE process of collecting subjective and objective data, analyzing and interpreting the data to develop an assessment, and then planning and implementing the program. Prevention activities are described for a typical client. Evaluation of both the program and the client outcomes also is described. The chapter ends with a discussion of the public health issues, including assurance of appropriate medication use, the time perspective, comments on the individual approach to prevention, and the relationship of the program to health disparities.

Public Health Issue: Obesity

Epidemiology of obesity

Individuals with a **body mass index (BMI)** of 30 or higher are generally considered to be obese; that is, they are at least 30 pounds over a body weight thought to be optimal for health for a 5′4″ person (BMI = weight in kg/height in m squared). The prevalence of obesity in adults has increased dramatically in the United States between 1990 and 2006. In 1990, the prevalence of obesity was less than 15% in all states; in 2006, the prevalence was more than 15% in all states. In two states, the prevalence was greater than 30%. One of the national health objectives for 2010 is to reduce the prevalence of obesity among adults to less than 15%, but the prevalence appears to be increasing instead of decreasing.[1] Approximately one third of adults in the United States are obese.

Risk factors for obesity

Obesity is caused by an imbalance between energy intake and energy expended; in other words, obesity is caused by eating too much and not engaging in adequate physical activity to use all the calories obtained from the consumption of food. About 26% of the U.S. population reports no leisure time physical activity.[2,3] Lack of physical activity is thought to be the primary causal factor for obesity in the United States.[1] Risk factors for obesity include educational level, socioeconomic status, and ethnicity. Generally, persons with lower levels of education and lower socioeconomic status are more likely to be obese than persons with more education and higher socioeconomic status. Black Americans, Hispanic Americans, and American Indians also are more likely to be obese than White or Asian Americans, although much of the disparity is eliminated when education and socioeconomic status are controlled in the analysis.

Obesity and preventable morbidity and mortality

Obesity has become a major cause of preventable morbidity and mortality in the United States. Obese persons are more likely to have hypertension, dyslipidemia, type 2 diabetes, coronary heart disease, stroke, gallbladder disease, osteoarthritis, and sleep apnea and respiratory problems as well as some cancers. Medical costs increase for persons who are obese; the cost of obesity to the nation was estimated to be $26 to $48 billion in 1998.[4,5]

Model Program

Obesity Prevention in a Latino Community

Background

Emily is a 25-year-old pharmacist who has been working for about 2 years as the only full-time pharmacist in the community health center in Gila, a town of about 20,000 located on the border between the United States and Mexico. The primary concern for Emily and other health care providers in the community is the very high prevalence of diabetes; about 40% of the adults over the age of 45 have type 2 diabetes. Because of the high level of poverty and low educational level of residents, persons with type 2 diabetes tend to be diagnosed late; many probably have had pre-diabetes or diabetes for more than 10 years. Thus, many individuals have a poor prognosis because their diabetes progresses rapidly and kidney failure ensues. This town is one of the smallest towns in the United States to have its own dialysis center. The high prevalence of diabetes puts an enormous burden on the local health care system.

Prevention at the Community Health Center
The community health center where Emily works has a separate division that is devoted to providing preventive services to clients. At a meeting Emily attended related to diabetes care, which included the director from the prevention division, several health center providers began discussing their wish that diabetes could be prevented so they did not have to watch their clients progress to kidney failure. The director from the prevention division suggested that they could use their highly successful **community health worker** program to prevent diabetes. A long discussion followed. Given that obesity is a risk factor for type 2 diabetes, the group decided that their focus should be on preventing obesity.

Committee for Obesity Prevention
A committee was formed to investigate a community health worker program to prevent obesity. The director of the prevention division would serve as chair and be primarily responsible for obtaining approval and resources for the program. The director thought that grant support would be needed since prevention activities in general are not reimbursable medical services and programs using community health workers are seldom reimbursable.

Other members of the committee began obtaining the data they would need to justify the service and design the program. Emily decided that she would participate even though her primary exposure to prevention was dispensing medications to reduce cholesterol and control blood pressure. Emily wanted to participate, in part, because of the commitment of other clinic staff to improving the health of the community. She knew that other staff had served on committees and worked with the public health department on several projects designed to improve community health, and she thought that she could contribute too.

Subjective Data

Key informants
The committee decided to begin their data collection with key informant interviews with other clinic staff, including the medical director and chief financial officer, as well as persons in the community who were concerned about health and knew about the health problems in the community. The nursing staff and the community health workers in the clinic also would be interviewed. Outside the clinic, interested staff at the local hospital would be interviewed as well as the director of school health nursing and the director of the public health department.

Key informant interview guide
The committee's first step was to develop a key informant interview guide. Fortunately, one of the nurses in the group had worked on a committee that used a key informant interview guide so she modified it and brought it to the group for comment. The final interview guide is shown in Figure 15.1. The committee then divided the interviews based on their time and availability. One nurse who commuted to the clinic from a neighboring town agreed to interview several of the clinic staff as she was not available

after hours for interviews. Emily agreed to interview several of the community health workers currently working in the prevention division.

Figure 15.1—Example Key Informant Questionnaire for Collecting Subjective Data about the Provision of Obesity Prevention Services

---

Key Informant Interview Guide: Prevention of Obesity

1. How are you or your agency involved in the prevention of obesity?

2. From your perspective, what do you think works best in your program?

3. What are the barriers to preventing obesity in this community?

4. Which one of these barriers do you consider to be the most important one?

5. What do you think could be done to prevent obesity in this community?

6. Can you suggest any other people I might talk to about the prevention of obesity?

Thank you for your help. Right now I do not have any more questions, but I may contact you in the future if other issues come up.

Informant Demographics

(Collect demographic data on a separate sheet of paper; informant demographics should not be associated with data.)

7. Sex: ___Female ___Male

8. Ethnicity: ___White ___Black ___Hispanic ___American Indian ___Asian ___Other

9. Affiliation: _____

10. Number of years at agency/organization: ____ years

11. Number of years lived in community: ____ years

12. Commutes from outside the community: ____Yes ____No

Literature on community health worker programs

A second issue that required subjective data was whether a community health worker program would be an appropriate method for preventing obesity in a minority, educationally, and economically disadvantaged population. Emily knew little about community health workers and volunteered to obtain information on the use of those health workers for prevention programs, particularly programs involving lifestyle change. Emily had developed a great deal of skill in reviewing the literature as part of her pharmacy program and thought that she could use those skills to justify a community health worker program for the prevention of obesity.

Objective Data

Community characteristics

The primary economic activity in Gila is related to the port of entry between the two countries located on the southern border of the town. Although the town is small, over 10 million legal border crossings and over 100,000 illegal crossings occurred during the past year. Much of the produce (about 70%) consumed in the United States from October to April entered the country through this port of entry; hence, residents employed in the produce industry are seasonal employees.

Population characteristics

The population is predominantly Hispanic (89%); the county where the town is located has the highest minority population among all counties in the state. Many are recent immigrants from Mexico and Central America. Of the population 5 and older, 51% live in homes where English is spoken poorly. The median income for the county is 23% below that of the state.

The general educational level of the community is low; only about 25% of adults have completed high school, and only about 10% of adults have a college degree. The birth rate is high —129 per 1,000 women; the rate for the United States is 17 per 1,000 women. The population is young because 35% is under the age of 14.

Community health center data

The clinic did not have the resources to conduct an extensive study on the prevalence of obesity and risk factors for obesity in the community. Instead, the committee would obtain objective data from the clinic, specifically from the prevention division if it was available and from secondary sources, for example, from data compiled by the state health department on the county or the community. Generally, minimal obesity-specific data was available to the community.

Data describing the women served by the maternal and child program of the community health center are shown in Table 15.1. The limited education and ethnic characteristics are evident in the data. Because the relative number of persons in the household is high (more than 5), a lifestyle program aimed at mothers would be expected to affect the lifestyles of several more persons in addition to the target individual. About 16% of the women reported being diabetic during their pregnancy, putting them at high risk for developing type 2 diabetes.

State health department data

Relevant data from the state health department is shown in Table 15.2. This data supports the description of the community as economically disadvantaged with high unemployment. State data also supports the health care professionals' perception that a significant amount of health care resources locally are directed to the treatment of diabetes because the community hospitalization rate for diabetes is more than 3 times the rate for the general population.

Table 15.1

Characteristics of the 82 Women Served by the Maternal and Child Program of the Community Health Center

Characteristic	Data
Age range	15–43
Marital status	43% married; 5% divorces; 51% never married
Ethnicity	90% Latino (primarily of Mexican origin); 7% Anglo; 3% Korean
Religion	85% Catholic; 8% Protestant; 7% no preference
Education	65% <12 years; 24% GED or high school diploma; 10% at least some college
Average number of persons in household	5.4
Diabetes with pregnancy	16%

Table 15.2

Relevant Community Data from the State Health Department

Characteristic	Gila Community	General U.S. Population
Income (% of population below 200% of federal poverty level)	61.5%	31.1%
Percent unemployed	15.6%	7.6%
Designation as health professions shortage area?	Yes	—
Hospitalization rate for diabetes	645	205

Assessment

Data analysis

Findings from the Key Informant Interviews

The findings from the key informant interviews are shown in Table 15.3. Several issues seemed important to the success of an obesity prevention program, including cultural norms, lack of resources in this economically disadvantaged population, and the difficulty in getting individuals to change their lifestyle. The current community health workers indicated that a program based on large, classroom-style training related to diet and exercise may be limited in value because lifestyle changes that are ethnically compatible and affordable would be needed.

Findings from the Literature Review

Emily's review of the literature described community health workers as members of the target population who have unique knowledge about the needs of the population and can establish links between the health care system and community members. Because the community health worker (CHW) is a member of the target population, he or she speaks the language and understands nonverbal communication as well as the local health beliefs, behaviors associated with health, and barriers that local residents encounter in attempting to access health care services. For example, Emily found an example of CHW experience with a mother who would not take her children for an eye examination and treatment even though one child was blind in one eye and partially blind in the other eye. The CHW took the mother and children to an appointment with the eye doctor. The doctor explained the procedure, and then the CHW explained it to the mother. Once the mother understood the procedure, she agreed to have her children treated.

The findings for the literature review on community health workers are shown in Table 15.4. Emily's conclusions from her literature review were that community health worker programs were an effective method of reducing health disparities. Community health worker programs worked well with disadvantaged and underserved populations and specifically addressed cultural issues by using workers from the local population. Thus, a community health worker program seemed like a viable option for preventing obesity.

Table 15.3
Primary Findings from the Key Informant Interviews

Date data collected: From ___June 1___ to ___Aug 1___

Total number of people interviewed: ___12___ Number of interviewers: ___3___

Finding	Comment
Difficulty in eating healthier foods on limited income and lack of knowledge of cooking healthy meals	Identified by all key informants
Cultural belief that women should not engage in strenuous physical activity or large amounts of physical activity; also that it was not considered safe for women to exercise by themselves outside	Identified by community health workers
Cultural preference for education and services based on personal relationships; advice on health was often sought from older female family members or community members	Identified by community health workers
Frustration expressed by several health care providers about getting patients to do what they "should" do	Majority (80%) of health care providers identified this issue
Cost of providing services to individuals with diabetes increases every year, but funds for prevention programs were problematic	Medical director and CFO of clinic
Difficulty in getting persons to change their lifestyle (i.e., eat healthy and exercise)	Considered by all key informants to be the most important issue
Belief that the role of health care providers was to treat obesity; prevention was too dificult	Belief expressed by one third of providers who were interviewed

Table 15.4

Summary of Findings on Community Health Workers

Type of Program	Finding
General community health worker programs[6]	CHWs are bridges between underserved populations and needed health and social services.
	CHWs provide health education that is specific to the client and the client's situation.
	Disadvantaged populations often need help acquiring basic needs (e.g., water service; CHWs assist with meeting those needs).
Diabetes prevention program[7]	"Lifestyle coaches" were used to implement diabetes prevention program that was individualized rather than intended for groups.
	A core curriculum of dietary modification and exercise was provided to all participants, but coaches were encouraged to individualize the program based on the barriers faced by each person.
	The program had served an ethnically diverse population by using coaches from corresponding ethnic groups.
State of evaluation; community health workers[8]	These authors reviewed the literature on CHWs and concluded that health disparities could be reduced by using community health worker programs.

Data interpretation

Assessment Summary

The objective and subjective data indicated that the target population had limited education and economic resources and that most members of the population were Hispanic. The information on community health workers indicated that they should be an effective method of working with participants in the program from the target population. The community health workers would share their language and culture; by providing services through home visits, the program would address issues related to the preference for personal relationships as well as build on women's role in the community as health advisors. The Committee for Obesity Prevention agreed that a community health worker program should be successful in this practice setting.

Planning

Plan

After reviewing the data and discussing the issue, the committee agreed that the most effective way to address the prevention of obesity through the clinic would be to build obesity prevention into the maternal child prevention programs that they offered. The committee felt that they could best address issues related to both culture and a disadvantaged population with a community health worker model.

Funding sources

The director of the prevention division had identified two sources of funding for the program: (1) a grant from the state health department and (2) through collaboration with the state university, a health sciences program. Two faculty members in health sciences had obtained a grant to develop an interprofessional training program. This training program could provide some support for the community health workers if students could team with the workers to learn about providing individualized prevention services to a disadvantaged minority population. Students working side by side with the community health workers would be advantageous because the student could assume responsibility for providing the education component of the intervention.

Program structure

The program would be structured around home visits by the community health worker–student team while students were in the community or by the community health worker when students were not present. Because students typically were in the community for 6–10 weeks and then were not present until the next group came, the program was structured so that new clients would be added while students were present. The student would be responsible for conducting a comprehensive assessment that included items related to income and residence; psychosocial problems such as communication with community resources; physiological problems (e.g., pain); and health-related behaviors, including nutrition and physical activity. The comprehensive assessment would address issues related to the inability to purchase healthy food as well as education about nutrition. Because the community health workers have expertise in community services, they could facilitate access to resources needed for health.[9]

Based on the outcomes of the assessment, appropriate interventions would be identified. The patient assessment model used a rating scale for knowledge, behavior, and status: 1 represented none or low (no knowledge, behavior not appropriate, or poor status), and 5 represented superior knowledge, appropriate behavior, or good health status.[9]

Implementation

Eligibility

Eligibility Criteria

Clients from the maternal and child program were eligible to participate. Initially providers wanted to include only clients who were overweight or obese, but a discussion of prevention persuaded them to include anyone in the maternal child program. All clients were low income and most were Hispanic with limited education, which increased their risk for developing obesity. Further, by definition, primary prevention is directed at individuals who are currently healthy.

Laura: A Typical Client

Laura is a 26-year-old married woman who has participated in other programs offered by the maternal and child health division of the community health center. Lorena, the community health worker who has interacted with her previously, states that Laura is of Mexican origin and Spanish speaking only. Laura moved to the United States 2 years ago and has lived in this community for a year. Laura completed the 10th grade in Mexico.

Laura's health history includes two pregnancies and two live births; she has a 6-year-old daughter and a 1-year-old son who was breastfed until about 9 months of age. The daughter weighed 8 lb. 10 oz. at birth; the son, 9 lb. 4 oz. During the pregnancy with her son, Laura was diagnosed with gestational diabetes, but she does not currently have diabetes. Laura is 5'4" tall and weighs 160 lbs. (BMI = 27.5).

Laura and her family have health insurance through the community health center, which covers primary care but no hospitalizations.

Client assessment

Nutrition

The nutrition assessment was purposely kept simple; previous experience had indicated that it was very difficult to get participants to keep a food diary. The Committee decided that rather than trying to get program clients to do something that seemed very difficult for them, a 24-hour recall would be done at each visit with the client. This data would be limited, but it also should be more reliable since the CHW could assist the client in recalling food intake.

Physical Activity

A form was used to assess stage of change relative to increasing physical activity. Then interventions were tailored to the stage of change. An example form is shown in Figure 15.2. The stage of change approach[10] recognizes that individuals must change their thinking and their goals related to physical activity, and these changes are recognized as success by both the individual and the provider.

Pedometers, which count the number of steps that an individual has taken, were used to facilitate increases in physical activity. A pedometer can demonstrate a low level of activity to an individual and also allow him or her to monitor activity levels and increase activity. For a healthy lifestyle, 10,000 steps (about 2 miles) is recommended daily.[10]

Laura: Lifestyle Data

Laura does not eat breakfast. A typical lunch is meatball soup with tortillas and coke. For dinner, Laura has about a cup of rice, a half cup of refried beans, grilled beef steak, flour tortillas, and salsa. For dessert, Laura has rice pudding. Laura snacks on chips and coke.

Laura *does* engage in some physical activity, primarily through walking her daughter to school. When Laura used the pedometer, she found that she walked about 4,000 steps a day, substantially below the 10,000 steps recommended. Laura was in stage 4 of the **stages of change** because she regularly engaged in physical activity, but she did not obtain an adequate amount of activity.

Because Laura is new to the community, she does not have a friend to share exercise workouts. Her husband also drives their car to work during the day, and no gym facility is located near her.

Interventions

Nutrition Education

Typical nutritional interventions included education, for example, the use of a place-mat with a plate drawn on it that describes appropriate portion sizes. A 2–3 oz. serving of lean meat is described as similar in size to a pack of cards and should constitute one fourth or less of the meal.[11] Another popular nutritional education activity was to demonstrate the amount of sugar in a soft drink by showing the client the number of individual packets of sugar contained in a single drink.

Figure 15.2—Example Tool for Identifying Stage of Change Related to Physical Activity

---

Assessing Your Stage of Change—Physical Activity

Most people who want to exercise regularly must go through several stages of change before they actually begin. It is easiest to change exercise habits if you can identify which stage of change you are in now and plan your activities accordingly.

Look at the stages below and decide which one best describes your situation.

Stage 1. Precontemplation (I haven't thought about it much stage.)

Persons in this stage typically believe one or more of the following:
- Exercise is really not that important. They can think of persons who don't exercise and are slim or persons who do exercise and are overweight.
- The benefits of not exercising outweigh the benefits of exercising.
- Past experiences with an exercise program may have been negative.
- They get enough exercise from their work or lifestyle.

Stage 2. Contemplation (I know I should exercise but….)

Persons may believe one or more of the following:
- Something should be done but hasn't been done yet; no specific plans have been made.
- The benefits of not exercising are at least as great as the benefits of exercising.
- No exercise or fitness goals have been established.

Stage 3. Preparation (You have plans to exercise within the next 4 weeks.)

Persons in this stage typically:
- Have an exercise goal that is focused on being able to exercise regularly as opposed to achieving a fitness goal.
- Have a specific plan. For example, they say that "I will try walking for 20 minutes on Saturday and Sunday before other family members get up."
- Believe that the benefits of exercising are greater than the benefits of not exercising.

Stage 4. Action (You are actually exercising several times a week.)

Persons in this stage typically:
- Are taking overt actions to change lifestyle, for example, walking around the block.
- Take small steps toward changing their lifestyle, for example, walking once this week and twice next week.
- May try several types of exercise before they identify one that suits them.

Stage 5. Maintenance (I exercise regularly at least 3 times a week.)

Persons in this stage typically:
- Have goals related to fitness, for example, "I want to be able to ride my bicycle 30 miles a week."
- Are concerned about the quantity and intensity of exercise that they engage in.
- Are concerned about lapsing or relapsing.
- Believe the benefits of regular exercise outweigh the benefits of not exercising.

Stage 6. Permanent Maintenance (Exercise is a part of my life.)

Persons in this stage typically:
- Change their fitness goals periodically.
- Change their exercise routine by alternating types of exercise.
- Experience periodic lapses; for example, they may not exercise at all for 2 to 4 weeks; however, they recognize that periodic lapses may be beneficial and that perfection is not necessary.
- Believe the benefits of regular exercise outweigh the benefits of not exercising.

Physical Activity

The pedometer used to assess level of physical activity also can be used to encourage clients to increase their activity; 10,000 steps or about 2 miles a day are recommended for a healthy lifestyle.

Planning

Seminars were held weekly for students to present their clients and the work that they had accomplished with the community health worker. Faculty from health sciences colleges as well as staff from the community health center attended the seminars. Faculty and staff made suggestions and helped student–CHW teams plan interventions for their clients.

Laura: Planning an Intervention

During the weekly seminar, several suggestions were made to the pharmacy student, Dustin, and community health worker, Lorena, who were the student–CHW team working with Laura. The dietitian with the community health center suggested that a demonstration showing how many packets of sugar are in a single can of coke might help Laura adopt a more nutritional drink. She also suggested that the food pyramid be reviewed with the client because she did not appear to be eating fruits and vegetables. The public health nurse suggested that the team look into whether the client was eligible to obtain food from the local food bank. Because the food bank received leftover produce from the produce industry, the client might be able to increase the fruits and vegetables in the family's diet.

Because Laura seemed to be in stage 4 of the stages of change model, Emily suggested that Laura should be complimented for her level of physical activity and encouraged to continue with it and to increase the number of steps she took over the next week.

Another community health worker commented on how important it was for this mother to model a healthy lifestyle for her children. One of the nursing students commented that Laura was at high risk for developing type 2 diabetes because of gestational diabetes that developed during her last pregnancy. Changes in lifestyle could delay or prevent the onset of type 2 diabetes.

Evaluation

Subjective data

The success of the program was reflected in the willingness of the clients to continue in the program when a second group of students arrived in the community the following semester.

Objective data

A total of 19 clients from the maternal-child program participated in the obesity prevention program; all were women with children, so changes in the mothers' knowledge and ability to live a healthier lifestyle could be expected to affect her children's lifestyle too.

To evaluate the program, the students calculated mean ratings for items in the client assessment and then these ratings after the students stopped working with the clients.[12] Most items for knowledge and behavior changed, on average, by 1—from 2 to 3 or from 3 to 4, indicating that knowledge and behavior were changed by the program. Health status changed less; on average, only 0.5 point, that is, from 2 to 2.5. The lack of change in the health status items probably represents the time required for changes in behavior to affect health status; for example, improvements in diet may not result in much weight loss in the 6–10 weeks that the students worked with the client.

Interpretation of program data

After reviewing program data at the end of 6 months, the committee concluded that the program seemed successful. Many clients had been served during the first 6 months; the clients seemed to like working with the CHW–student teams; and they were anxious to continue. Additionally, individual client data indicated that all clients had made at least some progress during the first 6 months.

Laura: evaluation of progress

Dustin and Lorena made a total of six visits to Laura while Dustin was in the community on his rotation. They assessed Laura's knowledge of nutrition and physical activity during the first visit and again at the last visit; they agreed that Laura had learned a lot about nutrition. On the first visit, she rated 2 and on the last, 4. On behavior related to nutrition, Laura was rated 1 on the first visit but 4 on the last because she had begun having a piece of fruit, corn tortilla with eggs for breakfast, and no coke because she drank water instead. For snacks, Laura ate jicama (a turnip-like vegetable) with chile pepper and lime juice. Laura also found a good source of nopales (green cactus that could be sliced in strips and eaten like green beans), which she served with dinner twice a week. However, Laura had not lost any weight. She had increased her number of steps from 4,000 to 6,000 and tried to make sure that she took her children to the park to play every day.

Dustin and Lorena felt like they had accomplished a lot in working with Laura, especially since the changes that Laura made in her lifestyle also would affect the lifestyle of her family. Lorena said that she would continue to visit Laura at least once a month until the next group of students arrived.

One of the other students commented that Dustin and Lorena had an "easy" client. Her client was not doing any type of exercise, and the client was in the pre-contemplation stage on the first visit and only in the preparation stage on the last visit. Emily said that she thought the client had made substantial progress; after all, the client had changed by two stages. The public health nurse agreed, and observed that the client might begin action with the next student. Lifestyle change is difficult, often slow, and progress should be celebrated.

Discussion

Assuring appropriate medication use

The community health worker program for the prevention of obesity described here includes student training as well as provision of services. The community health worker program was seen as a unique opportunity for health sciences students to learn to provide individual primary prevention services through a program that addressed the cultural issues of health care. The experience was offered to all health sciences students, including pharmacy students, even though the focus was on lifestyle change versus medication therapy. Medications are available to treat many of the outcomes of a poor lifestyle, for example, type 2 diabetes, hypertension, heart disease, and dyslipidemia, but medications are expensive and often associated with side effects. Hence, to use medications appropriately, pharmacists should be able to recommend lifestyle changes as alternatives to medications and to understand the issues related to lifestyle changes because of the difficulty people have making such changes.

Long-term perspective

The model program presented here illustrates that lifestyle changes generally require a long-term perspective. At the end of the student's experience in the program, the client had not lost any weight and another student's client had not begun exercising. Thus, programs aimed at changing lifestyle should have a long-term approach to the problem and not expect a single encounter or a few classes to result in dramatic changes. Use of a framework such as the stages of change also facilitates work in this area because it enables the provider to see progress even when the client has not made dramatic diet changes or adopted a high level of exercise.

Individual approach to prevention

This program represents the individual approach to prevention because changes in lifestyle were accomplished by working with individual clients. The effectiveness of the program could be increased if community-level activities related to lifestyle occur at the same time. For example, improvements in the sidewalks make it easier to walk and the availability of exercise programs based in schools make it easier for children to be less sedentary. The client in this example had access to the school and walked her daughter to school; she probably could have participated in an exercise class offered through the school but not one at a health club located in the suburbs.

Addressing health disparities

This model program describing a community health worker program for facilitating lifestyle change provides an example of how health care professionals can address prevention involving lifestyle for a disadvantaged minority population. If pharmacists and other health care professionals are going to effectively prevent severe disease, such as kidney failure, then they need to participate in programs like this community health worker program. Participation in these programs or similar programs also allows the pharmacist to become competent in providing culturally appropriate care.

Community health worker programs have been widely used, particularly in third world countries. Because these programs use local residents, the programs are adaptable to many different circumstances and seem to be an effective method of reducing health disparities. Pharmacists who work with disadvantaged minority populations may want to consider a community health worker program.

Chapter 15 Summary

This model program describing a community health worker program for supporting lifestyle change is an example of how practitioners can address prevention for a disadvantaged minority population. A pharmacist served on the community health center committee to develop the program and assisted with collecting the data and then planning and implementing the program. The program was structured around home visits by community health workers who provided education and assistance to clients to enable them to make lifestyle changes. The program involved health sciences students who provided most of the client education by partnering with the community health worker. Initial evaluation data indicated that the program was successful in enabling women from this disadvantaged minority population to change their lifestyles.

References

1. Centers for Disease Control and Prevention. Defining Overweight and Obesity. Available at: http://www.cdc.gov/nccdphp/dnpa/obesity/defining.htm. Accessed October 24, 2008.

2. Centers for Disease Control and Prevention. Overweight and Obesity: Introduction | DNPAO | CDC. Available at: http://www.cdc.gov/nccdphp/dnpa/obesity/index.htm. Accessed October 24, 2008.

3. Centers for Disease Control and Prevention. Overweight and Obesity: Economic Consequences. Available at: http://www.cdc.gov/nccdphp/dnpa/obesity/economic_consequences.htm. Accessed October 24, 2008.

4. National Center for Health Statistics. Prevalence of Overweight and Obesity among Adults: United States, 2003-2004. Available at: http://www.cdc.gov/nchs/products/pubs/hestats/. Accessed July 13, 2007.

5. Trust for America's Health. F as in Fat: How Obesity Policies Are Failing in America. Available at: http://www.healthyamericans.org. Accessed August 28, 2007.

6. National Rural Health Association. Community Health Advisor Programs. Available at: http://www.nrharural.org/pagefile/issuepapers/ipaper17.html. Accessed August 7, 2003.

7. DPP Research Group. The diabetes prevention program (DPP). *Diabetes Care*. 2002; 25(12):2165–71.

8. Nemcek MA, Sabatier R. State of evaluation: community health workers. *Public Health Nursing*. 2003; 20(4):260–70.

9. Martin KS, Scheet NJ. The Omaha System. Philadelphia, PA; 1992. Electronic version available at: http://www.omahasystem.org/. Accessed October 24, 2008.

10. Slack MK. Interpreting current physical activity guidelines and incorporating them into practice for health promotion and disease prevention. *Am J Health-Syst Pharm*. 2006; 63:1647–53.

11. The Portion Plate. Available at: http://www.theportionplate.com. Accessed March 3, 2008.

12. Slack MK, McEwen MM. The impact of interdisciplinary case management on client outcomes. *Fam Community Health*. 1999; 22(3):30–48.

Suggested Readings

Wing RR, Hill JO. Successful weight loss maintenance. *Annu Rev Nutr*. 2001; 21:323–41.
This is the seminal article on weight loss maintenance. Although many followup studies have been done, this original article provides a good understanding of the issues involved with weight maintenance and how individuals have managed those issues.

Jonas S. *Talking about Health and Wellness with Patients*. New York, NY: Springer; 2000.
This book is written for the health practitioner who is working with patients on lifestyle change.

Centers for Disease Control and Prevention. Obesity and Overweight. Available at: http://www.cdc.gov. Accessed October 24, 2008.
The CDC has a wide variety of information and materials available for promoting lifestyle change; anyone working in this area would want to review these materials.

The Portion Plate. Available at: http://www.theportionplate.com. Accessed October 21, 2008.
This is a handy tool to help clients learn portion size.

Martin KS, Scheet NJ. The Omaha System. Philadelphia, PA; 1992. Electronic version available at: http://www.omahasystem.org/. Accessed October 24, 2008.
The Omaha System is a community nurse's assessment and documentation system for home care and disease prevention. The assessment is comprehensive and includes economic factors, psychosocial factors, physiological factors, and health behaviors that work well for an interprofessional approach to care.

Chapter 15 Review Questions

1. **Identify examples of objective data that the committee used in the model program to establish a need for an obesity prevention program. (Select all that apply.)**

   (a) Prevalence of type 2 diabetes among adults over the age of 45

   (b) Hospitalization rate for diabetes

   (c) Prevalence of cardiovascular disease in the community

   (d) Incidence of gestational diabetes (diabetes with pregnancy)

   The correct answer is a, b, and d.

2. **Identify the risk factors for obesity that Laura had, the typical client in the model program:**

   - Lack of physical activity
   - High calorie diet
   - Women—gestational diabetes
   - Low level of education
   - Low socioeconomic status
   - Ethnicity

   The correct answer is all of the above.

3. **Identify one cultural issue and how it was addressed in the program.**

   Either of the two following responses is acceptable: (1) the cultural belief that women should not engage in strenuous physical activity. The program used pedometers to encourage clients to increase their amount of walking; or (2) the cultural belief that education and services should be based on personal relationships. This issue was addressed in the model program by using community health workers who made home visits so that the service would be personalized and the workers could form a relationship with the client.

4. **Identify the rationale for the pharmacist's participation in the model obesity prevention program.**

The role described for pharmacist participation in the model obesity prevention program was that of assuring conditions for appropriate medication use. For a person at risk for obesity and diabetes, the most appropriate approach is lifestyle change to a healthier diet with an appropriate number of calories and increased physical activity. Lifestyle change also increases the effectiveness of medications for weight loss and treatment of cardiovascular disease and diabetes; pharmacists should know how to intervene to promote a healthy lifestyle.

5. **A community coalition wants to hire a community health worker. Which of the following qualifications would the coalition want? (Select all that apply.)**

   (a) A trained health care professional with certification in health disparities

   (b) A person of the same race with a college degree

   (c) A member of the target population who has knowledge about health issues

   (d) A member of the target population who speaks the language, understands nonverbal communication, and knows the culture

Responses (c) and (d) are correct. A community health worker is a member of the target population who shares the same language and culture and understands the health issues of the population. Responses (a) and (b) are not correct; a health care professional or a person of the same race would be appropriate only if he or she was also a member of the target population.

Applying Your Knowledge

1. **Based on the progressive nature of obesity (individuals generally have normal weight, then become overweight, and finally obese), discuss when you think pharmacists should become involved in the treatment of obesity. Relate your discussion to the levels of prevention: primary, secondary, and tertiary.**

2. **Describe what subjective and objective data you would want to obtain to develop an obesity prevention program for college students. When thinking about the subjective data, identify possible key informants.**

3. **Could a pharmacist who practices in a community pharmacy implement a program similar to the community health worker program described here? Why or why not?**

Campus-Based Tuberculosis Service

■ ■ ■

Learning Outcomes

1. Describe types of data to collect for determining whether a campus-based tuberculosis service should be established and where to find such data.
2. Discuss steps to take during the planning and implementation phases to ensure acceptance of a new tuberculosis treatment and monitoring service on a college campus.
3. Explain the role of a formative program evaluation.
4. Discuss the pros and cons of various approaches to adherence in TB treatment.
5. Prepare an argument to support the role of pharmacists in TB control efforts.

Introduction

Finding new ways to reach populations at risk of disease or capable of spreading disease, if not treated, is always a concern in public health. Sometimes populations within a community that require extra attention are not immediately apparent. One of those groups is college students who are often in the community for only part of the year and tend to spend most of their time on campus where they are not readily visible to the community at large. This chapter explores how a community-level program that might be conducted by a health department can be adapted to high-risk students through a campus-based screening and monitoring service. After describing the epidemiology of tuberculosis (TB), the chapter will present a model program that focuses on students with latent tuberculosis. It also describes how the pharmacy at the student health service can promote adherence to the treatment regimen, which involves multiple medications taken over several months, and how to educate students with latent TB about their disease and the need to treat it. Because many of the high-risk students are from other countries, their cultural and health beliefs should be addressed. In addition, the pros and cons of using a voluntary adherence program will be explored. The early success and failure of the program will be assessed through a formative evaluation. Finally, the discussion section at the end of the chapter will consider the emerging resistance problem and mandatory medication administration programs.

Public Health Issue: Tuberculosis

Tuberculosis (TB), the White Plague or consumption, is an old disease that depends on crowded unsanitary conditions and people with deficient immune systems to survive and thrive. It is caused by infection with a microorganism, *Mycobacterium tuberculosis,* and can affect many organ systems in the body. The lungs are the most commonly affected part of the body, and it is through coughing that the microorganism becomes aerosolized and transmitted to others. A person infected with the mycobacterium may have latent TB (no symptoms and not **contagious**) or active TB (symptomatic and contagious).

Most TB cases begin as latent infections that are kept in check by a healthy immune system; however, when host defense mechanisms are reduced through immunosuppression or illness, the microorganism can begin to spread unchecked and an active case of TB develops. At that point, the person becomes contagious and can spread the disease to other people.

Eradication of the microorganism from the body requires months of treatment with several medications. For patients with latent TB, the only sign of disease may be their prescription vials of TB medication. Failure to fully treat with multiple antibiotics for the full 6- or 9-month regimen may result in an active TB case and promote the development of resistant strains of the microorganism. For current information on treatment guidelines for latent and active TB, check the professional information on the CDC web site.

With progress in improved sanitation, the use of quarantine and isolation, and the development of new effective medications, the prevalence of TB began to wane in the latter half of the 20th century. By the late 1970s, there was hope that TB would follow smallpox and soon be eradicated from the globe. However, in the 1980s the emergence of **HIV/AIDS,** a disease that suppresses the immune system provided the mycobacterium with an unforeseen opportunity to persist and expand to new populations around the world. After 20 or so years of believing that the disease was on its way to extinction, the **World Health Organization** declared a global TB emergency. Three principal factors are primarily responsible for the resurgence of TB as a global emergency: (1) emergence of antibiotic-resistant strains of *Mycobacterium tuberculosis*; (2) spread of acquired immunodeficiency syndrome (AIDS), which created a whole new population susceptible to TB; and (3) persistent economic and social conditions that reduce access to medical care.[1]

Epidemiology of tuberculosis

Today, it is estimated that one in three people worldwide is infected with TB and nearly 9 million infected people will develop the active form of the disease each year. This infection is the leading cause of death in HIV/AIDS patients and the leading cause of death from an infectious disease in the world.[2,3] In the United States, the incidence and prevalence of TB is actually declining with current rates similar to those seen in the 1950s. Because other regions around the world (e.g., nations in southern Africa, southeast Asian countries, and Russia) have very high rates of infection, international travelers and immigrants risk importing new cases to the states.[3] Identifying and treating cases of TB as well as reducing its spread is an example of the HP 2010 goal of reducing preventable morbidity and mortality related to infectious disease.[4]

Emergence of resistant strains

Like so many other infectious organisms, the *Mycobacterium spp.* has strains that are resistant to single and multiple drug therapies used to treat TB. The **multi-drug resistant** form of TB (**MDR-TB**), which is any strain that is resistant to the first-line antibiotic rifampicin, remains a threat. The **extensively resistant (XDR-TB)** form, which is any strain that is also resistant to any second-line antibiotic, is emerging as a threat in several regions around the world.[5] Resistance tends to emerge when an infection is not treated for a sufficient length of time or the antibiotic used to treat it is inappropriate. In countries where TB is widespread, a high incidence of counterfeit medications sold to treat it is adding to the problem.[6]

Length of treatment is a key issue for TB control because it is 6–9 months long depending on the situation and susceptibility of the microorganism to the antibiotics. Given the difficulty in getting patients to take an antibiotic for 7–10 days, the importance of convincing patients to complete 6 months of daily, multiple antibiotics (with nasty side effects) is not only critical but seemingly impossible.

Stigma of TB can affect patient behavior

Complicating identification and treatment of TB is the stigma associated with it. For many, the disease implies poor economic status and living conditions. Even possessing medical vials that are labeled with the names of drugs used primarily for treating TB can cause great embarrassment and concern. Some patients will remove the labels and risk getting confused about how to take the medicine rather than have someone see that they have TB medicine. In some cultures, a family member with TB will be sent away to avoid exposing other family members to the disease.[7]

Another factor adding to the stigma of a TB diagnosis is the link between HIV infection and TB. Many treatment guidelines now suggest testing for HIV infection in patients with latent TB infections because the co-existence of the two diseases is highly correlated, and the risks of developing the active form of TB and death are much higher in HIV-infected patients. So, a patient may opt not to be treated for TB because of the implied presence of an HIV infection too.[1,8]

Model Program

Campus-Based Tuberculosis Service

Background

This model will be a campus-based tuberculosis treatment and monitoring service run by the pharmacy. The idea for this fictitious model program was inspired by a real clinical pharmacy TB program at the student health service on the University of Montana campus and supplemented with details from published accounts of other campus screening or monitoring programs. [9–11]

Joe Lee is a fourth-year pharmacy student in his 20s who is currently on an advanced pharmacy practice experience (APPE) at the student health service on his campus. His major assignment for this rotation is to identify an unmet need of students who are clients at the health service. His preceptor has recommended thinking about public health issues in which pharmacy has traditionally had a limited role. Once his plan is prepared,

Joe will present it to the medical director and staff. If approved, Joe will be in charge of initial implementation. His classmates and the clinical pharmacists will continue his work after he leaves. Since Joe will return to the site in 4 months for his ambulatory care APPE, he will have a chance to evaluate the service. Joe decided to look into what might be needed for a TB medication service.

Objective Data

Campus characteristics
The campus is located in a modest-sized community of Riverette that lies in the Pacific Northwest about 50 miles from Portland, Oregon. The community boasts three major industries: a lumber and paper mill, electronics manufacturing, and tourism. The campus community swells the population count of Riverette to almost 280,000 when students arrive in the fall. Local residents embrace the outdoors lifestyle and enjoy a culturally diverse population that includes a large number of first-generation Americans of Chinese, Japanese, and Korean descents.

The State University campus enrolls around 18,000 students each year. It has a thriving graduate program with over 6,000 students in Master and Doctorate degree programs. It also boasts great diversity, with many foreign born students from across the globe, and a strong study abroad program that sends American students to over 50 countries throughout the year.

Student health service
Health care needs of students are provided by the on-site campus health service that includes a medical clinic, psychiatric care, urgent care services, 15 inpatient beds, nutrition counseling, rape and crisis counseling, and a pharmacy department with both dispensing and clinical services. Students may be referred to community clinics or hospitals, as needed, to appropriately treat their conditions. With the increasing number of nontraditional students, the clinic sees a variety of diseases including upper respiratory infections, birth control needs, and depression. The most common causes of the upper respiratory infections are viruses associated with the common cold, influenza, and secondary bacterial infections in the sinuses or pneumonias.

Student population
The average (standard deviation) ages on the campus for undergraduates and graduates are 21.5 (3.6) and 25.2 (6.3), respectively. The gender mix is 46% male and 54% female. The most predominant race on campus is Caucasian (32%) followed by Hispanic (21%), Asian-Pacific Islander (18%), African descent (14%), Mediterranean/Arab (10%), and Native American/Alaskan Eskimo (5%). Graduate students account for 76% of foreign-born students. The five countries with the most students on campus are Canada (28%), Serbia (22%), India (20%), Nigeria (17%), and China (13%).

According to a campus health survey conducted 3 years ago, students are involved in a number of risky behaviors that could impact their health. These include smoking cigarettes (32%), binge drinking (22%), driving under the influence (44%), inappropriate use of prescription medications (16%), poor nutrition and sleep habits (59%), lack of exercise (67%), and excessive consumption of caffeinated beverages (88%). The campus has also seen an increase in violent crimes with 32 cases of assault/sexual assault over the past 2 years.

Infectious disease has also increased with three cases of meningococcal meningitis diagnosed in the freshman dorm last year; two cases of **active tuberculosis** appearing in the graduate student population; and four cases of pertussis in the general student body. The recent SARS (Severe Acute Respiratory Syndrome) **epidemic** has focused the graduate programs on the need to protect its foreign-born and study-abroad student populations.

Local tuberculosis rates

In Riverette, the number of latent and active TB cases reported last year was 36 and five, respectively. This was an increase over the previous year in which 32 cases of latent and three cases of active TB were reported. Of the 57 students with positive skin tests, 21 had latent TB infections (LTBI) and one had active pulmonary TB. The rest had either a history of receiving the BCG vaccine, which is known to interfere with the skin test, or none of the risk factors for TB. The active case was neither the multi-drug nor extensively resistant form. Table 16.1 shows baseline data for the campus.

Table 16.1

Baseline Number of Incoming Students Screened and the Results

	Sept	Oct	Nov	Dec	Jan	Feb	Total
Number Screened	150	15	6	0	0	0	171
Number Positive	51	3	3	0	0	0	57
Number with LTBI*	17	3	1	0	0	0	21
Number with Active TB	0	1	0	0	0	0	1

*Positive skin test plus risk factors designated latent TB infection (LTBI).

Current TB programs

New cases of latent and active TB are identified through a campus-based mandatory screening program for students who come from high-risk countries or have high-risk contacts. Once identified, students with latent TB meet with the physician for an initial encounter where the infection and its treatment are discussed. The campus provides monthly supplies of medications in **self-administered therapy (SAT)**. If a student is deemed noncompliant, he or she is referred to the county health department for the **directly observed therapy (DOT)** program. When the student fills the prescriptions, the pharmacist provides counseling on the medications. No additional time is spent on adherence or education.

Students with active TB are immediately referred to the health department for treatment. The campus program for latent TB has not collected data other than missed appointments, but the medical director is concerned that many students are not beginning or completing the full course of treatment due to side effects and poor understanding of the latent infection.

The student health service provided medications for all but eight of the latent cases; the remaining students receive medications from the local health department or a private physician. The active case of TB is being treated through the health department.

The pharmacy at the student health service noted a discrepancy in the number of days between refills for students who are not using the DOT system. On average (SD), monthly supplies of antibiotics were filled every 48.5 (14.6) days. After 4 months, the number of students no longer refilling their TB medications was 48%. The clinic found a similar rate of attrition for appointments that were not kept (45%) after the first 3 months.

Subjective Data

Stakeholders as key informants

The medical director of the student health service expressed interest in providing more intense counseling and support for these patients. The clinical pharmacist found the idea interesting, and encouraged Joe to gather more information and prepare a plan for a TB service. The student health service and local health department received feedback from students who were being treated for latent TB; they said that they underestimated the seriousness of their illness and importance of taking their antibiotics for the full course of therapy (i.e., 6 months). They were extremely concerned about the approach of directly observed therapy (DOT) because their friends and classmates would figure out that they had TB. Others complained that their personal liberties and freedom were violated by programs that mandated visits to the health service every day or twice a week to receive medications. Three complained that the approach violated their **HIPAA privacy** because everyone knew that students who go to the health service through the west side door were going to the TB clinic.

Five students said they would remove the labels from their prescription vials so other students wouldn't know what they were taking. Students who were taking their medications religiously complained of uncomfortable side effects. Students with active TB were most likely to express fear and hopelessness. Students with latent TB did not seem to think they were at risk of developing MDR-TB or XDR-TB. Those with negative skin tests who were living in dorms thought they should be told if their roommate had TB, and most students thought casual contact would be sufficient for transmitting the disease. Students indicated interest in a campus-based program because it would be more convenient (Figure 16.1).

Figure 16.1—Categories of High-Risk Students

- Signs or symptoms of active TB
- HIV positive
- Close contact with someone with active TB
- Injected drug user
- Resided in or employed by high-risk settings (e.g., prison, nursing homes)
- Chronic disease that affects immune system
- Resided in high-risk country within past 5 years
- Local populations known to have increased risk

Literature on tuberculosis programs

Joe searched the medical literature to find models of TB medication services that he could adapt for use at the student health service. He quickly saw that compliance with the medication regimen was a problem due to the number of medications, nasty side effects, and the need to treat for at least 6 months. To ensure compliance, other health care workers had tried Directly Observed Therapy (DOT) or even incarcerating noncompliant patients in a local jail where they could receive daily treatment.[12,13] Often the failure to adhere to the treatment plan was an intentional action, not a misunderstanding or oversight, so counseling and support need to focus on an understanding of latent TB and the role of the therapy as well as identifying and overcoming any pre-existing notions or cultural influences related to the disease.[8] Also, studies that explored the growing problem with resistant strains of mycobacterium could affect the usefulness of the currently approved TB medications.[14,15]

Assessment

Data analysis

Scope of the Tuberculosis Problem on Campus
TB cases are increasing in the community, and the campus has a disproportionately high number of cases compared to the general population. A majority of the graduate students come from four of the five countries that have **endemic** TB. Adherence to therapy is assumed to be an issue since studies show that most people with latent TB do not complete a full course of antibiotics.

Interest in a Campus-Based Program
The community and campus have services that focus on dispensing medications and tracking cases. For patients who show poor compliance, there is the DOT program. At this time, no service is available for proactively monitoring compliance and educating patients about latent TB. The campus and community would benefit from an expanded clinical program that targets students with latent TB to improve compliance with the initial therapy. A dearth of information is also written in languages other than English.

Interest in a Pharmacist-Run Program
The medical director of the student health service is interested in having the pharmacy provide more intense counseling and monitoring of these patients so it can also evaluate the patients' adherence to therapy through their refill behavior and the presence of commonly encountered side effects. The clinical pharmacist at the student health service has expressed interest in creating a pharmacy-based TB screening and monitoring service for latent TB. Students taking the medications did not have a preference for a medical-, nursing-, or pharmacy-based service as long as it was on campus.

Interpretation of results
Results indicate a definite need and widespread interest in expanding the current services on the campus through a pharmacy-based service that will screen and treat students with latent TB. The service will need to be tailored for students who come from countries where TB is endemic or epidemic to ensure it is culturally and linguistically appropriate.

Planning

Scope of the service
Once Joe had decided to pursue a pharmacy-based support program targeting students with recently diagnosed latent TB to comply with their initial antibiotic treatment, he first proposed the idea to his preceptor, the medical director, and other health care

providers at the clinic. He also collected copies of forms currently in use at the student health service and contacted the health department to gather additional forms and information. Students with active TB would still be referred to the local health department for treatment.

Program protocol

Joe used the guidelines published by the American College Health Association (**ACHA**) and the Centers for Disease Control and Prevention (CDC) to revise the current screening and treatment protocol used at the student health service.[16,17] He scoured the literature to find examples of pharmacy-based TB services on college campuses.[9-11] Most of the literature focused on screening programs, not treatment programs, or they were based in other countries. The final protocol is shown in Figure 16.2. Because all the care would occur within the clinic, a standing order rather than a collaborative practice agreement was used to allow the pharmacist and the supervised APPE student to provide care per the approved protocol.

In addition to the protocol, Joe explored behavior change models to identify an approach that could be used to improve compliance. He settled on a **motivational interviewing** approach where the pharmacist would use questions to explore ambivalence and understanding of the treatment. What Joe didn't know was whether this approach would work with different cultures. His preceptor said they would try it and see how it worked. If needed, the approach could be adjusted as they go. In recognition of the significant number of students who spoke a language other than English as their primary language, Joe found medication and TB information sheets in Chinese, Japanese, and Korean at the Virginia department of health web site.

Since TB is a **reportable disease**, the health department would have to be notified when a student had a positive skin test. It was decided that the pharmacy would notify both the health department and medical director when a patient had latent TB. Students with active TB would be immediately referred to the health department for further testing and multi-drug treatment.

Physical space and staffing

The new pharmacy-based program would be housed in a counseling room that could be accessed from a doorway separate from the main clinic door. The counseling room contained a table and three chairs and a supply of TB and medication brochures in seven languages. Patient charts would be stored in the main part of the clinic and picked up each morning prior to a scheduled encounter. The service would be available through a twice-a-week clinic on Tuesday mornings and Thursday afternoons via appointments made with the receptionist at the clinic. Drop-in referrals from medical staff would also be accommodated as much as possible since a newly diagnosed student would be anxious to learn more about his or her condition and start therapy. Records for the TB clinic would be kept with the medical chart in the consults section.

Reimbursement plan

Billing for pharmacy services related to each encounter would be sent directly to the student unless there was a coincident encounter with a physician on the same day. The students would be charged a minimal fee of $15 per encounter. The last item on Joe's preparation list was the development of informational material and flyers that could be used to advertise the new service. Through an agreement with the health department,

Figure 16.2—Pharmacy-Based TB Screening and Treatment Protocol at State University

1. All incoming students must complete a TB risk assessment questionnaire.
   a. Pharmacy team will review questionnaires to identify students who are high risk and contact them to set up a skin test.

2. High-risk students will be required to have a TB skin test unless:
   a. They have documentation from another U.S. clinic or institution showing they have had one within the past 6 months;
   b. Currently being treated for active TB; or
   c. Prior vaccination with BCG is not a contraindication to a skin test.

3. Students with a positive skin test will be required to complete a chest x-ray to determine whether their infection is latent or active.
   a. Active cases (chest x-ray shows signs of infection) will be referred to the local health department for further testing and a multi-drug treatment regimen.
   b. Latent cases (chest x-ray is "clean") will continue working with the pharmacy team to begin isoniazid (INH) treatment to eradicate the microorganism and prevent conversion to an active case.
      i. INH dose: 5 mg/kg up to 300 mg po daily or 15 mg/kg up to 900 mg twice a week.
      ii. Duration of treatment: 9 months is preferred, but 6 months may be used in student with functional immune system and no fibrotic lesions on the chest x-ray.
      iii. If medical history indicates risk for liver disease, baseline liver function tests should be conducted and monitored monthly for the first 3 months.
      iv. If INH is not tolerated, may switch to rifampin 10 mg/kg up to 600 mg once daily for at least 120 doses within a 6-month period.

4. Students being treated for latent TB will be monitored for compliance with the treatment regimen, presence of hepatitis, and signs and symptoms of active TB disease.
   a. Monitoring will begin on a weekly basis for the first 2 months.
   b. Visits during the remaining months should be at least once a month, but may be more often if needed to ensure compliance.
   c. Directly observed therapy (DOT) of twice weekly doses may be started if compliance is a concern.
      i. Students requiring DOT will go to the student health service every Monday and Thursday morning between 8 a.m.–12 noon to take their dose while a member of the pharmacy team observes them.
   d. Each visit will be recorded in the consultation section of the chart.

5. Upon completion of the course of therapy for latent TB, students will be referred back to the clinic physician for a final assessment.

6. Students who complete treatment for latent TB 1 year but return home for the summer to an area that has endemic TB will be required to complete the risk assessment again.

Date approved:_____

Signature of Medical Director:_____

Signature of Clinical Pharmacist:_____

students could receive their TB medications free of charge at either the student health service pharmacy or the health department.

Implementation

Notifying stakeholders
Once all the forms, protocol, and standing orders were approved, Joe provided an inservice to the medical and nursing staff, the receptionist and support staff, and the pharmacy personnel to tell them about the new service. The service would begin the last week of Joe's rotation, so he would not get to see the full implementation of the service. Joe prepared a written set of instructions for students who would be involved in the service during subsequent rotations. He also distributed flyers announcing the service to areas of campus where the international students were likely to congregate such as the international studies building, dormitories, and graduate apartments. The service would receive all students with a positive skin test to discuss the results and let them know what to do next.

Referral system
With the first referral, Joe and his preceptor set up an appointment, met with the student, and began working on a care plan to help him or her successfully complete the 6-month treatment for latent TB infection. The results of the encounter were recorded in the consultation section of the chart. By the time Joe left the rotation, four students had been referred to the service and three of them had been seen and were started on their medications. No adverse reactions (to the medications) or noncompliance were reported at that time.

Evaluation

The preceptor recommended a **formative evaluation** during the first semester to double check the process and to see if the initial outcomes looked good. The outcomes they chose for latent TB infection cases were continued absence of disease symptoms and side effects, compliance with the treatment regimen, and understanding of the disease. They would also look at the structure of the service and its processes to see any trouble spots and possibly improve them.

Objective data
Six months after beginning the service, 48 students with latent TB infections had been referred to the pharmacy team. Of those, a total of 34 kept their appointments and met with the pharmacist or APPE student. During that time, one case of active TB was referred to the local health department for treatment. The number (%) of students dropping out of the program was 11 (32%). Table 16.2 shows the results of the screening program, while Table 16.3 shows the monitoring and treatment results.

Subjective data
Students enrolled in the pharmacy TB service were asked to provide feedback on the service after they had completed 6 months of treatment. The results contained comments indicating that the students thought it was a valuable service; they appreciated

having someone explain the disease to them; and they thought the information was easy to understand. The patients didn't like having to make another appointment and paying for the service. The pharmacist and the three APPE students noticed that many of the students with positive skin tests did not understand the disease. There were misconceptions about how it was transmitted, how someone could be infected without being sick, and why it was important to take all the medications for the entire time. Many of the students did not think it was a dangerous disease.

Table 16.2

Number of Incoming Students Screened and the Results with Pharmacy-Based Service

	Sept	Oct	Nov	Dec	Jan	Feb	Total
Number Screened	165	21	10	0	0	0	196
Number Positive	55	13	3	0	0	0	71
Number with LTBI*	29	11	8	0	0	0	48
Number with Active TB	0	1	1	0	0	0	2

*Positive skin test plus risk factors designated latent TB infection (LTBI).

Table 16.3

Results of First 6 Months

	Sept	Oct	Nov	Dec	Jan*	Feb	Total
Students with LTBI	29	11	8	0	0	0	48
First encounters	21	4	5	2	2	0	34
Total patients enrolled	**21**	**25**	**30**	**32**	**34**	**34**	**34**
Refused to participate	7	5	2	0	0	0	14
Total INH	21	24	26	28	28	28	28
Total rifampin	0	1	4	6	6	6	6
Side effects	1	6	4	4	0	1	16
Symptoms of TB	0	0	0	0	0	0	0
Prescriptions not filled	3	2	2	0	6	0	13
Converted to DOT	0	1	2	1	0	0	4
Lost to followup	5	1	0	1	4	0	11

*Winter break lasts until the third week of January, so many students are not on campus until January 24.

Analysis and interpretation

Compared to the previous program, the current pharmacy-based program works better for those students who continue with the service. Even after educational sessions, some students still believed TB was not a dangerous disease and did not feel compliance was important. Retaining the students in the service appears to be some problem, so the pharmacy teams need to look closely at their monitoring and education activities.

Discussion

Importance of treating latent TB infections

The importance of treating latent TB infections to prevent them from becoming the active form, which is also the contagious form, cannot be overstated. This leads to concern about the students who truly need treatment for their latent TB infection but either refuse to start it or fail to continue it for as long as recommended. Joe, the pharmacy student in the case study, did not seem to have a good plan for these patient behaviors. His options for determining why students who need therapy fail to seek it are somewhat limited.

The research literature may provide some clues as to the reasons, but measuring attitudes in groups of patients who refuse to be treated is often difficult. The attitudes toward treatment are often carried over to their refusal to answer questions about their behaviors, too. Some avenues worth pursuing may be to form focus groups of students who *are* participating to find out why they stay. Another idea may be to work with the international program to identify potential cultural or language barriers that persist in spite of efforts to reduce them.

Another population that has a higher-than-average risk of exposure to tuberculosis is health care workers. Naturally, those who work closely with infected patients are most likely to be at risk. Other caregivers, such as those in long-term care facilities or nursing homes, also have increased risks.

Resistant forms of tuberculosis

The emergence of resistant forms of the disease is another concern to the health care and public health communities. Most practitioners have been trained to treat TB and other infectious diseases with effective antibiotics. The loss of the effectiveness of first-line and second-line therapies opens the prospect of widespread disease. Until newer and more effective agents are found, health care workers may find themselves powerless to treat their patients and public health workers may retreat back to the old methods of isolation and quarantine. The use of TB sanitariums may re-emerge if resistant strains continue to spread. The impact of a surge of **resistant TB** strains could impact international travel and exchange programs found on many campuses in the United States.

Converting a campus program to the community

Although the campus-based protocol could be converted to a community-based pharmacy program, it would lack the mandatory requirement of risk assessment and skin testing possible with the campus program. A community pharmacist could offer the risk assessment, and those who volunteer to take it can be referred to the health department if their risk appears to be high. The community pharmacist can also watch for patients complaining of upper respiratory illnesses that include classic signs and symptoms of TB such as a persistent cough (>3 weeks) and/or bloody, rust-colored sputum. Other symptoms include night sweats, weight loss, and fatigue. Patients with symptoms that persist for several weeks should be immediately referred to a physician or the health department if they are also at high risk for TB (i.e., HIV positive). A pharmacist can identify the high-risk HIV and immune-suppressed patients based on their medications and suggest they get checked for latent TB.

Chapter 16 Summary

This chapter illustrates how a disease once thought to be almost eradicated took advantage of health and economic factors to become a global emergency. Although the United States has a declining rate of new cases, TB can return through many mechanisms. The model program described a service designed to reduce the risk of TB spread through a campus-based latent TB infection program for students from countries with high rates of TB. The program attended to linguistic, cultural, and access barriers through a pharmacist-run service that worked with students with latent TB infections and referred those with active TB to the local health department. By providing the service on campus, the pharmacy program improved access and compliance. Patients with latent TB who complete their full course of antibiotics will avoid the risk of developing active, contagious TB, which helps to reduce the spread of the disease. Given the recent trends in MDR-TB and XDR-TB, an ongoing need exists for services that promote adherence to a long and difficult treatment regimen as well as continuous monitoring to ensure the treatment regimen is indeed effective.

References

1. Gandy M, Zumla A. The resurgence of disease: social and historical perspectives on the "new" tuberculosis. *Soc Sci Med.* 2002; 55:385–96.

2. Division of Tuberculosis Elimination (DTBE). Centers for Disease Control and Prevention web site "Fact Sheet: A Global Perspective on Tuberculosis." Available at: http://www.cdc.gov/tb/WorldTBDay/resources_global.htm. Last reviewed/updated April 18, 2007. Accessed March 11, 2008.

3. World Health Organization. Chapter 1: monitoring the TB epidemic and progress in TB control in *Global Tuberculosis Control—Surveillance, Planning, Financing* (2008). Tuberculosis web page. Available at: http://www.who.int/tb/publications/global_report/2008/chapter_1/en/index.html. Accessed November 25, 2008.

4. Healthy People 2010. Objective 14–11. Reduce Tuberculosis. Available at: http://www.healthypeople.gov/document/HTML/Volume1/14Immunization.htm#_Toc494510241. Accessed November 25, 2008.

5. Centers for Disease Control and Prevention. Trends in tuberculosis incidence—United States, 2006. *MMWR.* 2007; 56(11).

6. Kelesidis T, Kelesidis I, Rafailidis PI, et al. Counterfeit or substandard antimicrobial drugs: a review of the scientific evidence. *J Antimicr Chem.* 2007; 60:214–36.

7. Mak WS, Mo PKH, Cheung RYM, et al. Comparative stigma of HIV/AIDS, SARS, and tuberculosis in Hong Kong. *Soc Sci Med.* 2006; 63:1912–22.

8. Stigma. Living and dying with tuberculosis web page of the WHO Europe web site. Available at: http://www.euro.who.int/features/2005/featuretb/20050317_14. Accessed November 24, 2008.

9. Colorado Department of Public Health and Environment. 2007 Guidelines for Tuberculosis Screening of College and University Students. Available at: http://www.cdphe.state.co.us/dc/TB/CollegeTBscreen.pdf. Accessed March 9, 2008.

10. Drummond J. Tuberculosis Recommendations for University/College Campuses in Missouri. Missouri Department of Health and Senior Services. Health Advisory August 7, 2007: Available at: http://www. dhss.mo.gov/BT_Response/HAdTBRecommendationsForUnivs8-7-07.pdf. Accessed March 9, 2008.

11. Norton D. Kirkwood Community College tuberculosis screening for international students. *J Am Coll Health*. 2000; 48(4). Published online at: http://www.ccid.kirkwood.cc.ia.us/memberactivities/exemp/ tuber.htm. Accessed March 9, 2008.

12. Munro SA, Lewin SA, Smith HJ, et al. Patient adherence to tuberculosis treatment: a systematic review of qualitative research. *PLoS Med*. 2007; 4(7):e238.

13. Burman WJ, Cohn DL, Rietmeijer CA, et al. Short-term incarceration for the management of noncompliance with tuberculosis treatment. *Chest*. 1997; 112:57–62.

14. Alexander PE, De P. The emergence of extensively drug-resistant tuberculosis (TB): TB/HIV coinfection, multi-drug resistant TB and the resulting public health threat from extensively drug-resistant TB, globally and in Canada. *Can J Infect Dis Med Microbiol*. 2007; 18(5):289–91 (commentary).

15. Centers for Disease Control and Prevention. Extensively drug-resistance tuberculosis— United States, 1993–2006. *MMWR*. 2007; 56(11):250–3.

16. American College Health Association. ACHA Guidelines: Tuberculosis Screening of College and University Students. November 2000. Available at: http://www.acha.org/info_resources/tb_statement.pdf. Accessed March 9, 2008.

17. Division of Tuberculosis Elimination (DTBE). Centers for Disease Control and Prevention web site "TB Guidelines." Available at: http://www.cdc.gov/tb/pubs/mmwr/maj_guide.htm. Accessed March 9, 2008.

Suggested Readings

Division of Tuberculosis Elimination (DTBE). Centers for Disease Control and Prevention web site "TB Guidelines." Available at: http://www.cdc.gov/tb/pubs/ mmwr/maj_guide.htm. Accessed March 9, 2008.

Tavitian SM, Spalek VH, Bailey RP. A pharmacist-managed clinic for treatment of latent tuberculosis infection in health care workers. *Am J Health-Syst Pharm*. 2003; 60(18):1856–61.

World Health Organization. Tuberculosis web pages. Available at: http://www.who. int/topics/tuberculosis/en/. Accessed March 9, 2008.

Chapter 16 Review Questions

1. **Describe types of data to collect for determining whether a campus-based tuberculosis service should be established.**

Joe used a combination of objective and subjective data to determine need. Rates of the disease on campus and in the community were gathered to see if a problem existed. Populations within the campus community were also identified so the service could focus on them. Joe also looked at other pre-existing services to ensure that the proposed service was actually needed and filled a void. Finally, Joe looked at the interest in having a pharmacy-based service on the campus.

2. **Describe steps taken by Joe Lee during the planning and implementation phases to get support and acceptance for the proposed latent TB infection monitoring service.**

Planning: Joe ran his ideas by the medical director of the health service and created a standing order for the clinic physicians to use. He probably got input from the physicians on the standing order to ensure they would accept and use it. For active cases, Joe's protocol had both the medical director and health department notified to keep everyone in the information loop.

Implementation: Joe presented an inservice to all the clinic staff prior to the initiation of the new program so that everyone was aware of it if they were asked. He also posted flyers to notify students that the new service was available.

3. **Based on the objective and subjective data gathered for the formative analysis, explain what you would keep the same and what you would change in the TB monitoring service. What other information would you collect to evaluate the service again in 6 months?**

Keep the same: Continue working with incoming and returning students from countries with endemic/epidemic TB each year, and continue providing intensive counseling and language-appropriate materials.

Change: Increase the number of languages for the reading materials, and improve followup methods for students who do not keep appointments.

Measure for next evaluation: Measure attitude and knowledge of the disease, and measure effectiveness of more aggressive followup approach.

4. **List two of the pros and two of the cons of having a pharmacy-based TB service based on the model described in this chapter.**

Pros: Monitor prescription fill and use more easily; build a better relationship with TB patients at your pharmacy; improve health outcomes of your TB patients.

Cons: Consider staffing and time resources when adding a new service; consider other patients' concerns about catching TB. You may lose patients if they do not perceive the service as helpful, confidential, respectful, or culturally appropriate.

Applying Your Knowledge

1. **Using the ideas for the TB service in the case study presented in this chapter, how would you design a pharmacy-based service for another infectious disease with a complicated long-term treatment requirement such as HIV/AIDS?**

2. **What would it take to eradicate TB from the globe? What are the barriers?**

Emergency Preparedness Planning and Response

Learning Outcomes

1. Describe types of data to collect for determining the risks of natural or manmade disasters in a community and where to find such data.
2. Discuss activities a pharmacist may participate in before, during, and after a disaster.
3. Explain the role of federal disaster response teams (e.g. DMAT) and how a pharmacist can contribute to the efforts of such teams.
4. List objective and subjective data to collect for evaluating pharmacy services during a response to a disaster.
5. Compare and contrast how pharmacy practice may differ between usual situations and disaster situations.

Introduction

Although infrequent in occurrence, disasters can overwhelm and disable a community when they do occur. Recent experiences with large-scale disasters have underscored the need to involve health care workers, including pharmacists, in preventing, preparing for, responding to, and recovering from disasters. Pharmacists can be involved as private citizens or as health professionals and their involvement can be at local, state, national, or even international levels.

This chapter begins with background on natural and manmade disasters and their impact on communities and then describes the efforts of one pharmacist to participate in a disaster response team. After looking at the local disaster risks and his current roles in the community, the pharmacist decides to seek a role on a regional medical response team that is part of a national system. The chapter follows his decisions to prepare for deployment and the actual deployment to a community devastated by a hurricane. Although the pharmacist and the experiences at the disaster care site are fictitious, they are based on published reports from actual disaster responses. Success of the response effort of the pharmacist's team and his personal sense of achievement are evaluated through objective and subjective data. The chapter ends with discussions about liability issues related to participating in a disaster response, other options for participating in planning or response, and new populations created from disasters that are vulnerable to disease.

Public Health Issue: Disasters

Each year natural and **manmade disasters** disrupt community infrastructure and economies and cause preventable injury and death. Although not specifically listed as one of
the 10 HP2010 goals, emergency response *does* help reduce morbidity and mortality due
to injury, infectious disease, and poor access to care and necessary supplies for survival.
Emergency response can be considered an integral part of the HP2010 goals when
viewed in this manner.

Epidemiology of disasters

According to the **United Nations' International Strategy for Disaster Reduction
(UN ISDR),** the most frequently occurring **natural disasters** worldwide are related to
hydrometeorological causes such as too much water (flooding, hurricanes, ice storms) or
too little water (droughts, lightning-sparked wildfires).[1] Almost 7,500 such disasters have
occurred since 1900. Geological events such as earthquakes and volcanoes are the next
most commonly encountered type of disasters; over 1,250 have occurred during the same
time period. They are followed closely by a third category of natural disasters, biological, which includes epidemics of infectious diseases at almost 1,100. The most striking
aspect of these statistics is the growing number of events in all categories. Compared to
1900, the number of weather, geological, and biological disasters in 2005 grew from 28
to 2,135, 40 to 233, and 5 to 420, respectively.[1]

   In addition to naturally occurring disasters, there are those caused by humans. Some
are accidental, such as a structure failure in a bridge or building collapse or a train wreck
that releases a toxic gas or liquid, while others are intentional acts such as terrorism and
arson-caused wildfires. Many natural disasters have a manmade element to them, too.
For example, poor farming practices combined with poor weather conditions may lead
to crop failure and famine; removing trees and vegetation from a hillside may facilitate
the development of a mudslide in a heavy rain. This means tracking human-caused disasters is not clean cut, but efforts to track terrorism-related disasters or attacks indicate an
increase in those activities in terms of scope and number over the past 100 years.[2]

Risk factors created by disasters

Ironically, although the number of natural disasters seems to be increasing, the mortality
rates appear to be remaining steady or even declining.[1] The UN ISDR report indicates
that the mortality created by various natural disasters can vary by continent. Between
1991 and 2005, the ISDR found that in Africa, where epidemics of HIV/AIDS, malaria,
and TB persist and war and poverty interfere with access to medical care or public health
interventions, biological disasters are the leading cause of death at 7.31 per 1 million
inhabitants. In Asia, the leading cause of death is geological events such as earthquakes
at 7.54 per 1 million inhabitants, while hydrometeorological disasters like floods claim
the most lives in the Americas at 6.23 per 1 million inhabitants and Europe at 4.77 per 1
million inhabitants.[1]

   Death is not the only result of disasters. In fact, it is just the "tip of the iceberg"
for considering the scope of impact of a given disaster. For every one person killed by
a disaster, probably hundreds of people are injured and thousands are directly affected
through loss of services, homes, businesses, and livelihood. The ripple effect can spread

to neighboring communities and states where hundreds of thousands of people can be indirectly impacted by a large disaster that affects demand and prices for services and products. Among these other impacts are the economic consequences that can lead to the demise of small local businesses, which leads to a loss of jobs and the long-term psychological consequences related to survivor guilt and post-traumatic stress disorders.

Emergency preparedness

Emergency response is only one part of an overall effort to reduce preventable deaths and disability; therefore, this chapter will use a more inclusive term called **all-hazards emergency preparedness**. Emergency preparedness covers a continuum of activities that include efforts to decrease the likelihood of a disaster occurring again; mitigation efforts to reduce the scope and magnitude of disasters that cannot be completely prevented; training and planning activities to ensure resources and personnel will be available and helpful during an actual disaster response; and long-term plans to recover after a disaster occurs. In short, emergency preparedness includes activities before, during, and after a disaster event.

Emergency preparedness is called "all-hazards" when the plans for a response focus on issues that require action such as loss of clean water supply or electricity rather than the cause such as an earthquake, explosion, or flood. This approach allows communities to prepare a master plan rather than a series of disaster-specific plans.

Roles for pharmacists

The involvement of health care professionals in emergency response is not new. Pharmacists have been volunteering for national teams since the 1960s.[3] If people are injured, then health care professionals will be involved in their care and recovery. This activity has led to the name, "**first receivers**," for those who are the first health care professionals to see disaster victims and their injured rescuers. In the initial phases of a disaster response, the clinic and hospital personnel are most likely to be the first health care providers to encounter the injured, so efforts to train and prepare have been focused on these sites and these providers.

With the increased awareness that some disasters may be manmade and intentional (i.e., acts of terrorism), health care professionals have come to accept that they may be the first to see and identify less obvious attacks such as intentional outbreaks of infectious disease or exposures to chemical agents. The retail pharmacist may be the first to see unwitting victims of a chemical or infectious disease exposure because initial symptoms are mild and the victims are self-treating. The realization that any health care provider in any location could become a **first responder** has led to an expansion in training and increased involvement of health care providers, including pharmacists, in planning, training, and preparation activities. Some of this training for pharmacists begins while they are still in school.

Model Program

Pharmacists and National Disaster Response Teams

Background

Lyle S. has been practicing as a pharmacist in Littlesburg, Ohio, for just over 8 years. He is employed full-time at a local pharmacy chain retail store where he is the assistant manager. His duties include the development of clinical services, which he has embraced enthusiastically. The store now boasts an immunization service, diabetes service, and medication therapy management service. In addition, free blood pressure readings are offered on demand. Now that Lyle has finally repaid all his student loans, bought the much desired new car, and acquired a mortgage for his first-ever home, he is interested in giving back to his community.

Local roles for pharmacists

After looking into several options, he signed up to become a volunteer for the Red Cross emergency services.[6] After completing the required training, he is now "on call" to help when local disasters occur. During the past year, he helped get shelter and supplies for five families after house fires left them homeless; twice he provided support (e.g., answering phones and serving hot coffee) to the local sheriff's search and rescue teams. In the pharmacy, Lyle offered the Red Cross emergency preparation lists for families to his customers too. Lyle began to wonder if his pharmacy knowledge would be especially useful in other ways to help in disasters. This case describes the options he considered, how he selected a way to become involved, and what he learned as a pharmacist during a mass casualty disaster.

Objective Data

Community characteristics

Littlesburg, Ohio, is larger than its name implies with just over 220,000 residents in the city and surrounding area. Originally a farming community, Littlesburg has increased its economic base with the addition of a nuclear power plant, community college, and two pesticide manufacturing businesses. The population echoes the national population in its distribution of gender, race, age, and education. Many families have lived in the area for multiple generations, and their devotion to the town and its history runs deep. The community boasts many churches serving a variety of religious denominations. The town also boasts an unsubstantiated link to the Civil War era Underground Railroad phenomenon and a vague undefined role in the creation of the nation in the late 1700s.

Local features of importance in disaster planning are the two rivers that flow through the town. The Jamison River, which flows through the middle of Littlesburg and effectively cuts it in half, is the larger of the two. Five bridges span the river, one of which is used by the interstate highway system. The Little Jimmy creek is much smaller and flows into the Jamison near the edge of the city limits. This creek has two small bridges across it. The gentle rolling landscape does not boast many high spots, and Littlesburg has a history of flooding during the spring when heavy rains and melting snow push the level of the river water above flood stage. The last major flood in 1928 took the lives of 55 residents, including 22 children who perished when their one-room schoolhouse was destroyed by a 6′ wall of mud and water. Since then, an earthen dam located just 5 miles upstream has been built, and flooding disasters have been greatly mitigated by the regulation of the water level in the river.

Other sources of potential danger include the interstate, where trucks hauling chemicals and explosive substances frequently travel, and the rail yard on the north end of town that still has freight trains filled with industrial wastes from the local manufacturers passing through three times a day. The nuclear plant, which is located downstream but upwind from Littlesburg, has a policy to neutralize and clean any and all wastes from its production. The pesticide plants are located at the other end of town, upstream on the Little Jimmy Creek, where yet-to-be-confirmed rumors are circulating of inappropriate disposal of production wastes.

The winter weather is another source of disaster for the community due to the high levels of snowfall, cold arctic air, and a tendency for freezing rain and fog to form during December and January. The ice storm of 1996–97 caused massive power outages when 2″ of ice coated both trees and power lines. On a happier note, the town of Littlesburg has not had a tornado since the 1800s and summers are pleasant with only moderate humidity.

Disaster data for the community

The last large scale disaster in Littlesburg occurred in the winter of 1996–97 when a freak ice storm coated the area with 2″ of ice. The resulting damage caused power outages in over 50,000 homes and businesses. This storm was followed by 5 days of brutally cold arctic air (–0° F) that hampered efforts to remove debris and downed power lines. Since the ice storm of 1997, one out of every five homes now has a gas-powered generator and two out of every seven has a wood burning stove. One half of all homeowners also keep candles and matches in their homes. The incidence of house fires during cold weather has quadrupled from three per year to almost 12. Most are due to unattended candles, but some are due to dirty chimneys or faulty wiring.

Current community programs for emergency response

Lyle discovered that the **local emergency planning committee (LEPC)** recently prepared an all-hazards disaster response plan. The plan is based on the characteristics of the community that put it at risk for natural and manmade disasters. They have been identified as flooding, ice storms, exposure to organophosphates or radiation, and bridge collapse. In reviewing the plan, Lyle could not see any discussion about pharmacy roles in a response. The plan discussed how it would receive and distribute the **Strategic National Stockpile (SNS)**, which is medications and medical supplies, but it assigned roles to physicians and nurses rather than pharmacists. The LEPC is working with county and state planners to provide a practice drill shortly. Lyle wanted to get involved in the planning, but felt he lacked the experience and knowledge to set up a mass dispensing or vaccination site.

While the LEPC is based on community agencies and their employees, volunteer organizations in Littlesburg also respond to emergencies. One such group is the local chapter of the **American Red Cross**. This organization has two branches—one for collecting blood and one for providing disaster support.[4] For disaster response, the Red Cross offers training to volunteers who want to assist with shelters, phones, and other tasks at local to national levels.

Subjective Data

Key informants

Most residents of the town do not give disasters a second thought and are happy to go about their daily lives working and building their community. When the rare disaster does occur, they are confident that their neighbors and the surrounding area will come to their aid, just as they would for them. When asked what type of disaster they are most likely to encounter, over 80% said winter blizzards and ice storms. They rate the likelihood of intentionally created disasters, such as acts of terrorism, as highly unlikely even though they are near a nuclear power plant that is not tightly secured.

The residents involved in the emergency planning and response activities for the community take a somewhat different view. They think disasters, though rare, will have a great impact on the community and firmly believe in working towards avoiding disasters (if possible) and preparing plans to minimize the impact (if disaster occurs). Many of these people are employed by traditional first responder agencies such as the city police, fire department, and hospital-based **emergency medical services (EMS)**.

Health care workers, including pharmacists, seem to represent middle ground in terms of their perception of risk and prior involvement in responses. Those who were in town during the 1996–97 ice storm are adamant about the need for involvement as well as newer employees who come from other parts of the country where they experienced disaster response firsthand. Administrators, especially the Chief Financial Officer, accept risk but have a hard time justifying training or additional equipment and supplies in their operating budgets. As a result, health care workers interested in a larger role in response have been seeking involvement outside of their employment.

During the 1997 ice storm, Lyle noticed how many residents forgot to take their medications with them when they were **evacuated** to shelters and how pharmacies could not provide medications because their computer systems were unable to run without electricity. The legality of having other pharmacists, such as Lyle, provide medications was not clear. Even after the Governor declared a state of emergency, no one could tell Lyle and other pharmacists if they could provide "unauthorized" refills of chronic medications like digoxin and Coumadin®. Luckily, the local emergency department physicians provided one-time prescriptions to ensure patients had medications, but that system took 3 days to organize.

Literature on pharmacy and disaster response

Lyle discovered that national emergency response teams consisting of health care workers, including pharmacists, were being formed.[5] These teams had existed for many years, but were now reaching out to include more health professions. The difference between these teams and local response groups was the opportunity to help disaster victims anywhere in the United States. Lyle saw this as an opportunity to gain the knowledge and experience he would need to become an active participant in the local disaster planning and response.

Lyle found a web site for the **National Disaster Medical System (NDMS)** describing two response teams that used pharmacists.[5] The NDMS is located in the office of the **Assistant Secretary for Preparedness and Response (ASPR)** in the **Department of Health and Human Services (DHHS)**. The **National Pharmacist Response Team (NPRT)** was specifically focused on pharmacists, technicians, and students for mass dispensing and vaccination efforts. The **Disaster Medical Assistance Team (DMAT)** consisted of a mix of health professions and usually had one pharmacist.[5] Responders are now limited to participating in one or the other response teams. Since the DMATs were deployed for disasters, Lyle chose to pursue the DMAT option.

The DMATs are organized within states and divided into three national regions—East, Central, and West. The various DMATs are identified by a state and number designation. Lyle learned that DMATs must each be sponsored by a public or private organization and have sufficient resources to sustain themselves and serve patients for 72 hours. The DMAT must be able to deploy immediately when called and work in temporary or permanent patient care sites.

Assessment

Data analysis

Findings from Community Review
Littlesburg, like any community, has many sources and features that may be the cause of a natural or manmade disaster. Unlike many communities, the local agencies have drafted a disaster plan and begun training and practice drills. Unlike Lyle, many residents are not concerned with the prospect of a disaster and do not seek to prepare or gain additional training.

Findings from the Literature Review
The review of the literature revealed the existence of national emergency response teams that pharmacists can join with a license in good standing. These teams may respond to emergencies anywhere in the United States and for any type of disaster.

Interpretation of results
Locally, no additional activities are available in which Lyle can participate to increase his knowledge and skills in disaster response or add to existing programs. Lyle's decision to join a national team of health care responders will provide him with training and experience he can bring back to his own community to help the local plan and response. His skills with mass dispensing clinics will fill a gap in services.

Planning

Gathering information about DMAT
Lyle found the regional DMAT in Ohio, the OH-1 DMAT. Formed in the mid 1980s by a physician, the OH-1 DMAT has grown to a stable size of around 120 practitioners and support personnel; it has a long history of involvement in local and national response efforts beginning with Hurricane Andrew in 1992. According to the Ohio DMAT's web site, the group was looking for pharmacists for the team.[6] Lyle responded to the call and was referred to the DHHS NDMS web site for registration and training information.

Personal planning for participation
Planning to become part of a national emergency response team required serious consideration of personal and professional responsibilities at home. Lyle began his planning by getting more information about the time commitments and requirements to participate in a national response team. He first discussed the idea with his family to see if they had any strong objections, and then he discussed his interests with his boss to ensure that he would be able to attend training sessions and be able to respond if called.

Training and applying for a regional team

The training consisted of two main parts: online distance learning modules and a practice drill. The learning modules used as part of the training are updated and managed by the federal DMAT program, while the practice drills are a combination of national and local training events. The training includes several modules on the **Incident Command System (ICS)**, which is used to organize all types of disaster responses.[7] Lyle was actually familiar with the organizational strategy after spending two summers in Idaho as a fire fighter. The ICS has been used for years in forest fires. In addition, Lyle had a physical exam to ensure he was physically fit for a rigorous response effort and updated all his vaccinations to include coverage recommended by the DMAT program.

Preparing for deployment

After training and attending to his physical needs, Lyle prepared a deployment plan with his boss and provided training for two of his colleagues about tasks they would cover during his absence. His preparations caught the attention of another pharmacist and a technician who both decided to look into the program.

Once Lyle had been accepted for the OH-1 DMAT training, he decided on the best times to attend training and be on call to respond to a disaster. Although Lyle is single, he does have two dogs, Wally and Buster, who will need care while he is gone. One of his co-workers, who also has a dog, said she would be able to care for both pups. Lyle's boss said he would handle or delegate the assistant management duties as needed, when Lyle was gone, since it sounded like an important activity. Lyle also had to consider how he could automatically pay bills, including his new mortgage payments, to ensure that he would not become delinquent while away.

Preparing for deployment involved finding out what kind of supplies and equipment he would need during a 2-week response. Planning what to bring and how to pack reminded Lyle of his childhood when he went backpacking in Wyoming and Montana. The deciding factor is to bring only what you can use. By planning for no food, water, or electricity, the DMAT volunteer will be prepared for just about anything during the first 72 hours. The MI-1 DMAT (Michigan) guidelines for packing suggest using two bags: a large duffel bag with wheels to hold most of the clothing, food, equipment, sleeping bag, and personal items; and a small backpack with one change of clothing, medication, water, some food, and a book for entertainment.[8] Placing items in zip-lock plastic bags protects them from moisture, and extra empty plastic bags will come in handy once at the site. Clothing must be appropriate to the weather conditions—cool in summer or warm layers in winter. Good sturdy shoes or boots will be needed since all volunteers will spend a lot of time on their feet. A second pair of shoes such as trainers will be used during down time. The bag and backpack should be packed and ready to go.

In addition, Lyle had heard or read other advice from volunteers. One person said to remember extra batteries for the flashlight, while another recommended bringing a container of baby wipes. Apparently, the baby wipes come in handy when shower or bathing facilities are non-existent. Lyle opted to pack non-perishable, freeze-dried food and dry food for the first several days. He was going to bring a laptop computer, but figured it was too heavy; if there was no electricity, it would run for only a couple hours on batteries. In the end, he left it out of the duffel bag and brought a paperback novel instead.

Implementation

Deployment

For Lyle, implementation of his new service would be deployment to a disaster site, and his first response experience would be a memorable one. In late August 2005, he saw on the news that a large hurricane was heading for the Louisiana/Mississippi coast. He double checked his bag and backpack and let his boss and doggy-sitter know that he would probably be called to help. The call came the next day, and Lyle drove across Ohio to meet part of his team at the airport where they flew to an airport in Mississippi. From there, they met up with the rest of the team who had driven trucks filled with medical supplies to create a convoy. It would drive to their assigned site, an abandoned high school, in southwestern Mississippi. Their job was to create a new care site to **triage**, treat, and transport patients as needed. Within 72 hours, they would receive additional support from the U.S. Army and a portion of the Strategic National Stockpile.

Lyle was joined in the pharmacy component of the DMAT by another pharmacist, Brenda, and a pharmacy technician, Claire. He heard there would be four volunteers from the local community who would also help with set up and initial work. During the drive to their assigned site, team members were assessing the types of medical needs they were most likely to encounter. For a hurricane, they assumed blunt force injuries like broken limbs and lacerations would be common as well as dehydration due to lack of clean drinking water, infectious diseases spread by contaminated water and food (e.g., hepatitis), psychological trauma, and heat-related illness. The convoy stopped to refill water bottles and have one last warm meal about 4 hours before arriving at "their" school.

First 24 Hours

The team had to do all of its own work, including cleaning up the rooms where the supplies would be unloaded and stored. It took the team almost 6 hours to completely unload all the trucks. Items were placed in their approximate final locations, although some refinement was needed. The pharmacy was set up in the old art room; the clinic to receive patients was located in the gym; and the team took over a smaller workout room next to the showers for its dormitory.

The building had sustained minor damage on its south side so that section of the building was closed off. The building had running water but no electricity or heat. The team used flashlights and daylight to illuminate their work. They located containers that could be filled with ice to store the vaccine when it arrived. Because it was so hot, ice was also used to treat patients suffering from heat-related illness as well as for cold compresses.

Without electricity, the pharmacy had to be organized using paper files and handwritten information. The team had thought to pre-print labels and use small zip-lock plastic baggies for dispensing. Preparing sterile intravenous medications would be a challenge since they would not be able to run a laminar airflow hood. The medication supply consisted primarily of intravenous fluids and antibiotics, oral antibiotics, narcotic pain relievers, an anti-anxiety medication, and vaccines. Other medications, such as those the victims may have lost or left behind when they were evacuated, would have to be obtained from pharmacies in the surrounding area.

In the gym, the team prepared an intake station near the doors to control the incoming flow of victims and allow the intake team to triage them into those who need immediate help and those who can wait. Triage optimizes the use of limited medical resources. Originally designed to help determine who should be given priority in transporting from the disaster site to a care site, triage can be thought of a general approach to sorting disaster victims into (1) those who are beyond saving, (2) those who can be saved with immediate intervention, (3) those whose injuries are not immediately life-threatening and can wait, and (4) those whose injuries do not require medical care. At the DMAT site, the intake team will determine the nature of the victims' injuries and send them to the appropriate treatment area. The gym at the school had a waiting area for minor injuries, an immediate care area for serious injuries, and a stabilize-and-transport area for those with potentially life-threatening injuries. Initially, no system was in place for helping victims who had lost medications for chronic conditions because it was not deemed a critical or large-scale problem. This floor plan meant the pharmacy team would receive some patients directly from the intake station and others from the immediate or delayed care areas after they had been seen by a physician or nurse.

First 72 Hours

During the initial 3 days, the pharmacy dispensed antibiotics and pain medication, administered vaccines, prepared intravenous fluids and medications, and tried to find medications for chronic conditions. By the third day, the pharmacy team was getting creative in its substitutions for chronic medications. They had the approval of the medical officer who fully understood their predicament. They had local volunteers assist each day. In addition, three helicopter pads were used to bring injured victims rescued from rooftops and transport seriously injured people to a surgical site in a nearby community.

On the third day, a small party of DMAT volunteers went to nearby pharmacies and hospitals to secure additional supplies since their replacement items had not yet appeared. At one point, they were near a very devastated area. Lyle was struck by the extent of the devastation. Not even a street sign was available to help them find their way to the area hospital where some spare morphine was waiting. If it hadn't been for the help of a survivor from the neighborhood, they would have been hopelessly lost.

By the third day, the DMAT team was joined by troops from the Army but their portion of the Strategic National Stockpile had not yet arrived. On the fifth day, a 10-day supply of narcotic pain relievers and antibiotics arrived and replenished the almost depleted supplies. On the fourth day, the DMAT team was asked to send a small contingent of volunteers to four nearby **Red Cross shelters** to begin immunizing against water-borne illnesses.

Throughout the effort, Lyle and the pharmacy team had to scramble to provide additional medications for chronic conditions. They opted to fill a 3-day supply in the hopes that the person would soon be able to get evacuated to another site where he could receive a full supply of the lost medications.

Rumors and Other Distractions

Reports coming in via battery-operated radios and cell phones included news of looting and shooting in areas of New Orleans and other devastated communities, an increasing body count as more victims were found, and ongoing problems with evacuating people to emergency shelters. The weather remained in the 90s with high humidity, and ice was becoming a rare and valuable commodity. There were reports of killings related to fights over bags of ice. Lyle was astounded to think that they might have to put the water bottles and ice in the locked room where the narcotics were currently being secured. There were also reports of water-borne and food-borne illnesses spreading in other coastal communities. Lyle couldn't help but compare the conditions to a third-world country during war as he researched information on the symptoms and treatment of cholera, diphtheria, and botulism.

Second Week

The DMAT team spent its second week at a critical care hospital about 100 miles north of their initial site. They provided additional manpower and support for the facility as it dealt with the influx of critically injured patients. In this setting, the routine was more similar to a normal work load except for the large number of patients. The hospital opened two additional care sites to handle the overflow of injured patients while maintaining care of its current patients. In addition to the hospital work, Lyle and his pharmacy team visited two Red Cross shelters to meet with evacuees who were in need of medications for chronic use. By this time, contingency agreements were in place to allow dispensing for prescriptions from other states and emergency fills on medications for chronic conditions regardless of ability to pay. A temporary emergency pharmacy had also opened in the area, and Lyle was able to provide them with a list of patient names and medications for the shelter residents.

Debriefing

After 14 days in the region, the DMAT team was relieved by a new team. On their return trip to Ohio, the team stopped to debrief in the comfort of an air-conditioned building with lights, hot showers, and warm meals. During the session, the members discussed their successes and frustrations and shared stories and reactions. They also discussed some of the potential delayed psychological effects they were likely to experience and planned a followup phone conference to check on each other in 2 weeks.

Evaluation

The full evaluation of the DMAT and its site would be conducted after the team had returned home; however, some formative evaluations were conducted to help the team adjust its efforts and revise some of its strategies during its response. That data is reported here.

Objective data

The DMAT site served a total of 15,200 patients in the first 72 hours. On the first day, 4,500 patients were treated, most of whom had minor injuries that were quickly resolved. By the second day, more seriously injured patients were delivered via automobile and helicopter. That day, about 6,050 victims were triaged and treated as needed. By the third day, another 4,650 patients were seen. Most were suffering from traumatic injuries, heat exhaustion and dehydration, and infection. Many had underlying chronic conditions that were not currently being treated including hypertension, diabetes, heart disease, and arthritis. At the site, 98 deaths were reported due to lack of sufficient transportation for some of the more critically ill patients.

The DMAT used 92% of its narcotics, 91% of its antibiotics, and 46% of its vaccines within the first 72 hours. The vaccination clinic provided immunizations for almost 8,200 people in surrounding shelters during the first week. They did not track the amount of water or ice consumed by patients or used as part of the storage or treatment effort.

Subjective data

The DMAT volunteers experienced several strong emotions when faced with the enormous task of providing care for another 15,000 victims. Annoyance at the lack of electricity and air conditioning that they felt when setting up the clinic was dwarfed by the stunned faces of victims who had lost all their possessions and hadn't had food or water for almost 2 days. Their gratitude for the simplest gesture and help kept the medical volunteers going for long 16-hour shifts. By the second day, the endless lines of injured and sick began to wear on the volunteers. Some said they began to feel like life would never be normal again. The sad stories of loss, families separated and pets abandoned, looters and shootings, delayed rescues, and despair accompanied the process. A month after returning home, a number of volunteers reported difficulty sleeping and some depression. In spite of the difficulties, all the volunteers said they would go again.

The delay in getting the SNS supplies replenished added to the stress of having to decide which patients would receive a medication. Lack of access to basic equipment, supplies, or even electricity made every procedure and encounter more difficult. The need for better communication and organization at a higher level became apparent within the first 4 days.

As hard as the work was, many team members admitted that they had a difficult time leaving a place with so much need. Once they had actually left, they just wanted to get home and resisted stopping for a debriefing session. This session was the idea of several experienced team members who were concerned about unspoken emotions and concerns. At the end of the session, team members all agreed it was a good way to clear the air and record their observations, frustrations, and lessons learned.

Analysis and interpretation of response

The DMAT was able to arrive and set up its clinical services quickly and effectively. Its presence provided care for 15,200 victims of the hurricane. The supplies were sufficient for the 72-hour window, but delays in replenishing the supplies led to desperate attempts to locate items in nearby areas, some of which were dangerous due to hurricane and flood damage. Better communication and organization at the federal level is needed for a response of this magnitude. All the volunteers experienced emotional and physical effects, but it would not deter them from going on the next deployment.

Lyle's personal assessment

Now that Lyle has some first-hand experience with disaster response, he could be an even more valuable member of a local disaster planning group. He should consider approaching the Littlesburg LEPC and asking to be added to their group. He could be especially helpful in planning the mass casualty dispensing clinics for the community and county. These mass care sites are critical for disasters where surviving pharmacies, clinics, and hospitals will be quickly overwhelmed by the large number of individuals seeking care. To deal with the sudden increase in patients, something referred to as "surge capacity," many communities have plans to provide alternative treatment sites and mass dispensing clinics in addition to the usual care facilities. Lyle could think about becoming involved in this type of planning and training, too. His experience with the large field clinic in Mississippi will give him a good idea for organizing the floor plan and coordinating the flow of patients through the care site. Lyle's knowledge of his own community, including buildings and general traffic patterns, will help him adapt mass dispensing clinic plans to Littlesburg. Finally, he should also offer to share his experiences and knowledge with other pharmacists and pharmacy students to increase their interest in disaster response and planning.

Regardless of Lyle's intentions to continue his work in emergency preparedness, he must plan to be proactive. Outside of the pharmacy profession, emergency preparedness efforts typically don't include pharmacists. Even groups that include pharmacists in their work tend to limit their roles to dispensing. The good news is that most planning groups come to value pharmacists as they work with them and gain an appreciation of their contributions.

Discussion

Options for participation

Lyle had other options to help with the Hurricane Katrina response such as training to become an emergency volunteer for the American Red Cross. In that capacity, he would provide general support at evacuation shelters closer to the disaster or help with other Red Cross services. This approach would probably not use his pharmacy expertise, which is something he specifically wanted to do. Another option for Lyle would have been to fill in for other pharmacists who were deployed, which works most easily when both pharmacists are employed by the same organization. In Lyle's case, his colleagues covered for him during his 2-week deployment in which he spent his last week covering for pharmacists at a hospital located near the disaster site.

Lyle could also have opted to become part of the National Pharmacy Response Team (NPRT) instead of a DMAT. As a federal response team, he would have had similar training, application to regional team, and equivalent credential requirements as the DMAT experience. The NPRT may be more focused on establishing dispensing services for displaced and evacuated victims rather than primary care, but the scope of the roles can easily overlap between DMAT and NPRT during the initial response.

Liability and employment issues

Prior to leaving, Lyle looked into two important professional issues: covering his absence from work and professional liability. As a member of a regional DMAT, Lyle is considered a temporary employee or agent of the federal government. This status allows him to receive compensation (i.e., wage) and reimbursement for travel and *per diem* expenses. His current license in Ohio is recognized in all states as legal while he is working for the federal group. He also has liability protection through the **Federal Tort Claims Act (FTCA)** as long as he provides care to victims in good faith (i.e., to the benefit of the patient as much as possible in a situation and with potentially limited resources) and within an acceptable scope of practice. In addition, most states recognize the unusual situation created by disasters and will offer **"Good Samaritan" laws** as protection for volunteer responders (i.e., not employed by state or federal government) who act in good faith and within acceptable practice. Acts considered appropriate or acceptable scope of practice within a disaster response may be interpreted more broadly from the usual standards, but they should not be intentional acts to harm or take advantage of victims. Unusual practices, such as allowing hospital emergency departments to refuse new patients and send them to an alternate mass care site, are legal in an emergency as long as the disaster plan spells out when such sites can be used and when hospital emergency departments can send patients to them. In normal circumstances, it is generally illegal for hospital emergency departments to refuse care.

Another issue deployed medical volunteers or NDMS participants may face is ensuring that they will not lose their job because they are deployed for several weeks. It makes sense that this issue should be discussed up front with the employer, but a federal law also protects citizens who take time away from work to provide services for the countries. The employment protection for privately employed pharmacists like Lyle who deploy with a NDMS team comes from the **Uniformed Services Employment and Reemployment Rights Act (USERRA)**. If a response team member is already a federal employee, such as an **IHS** or **PHS** pharmacist, then the deployment is considered part of his or her existing job.[9,10]

Populations made vulnerable by a disaster

Another issue created by disasters, which is people rendered vulnerable by the disaster and its aftermath, is one that can be easily overlooked when planning for response and recovery. Within any community at any time are subgroups of the population with unmet health needs. In a normal situation, these people typically are economically or educationally disadvantaged, very young and very old, disabled, or culturally different from the general population. Communities often have services and programs designed to improve access to care and reduce health risks for these populations. Unfortunately, during a disaster, especially one that creates a lot of destruction of buildings and services, these safety net services are no longer available. Therefore, planning needs to consider how the loss of services and infrastructure will affect groups especially vulnerable to health risks. For example, older residents who can no longer drive may use bus services to go grocery shopping and run errands. Some may receive their meals through a "meals-on-wheels" type of program and have their prescription medications delivered or mailed to their homes. For some, home maintenance may be foregone because of expense or inability to perform needed tasks. Retirement funds may become insufficient due to inflation and the rising cost of living, and the older residents may have to reduce heat or turn off the air conditioner. Many older residents become less social, and their family networks are spread across the country with no one living nearby. In a sudden, catastrophic event where all local services grind to a halt, the older resident may quickly find him- or herself isolated without phone service, heat or water, no transportation, and no information about what is happening or where to go for help. This scenario could also impact younger adults and children, so age is not the only factor in creating a vulnerable population. For some, language and cultural barriers could further hinder understanding and subsequent ability to act in a manner that reduces health risks. Imagine not understanding a simple order to boil water due to a language barrier or poor understanding of how microorganisms can spread disease.

Another group of individuals not usually considered vulnerable in normal circumstances are health care workers. In the case of a chemical or biological disaster, this population has a much greater risk of contamination, illness, and death because of their role in rendering care. Most disaster plans recognize this risk and provide guidelines for decontaminating and isolating victims to control the spread of the disease or exposure.

Chapter 17 Summary

This chapter described the activities of one pharmacist who becomes part of the national disaster response M (NDRM) system through a disaster medical A team (DMAT). Already involved in local response efforts through his Red Cross Disaster Services training, the pharmacist sought an avenue where he could apply his pharmacy knowledge. The structure of the national response team was described as well as the training and deployment planning each team member must complete. The actual experiences gained through deployment are described in the implementation section. Throughout the deployment implementation and evaluation, the myriad of issues and concerns a pharmacist faces while participating on a national response team are described. The pharmacist has federal liability and employment protections in place because he was deployed as part of a federal team. Upon returning to his community, the pharmacist brings knowledge and skills related to mass dispensing clinics that can be incorporated into local plans.

References

1. United Nations International Strategy for Disaster Reduction (ISDR). Disaster Occurrence 1900–2005, UN ISDR web site. Available at: http://www.unisdr.org/disaster-statistics/occurrence-trends-century. htm. Accessed December 2, 2008.

2. U.S. Department of State, Country Reports on Terrorism (updated April 30, 2008), National Counterterrorism Center: Annex of Statistical Information web site. Available at: http://www.state.gov/s/ct/rls/crt/2007/103716.htm. Accessed December 2, 2008.

3. Cohen V. Organization of a health-system pharmacy team to respond to episodes of terrorism. *Am J Health-Syst Pharm.* 2003; 60:1257–63.

4. American Red Cross web site. Disaster Services and Blood Services links. Available at: http://www.redcross.org/index.html. Accessed March 3, 2008.

5. National Disaster Medical System, U.S. Department of Health and Human Services. Web site available at: http://www.hhs.gov/aspr/opeo/ndms/index.html. Accessed March 3, 2008.

6. OHIO 1 DMAT web site. Available at: http://www.oh1dmat.org/blog/. Accessed March 2, 2008.

7. Emergency Management Institute of FEMA. IS-100: Introduction to Incident Command System, I-100. Available at: http://www.training.fema.gov/emiweb/is/is100.asp. Accessed March 3, 2008.

8. How to Pack. Michigan 1 (MI-1) DMAT web site. Available at: http://www.mi1dmat.org/How%20 to%20Pack.htm. Accessed March 3, 2008.

9. Uniformed Services Employment and Reemployment Rights Act (USERRA). Available at: http://www.hhs.gov/aspr/opeo/ndms/join/userra.html. Accessed March 3, 2008.

10. Federal Tort Claims Act. While deployed, DMAT members are considered federal employees, which entitle them to coverage by the Federal Tort Claims Act. http://www.fas.org/sgp/crs/misc/95-717.pdf. Accessed March 3, 2008.

Suggested Readings

Bratberg J. Hurricane Katrina: pharmacists making a difference. *JAPhA.* 2005; 45(6):654–8.

Gavagan TF, Smart K, Palacio H, et al. Hurricane Katrina: medical response at the Houston Astrodome/Reliant Center Complex [CME topic]. *Southern Med J.* 2006; 99(9):933–9.

Velazquez L, Dallas S, Rose L, et al. A PHS pharmacist team's response to Hurricane Katrina. *Am J Health-Syst Pharm.* 2006; 63:1332–5.

Vankawala HH. Medical triage at its most basic [on the front lines of Hurricane Katrina]. *Emerg Med News.* 2005; 27(10):1–12.

American Red Cross Disaster Services web site. Available at: http://www.redcross.org/services/disaster/0,1082,0_319_,00.html.

National Disaster Medical System (NDMS) web site. Available at: http://www.hhs.gov/aspr/opeo/ndms/index.html.

Centers for Disease Control and Prevention (CDC) Emergency Preparedness and Response web site. Available at: http://www.bt.cdc.gov/.

Federal Emergency Management Agency (FEMA). Emergency Management Institute (EMI) web page. Contains training materials for incident command systems. Available at: http://www.training.fema.gov/.

Chapter 17 Review Questions

1. **Describe two natural and two manmade disasters that could potentially occur in Lyle's community of Littlesburg, Ohio.**

Natural disaster risks: ice storms and other winter weather, flooding rivers, winter.

Manmade disaster risks: chemical spills from pesticide plants or release of radioactive substances from nuclear plant, bridge, or earthen dam collapse; spills from passing trains or trucks on the interstate.

2. **Discuss the activities that Lyle, in his professional capacity as a pharmacist, could participate in before, during, and after a disaster.**

Before: plan for pharmacy or community response, train to be a responder, improve knowledge of risks and their treatments, prepare a family or personal emergency kit and plan.

During: work with other responders or receivers, deploy with response team, fill in positions vacated by others who are deployed, offer both personal and professional skills, continue normal operations as much as possible, monitor for outbreaks of disease or other health risks created by loss of infrastructure.

After: work to return to normal routine, review how well efforts worked, replace used supplies and prepare for next disaster, monitor self and others for long-term psychological and behavioral effects.

3. **Using Lyle's experience, explain the role of federal medical teams (e.g., DMAT) in disaster response and ways that a pharmacist can contribute to the efforts of such teams.**

Role of federal teams: These groups of health care professionals are often tasked with creating new care sites to handle the surge of injured or exposed victims. Some groups like DMAT have a variety of disciplines to ensure a range of services can be provided, while others like NPRT have a more focused mission related to pharmacy services and pharmaceuticals. Both require training and participation in drills to ensure preparedness to respond.

Pharmacist contributions: These efforts include setting up dispensing clinics, providing information to victims, and supporting other health care professionals. Pharmacists could be involved in triaging patients by their need for treatment or post-exposure prophylaxis. They should be able to receive, store, secure, and monitor medication supplies.

4. **Give two examples each of objective and subjective data used to evaluate pharmacy services provided by Lyle's DMAT team.**

Objective data: number of patients seen each day, number of medications used by category, number of types of diagnoses by general classes.

Subjective data: satisfaction with and perceived effectiveness of the services by victim and health care provider comments, feelings of response team after completing the 2-week deployment.

5. **Describe how Lyle's practice of pharmacy during his disaster response in Mississippi probably differed from his usual routine at his Ohio practice site.**

The first difference of note is the physical working environment. During the response, Lyle did not have computer support, electricity, or running water. He had to improvise with ice to store refrigerated items like vaccines and use water sparingly. He worked longer hours than a typical 8–10 hour shift and served many more people. It sounds like he had to improvise with the records system too—using paper and pencil to record information and track the distribution and dispensing of the inventory. He also had to organize the supplies from the SNS and participate in a search for more resources from local sources. In the second week, he practiced as a pharmacist in a hospital rather than a retail setting. It was another difference between his usual routine and the response routine.

Applying Your Knowledge

1. **Consider the community where you now live or the one where you grew up. What are the risks for a natural or manmade disaster in that community?**

2. **How can pharmacists be involved in mass dispensing or mass vaccination clinics?**

3. What is the plan in your state and county for receiving and distributing the contents of the Strategic National Stockpile during a disaster? How can pharmacy students be involved in the process?

4. Locate a hospital, county, state, or national disaster plan—either an all-hazards plan or one for a specific disaster (e.g., influenza pandemic). Look at the plan and describe the types of problems that are identified and addressed. Is there anything else you would add?

5. Look at your state's emergency declaration wording. Does it cover emergency dispensing by pharmacists? Does it specifically ban it? What options would you have for providing medications and pharmacy services if all of the existing pharmacy resources in your community were severely damaged or eliminated during a disaster?

Domestic Violence Prevention: Improving Services for Perpetrators

Learning Outcomes

1. Identify one example each of subjective and objective data to collect for determining the need for a program to address services for domestic violence perpetrators.
2. Identify three risk factors for domestic violence.
3. Differentiate between individual and population level risk factors for domestic violence.
4. Identify at least one measure that would appropriately evaluate a community forum.
5. Discuss the rationale for pharmacists' participation in efforts to address domestic violence.

Introduction

Public health is aimed at improving health and preventing illness. Because health determinants operate at the level of the person and the community, efforts to improve health and prevent illness must occur at both levels. For health issues like domestic violence, a comprehensive approach is required for prevention because treating the victim after an incident does not address the causes of domestic violence. Pharmacists who want to become involved in addressing the causes of poor health that result from domestic violence must be willing to address the determinants of health at the community level.

This chapter begins by discussing the epidemiology, health consequences, and risk factors for domestic violence. Then the activities of a community coalition, which includes a pharmacist, are described. The coalition is formed to address how perpetrators of domestic violence are treated in the community. The example uses the basic SOAPE framework of the public health process: subjective data, objective data, assessment, planning and implementation, and evaluation. The example begins with background on the community and its efforts to address domestic violence and then describes a community forum for stakeholders involved in providing services for perpetrators of domestic violence. The chapter ends with a discussion of pharmacists' roles in health co-alitions such as the domestic violence coalition, characteristics of community health and the relationship of health determinants to the health care system, and the importance of addressing population (community) as well as individual level health determinants.

Public Health Issue: Domestic Violence

Epidemiology

Domestic violence, also known as intimate partner violence, involves intimate relation-ships characterized by abuse; it includes physical abuse, sexual abuse, threats of either physical abuse or sexual abuse, and emotional abuse. Domestic violence is a significant public health issue. Some 4.8 million women and 2.9 million men experience domestic violence annually in the United States. Additionally, in 2004, domestic violence resulted in 1,544 deaths; of these, 75% were women and 25% men. The cost to society is high—domestic violence resulted in an estimated cost of $8.3 billion in 2003. Most costs, 70% or $5.8 billion, are attributed to increased medical and mental health expenses. The remaining 30% or $2.5 billion results from the indirect costs of lost productivity.[1,2]

Health consequences

The consequences of domestic violence can be physical, psychological, social, and behavioral. Victims of domestic violence may experience physical injury such as bruises, broken bones, headaches, gynecological disorders, and gastrointestinal disorders. Chil-dren may be included in the violence; children of abused mothers are 57 times more likely to have been injured if their mother is being abused than are children in non-abusive households. Psychological consequences include reduced self-esteem, depression, and symptoms of post-traumatic stress disorder. Social consequences include inability to access services, strained relationships with employers, and social isolation from family and friends. Women with a history of domestic violence are more likely to engage in be-haviors that are detrimental to health including high-risk sexual behavior, smoking, illicit drug use, unhealthy eating behaviors, and overuse of health services.[1,2]

Risk factors

Risk factors for experiencing domestic violence include a history of abuse; being younger than 35; being single, divorced, or separated; being of a lower socioeconomic status; substance abuse, including abuse of medications and prescription drugs; smoking; and problem drinking (four or more drinks on one occasion in the past 30 days). Of the general population, about 25% of women report having experienced physical or sexual abuse in their lifetime. For women, being pregnant, having a physical disability, or being elderly and frail increase the risk of domestic violence.[1,2]

Risk factors for perpetrating domestic violence include psychological factors, rela-tionship factors, community factors, and societal factors. Psychological characteristics such as antisocial or borderline personality, low self-esteem, and poor impulse control are associated with domestic violence as is a history of violence in other situations or having been a victim of abuse. Relationship factors include marital conflict, economic stress, unhealthy relationships such as dominance or control over others, and economic stress. Community factors include poverty, low social capital (lack of institutions or norms that shape a community's social interactions), and weak community sanctions against domestic violence. Societal factors related to beliefs about gender roles also can increase risk for domestic violence in a community.[1]

Model Program

 ### A Community Forum on Services for Perpetrators

Background
Lena is a 28-year-old staff pharmacist in a 150-bed community hospital in Grangewood, a city of about 86,000. It is located in a suburb of a metropolitan area of about 2.5 million in the Midwest. Lena has been working with the emergency department (ED) to reorganize stock medications and review the formulary to reduce the number of special requests for out-of-stock medications. It is a particular problem when the ED is very busy. The process required a substantial amount of data collection and data analysis to identify and implement new procedures. Lena's ability to collect and analyze data became known; therefore, she was asked to retrieve and analyze data related to victims of domestic violence seen in the ED. A domestic violence coalition, formed with the objective of improving services for victims, requested the data. The coalition was trying to evaluate the outcomes of their efforts. The data they were analyzing was collected on domestic violence following the development of new protocols, including data collection requirements, now used in the ED. The group wanted to determine the status of treatment for domestic violence now that the protocols had been used for several years.

Domestic Violence Coalition
The coalition consisted of eight to 10 community members, primarily involved in health care, who were trying to improve the treatment of domestic violence victims in the community. The coalition had worked hard over the past several years and felt like they had greatly improved services for victims. They had helped revise the domestic violence protocols used by the county; increased the number of women who were routinely screened for domestic violence; and enhanced several programs serving the victims.

Lena had been invited to a meeting of the domestic violence coalition. At first, she hesitated because pharmacists don't usually get involved in social problems. However, other coalition members assured Lena that they did not have specific training in domestic violence. Their training and work were related to their professions; however, they all had an interest in improving the health of community members. Anyone who shared their interest in community health was welcome.

Services for Perpetrators
At the last meeting of the domestic violence coalition, Lena and several members discussed treatment of **perpetrators**. A counselor from a local guidance center had the impression that not much happened to perpetrators. The counselor did not believe that perpetrators were participating in counseling programs, and he wondered why. The coalition members also discussed how treating the victims of domestic violence addressed only half the problem. The coalition decided to investigate the treatment of perpetrators of domestic violence to determine what services were available for them and if services needed to be or could be improved.

Subjective Data

The first thing that the domestic violence coalition decided was to collect data on the services available for perpetrators and information about how they were treated in the community. The members of the coalition had to admit that they really did not know how perpetrators were treated. Coalition members would collect both subjective and **objective data**; the **subjective data** would reflect the opinions of the **stakeholders** in the community on the treatment of perpetrators, and the objective data would reveal how many perpetrators currently were receiving treatment in the city and the county. The assessment process would allow all members of the coalition to develop a common understanding of the problem so that they would be able to identify aspects of the perpetrators' treatment that might be amenable to change.[3]

Key informant interviews

To collect subjective data, interviews were conducted with **key informants** in the community. Key informants included anyone in the community who had an interest in or who was involved with the treatment of domestic violence victims or perpetrators. Lena said that she would be glad to help with collecting the interview data. She agreed to interview someone from the city police department to determine what happened when the police received a domestic violence call and, specifically, what happened to the perpetrator. Another coalition member would interview someone from the county sheriff's office, and a third person would interview the director of the guidance center.

The decision to collect data from law enforcement and from the justice system, which did not provide health care and didn't seem to have much to do with health, caused discomfort for several members of the coalition. Based on the understanding that health resulted from factors other than health care services, members decided that they needed to know how law enforcement and the justice system contributed either positively or negatively to the health problem of domestic violence. Then the coalition could decide if they could do anything related to perpetrators outside the health care system.

Key informant data

Coalition members used the form in Figure 18.1 to collect the data from the interviews. This tool was designed to obtain data on how each agency was involved in the treatment of domestic violence perpetrators as well as what the interviewee thought were the strengths and weaknesses of the program.

The interview with the director of the counseling agency indicated that he thought few perpetrators were being appropriately treated in the community. Although the guidance center offered anger management classes to perpetrators of domestic violence, few of them were referred for counseling; of those referred, few completed the counseling program.

Figure 18.1—Example Opinion Survey for Collecting Subjective Data about the Treatment of Perpetrators of Domestic Violence

---

Community Opinion Interview Guide: Perpetrators of Domestic Violence

1. How are you or your agency involved in the treatment of perpetrators of domestic violence?

2. From your perspective, what works best in your program?

3. What are the problems with the treatment of perpetrators of domestic violence in your community?

4. Which one of these problems do you consider to be the most important one?

5. What do you think could be done to improve the treatment of perpetrators in your community?

6. Can you suggest any other people with whom I might talk about the treatment of perpetrators of domestic violence?

Thank you for your help. Right now I do not have any more questions, but I may contact you in the future if other issues come up.

Informant Demographics

(Collect demographic data on a separate sheet of paper; informant demographics should not be associated with data.)

7. Sex: ___Female ___Male

8. Ethnicity: ___White ___Black ___Hispanic ___American Indian ___Asian ___Other

9. Affiliation:_____

10. Number of years at agency/organization: ___years

11. Number of years lived in community: ___years

12. Commutes from outside the community: ___Yes ___No

Interviews of the key informants from the sheriff's office, the city prosecutor, the city magistrate judge, the justice of the peace, and the county attorney revealed that perpetrators are referred to three different courts: the city court presided over by the city magistrate, the justice court presided over by the justice of peace, and the superior court presided over by a superior court judge.

Objective Data

Community characteristics
Grangewood's location as a suburb of a larger metropolitan area has strongly influenced the characteristics of the community. The town was originally a stop on the railroad to the metro area where produce and other foodstuffs were transported to the metro area. In the past 30 years, the community had changed from a primarily agricultural focus to a mix of residential developments and smaller manufacturing plants located near the toll road and the railroad. The community's agricultural heritage was still evident. New housing developments were built in corn fields, and anyone traveling away from the town and the metro area is immediately engulfed in corn fields.

The original town now constitutes the Old Town, while several new shopping centers and office complexes have been built in the newer areas of the city. The hospital is relatively new and is located away from the commercial and industrial areas close to several of the newer subdivisions.

The primary and secondary school systems are generally quite good, but the nearest college is a junior college in a neighboring suburb. For most residents, training for a profession or skilled occupation requires relocating or commuting to the metro area.

Population characteristics
The population is predominantly white (78%), and so is the county where the city is located. A small black population, about 10%, has resided in the area since the construction of several manufacturing plants and growth of the service industry. Recent immigrants from the Middle East and the former republics of the old Soviet Union make up the other 12% of the population. At least half the population is relatively new to the city; they have been living there for less than a generation so their parents live elsewhere and their children have not yet become independent adults. Despite the size of the city, few young adults live there. Most are either attending college somewhere else or otherwise being trained for careers outside the city.

Unemployment is relatively low, about 5% for the past year. However, the **median income** for the city is 8% below that of the state because much of the employment is in low-paying service jobs. About 16% of the population has incomes less than 200% of the **federal poverty level**.

The general educational level of the community is average—about 25% of adults have a college degree, another 10% have completed some college, and the high school graduation rate is about 85%. The population is relatively young, with most of the population working-age adults; however, the population of older women is significant.

Community data on treatment of perpetrators
Objective data was collected on the numbers of domestic violence victims and perpetrators in counseling and on the numbers of victims using legal aid. One of the local guidance centers reported 83 domestic violence victims were referred for services last month, but only five perpetrators were known to be in counseling. Of the last 700 people using legal aid, about half have domestic violence issues but counseling groups for perpetrators include only 18 to 25 people at a time. The city attorney's office reported that some perpetrators were able to avoid counseling for as long as 5 years.

Assessment

Data analysis

Findings from Key Informant Interviews
Three different types of agencies were identified as being involved in the treatment of perpetrators: law enforcement, criminal justice, and health care. (Health care participated primarily through counseling services.) Particular problems seemed to occur when perpetrators were placed on unsupervised probation or were referred to counseling without concurrent probation. Non-compliance with sentencing typically was not detected until the individual was involved in a subsequent violation or crime. However, perpetrators sentenced to probation were followed by a probation officer who made sure that the individual was compliant.

In general, perpetrators were treated differently depending on the discretion of the officer who responded to the domestic violence call, on the discretion of the city and county attorneys, and on the discretion of the judges who ruled on individual cases. For example, if a perpetrator appeared before the justice of the peace and did not abuse drugs or alcohol, he typically recommended that the perpetrator be released to unsupervised counseling.

Interviews of representatives of the different agencies also revealed that there was no general knowledge of what each agency did related to perpetrators of domestic violence and how their actions related to the actions of other agencies. Thus, the city and the county did not seem to have a coordinated plan about processing perpetrators through the system and requirements for doing so. Further, agencies did not seem to have a method of tracking perpetrators and assuring that they completed their mandated treatment.

Data interpretation

Assessment Summary
The findings from the key informant assessment are summarized in Figure 18.2. In general, perpetrators of domestic violence were not receiving treatment either because they were not compliant with sentences or because they were dropped from the justice system at the discretion of an officer, attorney, or judge. Further, a lack of coordination seemed to exist among agencies that dealt with perpetrators of domestic violence.

The findings from the objective data documented that perpetrators were not receiving services even if the services were mandated by the courts.

Figure 18.2—Framework for Analyzing Data Obtained through the Opinion Survey on the Treatment of Perpetrators of Domestic Violence

Summary of Opinion Survey Data

Date data collected: From __Feb 2007__ to __May 2007__

Total number of people interviewed: __25__   Number of interviewers:__6__

Rank	Issues Identified	Number of Persons Identifying Issue	Percentage of Persons Identifying Issue
1.	Perpetrators do not attend counseling	5	20%
2.	Primary determinant of treatment is at the discretion of individual officers, attorneys, or judges	11	44%
3.	Services among agencies were not coordinated	13	52%
4.	Perpetrators who failed to adhere to sentencing guidelines were not identified in a timely manner	8	32%

Planning

Plan

The coalition met and reviewed the findings from the assessment. A group discussion followed as they attempted to define the next step in addressing the treatment of domestic violence perpetrators. Changes to the current system of treating perpetrators depended primarily on the law enforcement and the justice systems; hence, any attempts to modify the process would require involvement from those agencies. The coalition decided that the best place to begin would be a forum in which their findings about perpetrator treatment were presented to stakeholders from law enforcement and the justice system. Through a forum, the members of the coalition could describe the current situation to stakeholders and discuss options for improving treatment.

The coalition members decided to meet every other week until the forum was held. The plan was to have an update on the progress of planning for the forum and to work on the presentation for the forum.

The domestic violence coordinator from the county health department agreed that the services of her office could be used to make the arrangements for the community forum. The judge of the superior court offered the courtroom as a meeting site for the forum. The coalition members, including Lena, prepared charts on newsprint to present a summary of their findings. Stakeholders from the justice system were identified, and invitations to the forum were extended.

Forum agenda

An agenda was developed and sent to everyone invited to the forum. As listed on the agenda, everyone introduced themselves and identified the agency that they represented (see Figure 18.3). The presentation would begin with a brief history of the domestic violence coalition, its activities over the past several years, and the impetus for addressing issues with the perpetrators of domestic violence. The findings of the domestic violence coalition related to the treatment of perpetrators would be presented, followed by an open discussion of the route taken by the perpetrator through the system. At this point, attendees would have an opportunity to correct information or to enhance the information provided. If needed, a discussion of the strengths and weaknesses of the current system would be facilitated. The last item on the agenda would be the development of an action plan.

Figure 18.3—Agenda for Forum

Agenda: Forum on the Treatment of Perpetrators of Domestic Violence

1. Introduce attendees (attendees introduce themselves and identify the agency that they represent)

2. Review purpose of the forum

3. Present findings from subjective and objective data collection; include flow chart of how a perpetrator entered and went through the system; obtain feedback on the accuracy of the flowchart

4. Facilitate discussion of how perpetrators were treated

5. Develop action plan

6. Thank everyone for attending

7. Adjourn meeting

Implementation

Forum setting and attendees

The forum met on a Thursday morning when court was not in session. Eight members of the coalition attended; fortunately, Lena was able to trade her weekday hours for some weekend hours so that she could attend the meeting. Stakeholders from the justice system and law enforcement included the county attorney, the superior court judge, the city attorney, two representatives from the police department, and a deputy from the sheriff's department. From the health care system, the director of the guidance center attended and so did a nurse from the hospital emergency department and the director of nursing services at the clinic. Two persons also attended from a non-profit organization that provided court-mandated educational sessions for domestic violence, substance use, and alcohol abuse.

Conduct of the meeting

The actual meeting did not require a lot of facilitation. After the presentation, attendees pointed out gaps in the information, expressed frustration with what their agency was able to accomplish, and clarified their understanding of the process. A consensus emerged: a case-manager position or something similar was needed to ensure that paperwork was transferred in a timely manner and that perpetrators did not "fall through the cracks."

Action plan

Four actions were identified for community agencies to minimize the perpetrator's ability to manipulate the system, including:

- Add a case management position to the system. This position would assign a specific person to track perpetrators through the system to assure coordination and reduce time to follow up if the perpetrator does not comply.
- Address the issue of prosecutorial discretion. Currently, perpetrators may not be held accountable based on the judgment of the arresting officer, the attorney, or a judge.
- Improve support for the victim services program. This program is essential to encouraging victims to testify; if the victim fails to testify, there may be no consequences to the perpetrator.
- Modify the police data form so that domestic violence is clearly documented.

The attendees decided to meet again the following week to discuss a case management position and its possible location. The agenda for the next meeting also would include a discussion about possibly getting a grant to hire someone for the paperwork processing related to domestic violence. The general consensus was that perpetrators should be held accountable for their actions and that the ultimate goal was to prevent domestic violence incidents.

Evaluation

Subjective data

In their planning meetings, the coalition members also discussed how they would evaluate the outcomes of the forum. Because the forum by itself would not directly affect a perpetrator or a victim of domestic violence, measures of change in health status would not be appropriate for this intervention. Lena, who had helped with evaluation of other domestic violence activities, suggested that the forum be evaluated by its outcomes and by the number of agencies invited that actually sent a representative and participated meaningfully in the discussion. The forum would be considered successful if all invited agencies sent a representative, if attendees participated in the discussion, and if an action plan was developed to address how perpetrators of domestic violence were treated.

Data from the meeting indicated that all invited agencies had sent representatives, discussion had been substantial, and the group clearly had an action plan for addressing the issues related to perpetrators of domestic violence.

Objective data

A representative from the domestic violence coalition continued to attend the followup meetings related to perpetrators and reported back to the coalition that a case manager had been hired within 6 months. Followup with the director of the guidance center also indicated that the number of perpetrators of domestic violence treated at the center had increased from 5 to 43 since the forum.

Interpretation of data

When the coalition met and reviewed the evaluation data, they considered the forum a success. In fact, they were more successful than originally anticipated; within 6 months, a case manager had been hired and the number of perpetrators in treatment had increased. It seemed like community stakeholders had been ready to address the issue but just needed someone to collect the relevant data and convene a meeting.

Discussion

Pharmacists' role in community health

The characteristics of the coalition activities that are likely to be most noticeable to a pharmacist or a pharmacy student are the absence of medications or medication therapy. Furthermore, most of the current activities of the coalition involved law enforcement and the justice system, which are not considered part of the health care system. Hence, one might ask if participation in a domestic violence coalition is appropriate for a pharmacy practitioner. Based on the discussion of the determinants of health within the ecological framework, pharmacists could have roles relating to medications, assuring conditions for effective medication use, and assuming responsibility to address health issues in the community.

Medication-Related Role

The direct role of pharmacists related to medications and domestic violence are connected to the relationship between substance abuse, including medications, and the risk for domestic violence. Pharmacists could become involved in prevention of substance abuse or the treatment of substance abuse, including efforts to assure that treatment is available for such abuse.

Role Related to Appropriate Use of Medications

The second part of the rationale for pharmacists' participation in domestic violence prevention is to assure that medications are used appropriately. Using medications to treat the effects of domestic violence should be a part of a comprehensive approach that includes prevention rather than a substitute for prevention. In a community where a strong system is not in place for treating perpetrators of domestic violence, the community can expect to see perpetrators with multiple offenses. This is an alarming trend because the more times a single victim experiences violence, the more likely that victim is to suffer severe consequences such as broken bones or death.[1,2] To restrict the pharmacists' role to one directly involved with the drug product is to deny them the opportunity to promote health as well as to treat disease.

Role Related to Responsible Promotion of Community Health

The third part of the rationale for pharmacists' participation is that all community members have a responsibility to promote the health and well-being of their community. Pharmacists, like other health care professionals, have increased responsibility based on their education and training; they have advanced knowledge of health and the factors that promote health, which can be used to improve the health of their community.

Characteristics of community health interventions

Long-Term Nature of Community Health

The domestic violence example illustrates the long-term nature of many community health activities. The domestic violence coalition had worked for several years to improve the services for victims and then another year was required to make substantial changes in the treatment of perpetrators. Participants in community health should not expect to see all related problems solved with a single community forum; rather, they can expect changes in the community to take time. In this example, the work that the domestic violence coalition had completed for victims might have facilitated their work with perpetrators. The coalition already had provided numerous educational programs and activities related to domestic violence; hence, most community agencies understood domestic violence as a health problem and agreed that prevention of it was important to the community. If little had been known about domestic violence as a health problem in the community, then educational interventions would have been needed.

Incremental Nature of Community Health Interventions

The example also illustrates that the entire problem does not need to be addressed at once. This community did not try to solve all the issues with domestic violence in their community at one time. A coalition was formed and worked for several years on improving services to victims of domestic violence before they began to address services to perpetrators. The segmented approach to the problem probably increased the chances that the coalition would be successful; most members of the coalition were essentially volunteers and were participating because of their interest in community health. Volunteers typically are busy and cannot devote a lot of time to a new activity. Addressing one issue at a time permitted these volunteers to accomplish their goals.

Health Determinants and the Health Care System

The domestic violence example illustrates another characteristic of community or public health; improvement in community health may involve agencies or organizations that are not involved in health care delivery. The justice system and law enforcement are not involved in the provision of health care yet, for domestic violence, their involvement was essential to addressing the problems with the treatment of perpetrators. Therefore, someone interested in community health needs to be prepared to work with community members outside the health care system.

Four types of risk factors for domestic violence were listed in the introduction to this case: psychological and relationship factors as well as community and societal factors. The health care system with a focus on providing services to individuals can address only the first two risk factors. To address community and societal factors, action at the community level is needed. The community forum and resulting changes in the local system for treating perpetrators addressed two of the risk factors, community and societal factors. Community sanctions against domestic violence were strengthened, and social capital was increased. Social capital involves the interactions among systems; by conducting the forum and increasing the cooperation among the law enforcement, justice, and health care systems, social capital was increased.

Chapter 18 Summary

This model program, describing a community coalition to address treatment of the perpetrators of domestic violence in the community, provides an example of how health care professionals (e.g., pharmacists) can address community level risk factors. Some examples are community sanctions and social capital related to a health problem outside the health care domain. The pharmacist was a member of a domestic violence coalition that collected subjective and objective data; then, based on the assessment findings, conducted a community forum including stakeholders from the law enforcement and judicial systems to address the issue of how perpetrators of domestic violence were treated. The forum's activities resulted in actions within the law enforcement and judicial systems to improve the use of the health care system and its services by perpetrators. Presumably, the concerted actions of all systems will reduce the incidence of domestic violence, particularly repeat offenses, and improve the health of community members.

References

1. Centers for Disease Control and Prevention. Intimate Partner Violence Prevention. Available at: http://www.cdc.gov/ncipc/dvp/IPV/. Accessed October 29, 2008.

2. Stillman JS. Domestic Violence. ACP Medicine. Available at: http://www.acpmedicine.com/learnmore.htm. Accessed October 30, 2008.

3. Anderson ET, McFarlane J. *Community as Partner*, 4th ed. Philadelphia, PA: Lippincott Williams & Wilkins; 2004.

Suggested Readings

Anderson ET, McFarlane J. *Community as Partner*, 5th ed. Philadelphia, PA: Lippincott Williams & Wilkins; 2008.

This most recent edition of the book contains new examples of community health activities described in the fourth edition. This book was written for nurses, but the approach is readily adaptable to interprofessional teams or other health professions interested in promoting the health of their community.

Centers for Disease Control and Prevention. Intimate Partner Violence Prevention. Available at: http://www.cdc.gov/ncipc/dvp. Accessed October 29, 2008.

The CDC has a substantial amount of information available on domestic violence, including references to studies conducted on methods to prevent as well as procedures for treating victims and perpetrators.

1. Identify one example each of subjective and objective data to collect for determining the need for a program to address services for domestic violence perpetrators.

Any of the following would be an example of subjective data:

- The opinion of an individual informant about the reason that perpetrators are not in counseling services.

- The opinion of an individual informant about the reason that perpetrators are not held accountable for their actions.

- Any type of opinion expressed by an informant related to the cause or the treatment of perpetrators of domestic violence.

Any of the following would be an example of objective data:

- The number of perpetrators currently in counseling.

- The percentage of perpetrators who complete their counseling.

- The number of perpetrators compared to the number of victims of domestic violence.

- Almost any number that reflects incidence or treatment of perpetrators of domestic violence.

2. Identify three risk factors for domestic violence.

Any of the following individual risk factors would be acceptable responses:

- History of abuse
- Younger than age 35
- Being single, divorced, or separated
- Lower socioeconomic status
- Substance abuse, smoking, problem drinking
- For women: being pregnant, having a physical disability, being elderly and frail

Any of the following community risk factors would be an acceptable response:

- Poverty
- Low social capital (lack of institutions or norms that shape a community's social interactions)
- Few sanctions against perpetrators of domestic violence
- Beliefs about gender roles

Any combination of three individual and community risk factors would be acceptable.

3. **For the risk factors given in question #2, identify which are individual risk factors and which are community risk factors. If you listed only one or the other, provide an example of the missing type of risk factor.**

   See response to question #2. Any combination of individual and community risk factors listed would be an acceptable response.

4. **Identify at least one measure that would appropriately evaluate a community forum.**

   Any of the following would be an acceptable response: number of attendees, level of participation by attendees, level of participation in the discussion by attendees, whether or not an action plan had been developed, and whether a followup meeting date had been identified.

5. **Discuss the rationale for pharmacists' participation in efforts to address domestic violence.**

   Any of the three rationales provided in the chapter are acceptable, including:

   - The relationship between substance abuse and domestic violence, including prevention of abuse or appropriate treatment of abusers.

   - Assurances that medications are used appropriately, that is, not used to treat injuries or disease preventable by taking action.

   - The responsibility of pharmacists, as highly trained health professionals, to promote the health of their community.

Applying Your Knowledge

1. **One of the ways that Lena contributed to the domestic violence coalition was through her knowledge of data collection and analysis, which is not directly related to drug therapy. Do you have a similar skill that you could contribute to a group like the domestic violence coalition?**

2. **Suppose a community pharmacy determined that a number of their patrons had problems obtaining their prescriptions from the neighborhood pharmacy. A pharmacy delivery service might be of great service to the patrons, but most were low income and likely could not afford to pay for the service. Could you form a coalition to address this issue? Why or why not?**

3. **Most members of the coalition formed to address domestic violence described in the case example were volunteers, that is, participation was not part of their usual professional duties. Should identifying treatment issues for victims or perpetrators of domestic violence, or of similar health issues, be the responsibility of government (local, state, or national)? Why or why not?**

Glossary

Abstinence program: Programs that require a person to completely stop using or doing something. These programs often are encountered in discussions of how to treat substance abuse or addiction.

Adverse drug reaction or event (ADR or ADE): Reactions to a medication, often severe and unpredictable, that can be life threatening or cause permanent damage.

Advisory Committee on Immunization Practices (ACIP): An advisory group for CDC that consists of medical and public health personnel who use the latest information to prepare recommendations for immunization schedules for various age groups and populations.

American College Health Association (ACHA): National organization comprised of institutional and individual members who provide health care to college students.

American Pharmacists Association (APhA): A national organization that represents individuals such as pharmacists and pharmacy technicians to improve and promote safe and effective medication use and patient care.

American Red Cross: A private organization that provides two types of services—blood collection and disaster services. It is part of a larger international organization called the **International Federation of the Red Cross and Red Crescent (IFRC)**.

Analytic epidemiology: A branch of epidemiology that uses comparison groups to establish potential cause and effect relationships. Not considered as conclusive as experimental or interventional epidemiology, analytic epidemiology may be the only option to study certain exposures and subsequent disease formation.

[Office of the] Assistant Secretary for Preparedness and Response (ASPR): The principal advisory group for the HHS Secretary on public health emergencies, including bioterrorism. Office of the ASPR was formerly called the Office of Public Health Emergency Preparedness.

At-risk populations (or individuals): For a given disease or injury, the person or population with an increased likelihood of being exposed, injured, or disadvantaged than the general population.

Baby boomers: Adults who were born following World War II (1946–1960).

Beneficence principle: One of four guiding principles for bioethics. It speaks to acting in a manner that is beneficial to others.

Bioethics (bioethical principles): Field of philosophy that considers how values and morals are manifested in behaviors in health care and biomedical research. Bioethics serves as a foundation for pharmacy ethics.

Board of Health (or Health Board): Local or state level organization that consists of members who represent various aspects of the population, including expertise on health. Usually an appointed position, these boards provide oversight and guidance to state and local health officers and departments.

Board of Pharmacy: Body that provides oversight of the licensure and practice behaviors of pharmacists, pharmacy technicians, and pharmacies within a state. The board is responsible for licensing practitioners and sites as well as monitoring practice. Members are usually appointed by the governor.

Booster (vaccine booster): Shot given for vaccines with antibody counts that tend to diminish over time. The booster shot helps the body ramp up the antibodies to a protective level.

Case definition: A description of the symptoms, lab tests, and behavior of a disease used in disease surveillance and epidemiology to standardize how illnesses are labeled and counted.

Case law: The interpretation and further refinement of understanding of laws that occurs as court decisions are appealed and the court judges outline their arguments and interpretations for others.

Case report: A type of descriptive epidemiology that details the occurrence of an illness or injury from exposure to endpoint. Case reports are often the first indication of a cause-effect relationship between an exposure and disease and can inspire further research on the issue.

Case series: A type of descriptive epidemiology that consists of more than one case report. The case series is used to begin looking for potential patterns and similarities among various cases.

Case-control study design: An analytical epidemiology design that is used to study rare diseases. Subjects for the study are identified on the basis of their disease status and then retrospective data about exposures to disease-causing factors are collected.

Causal factors: Things that directly or indirectly contribute to the development of a disease. These factors are often described with a **causal pathway** to show relationship with disease and other causal factors.

Census Bureau: Colloquial term used to refer to the United States Census Bureau. The U.S. Constitution requires that the population of the United States be enumerated every 10 years.

Center for Drug Evaluation and Research (CDER): The center within the Food and Drug Administration that exists to ensure safe and effective medications are available for use in the United States. CDER regulates over-the-counter and prescriptions products as well as health products such as fluoride toothpaste and sunscreen products.

Centers for Disease Control and Prevention (CDC): One of the major operating components of the HHS with a primary role in providing and supporting public health activities.

Code of ethics (professional codes of ethics): Explicit list of the principles that guide ethical practice of a profession. Pharmacy has its own code of ethics called "**Code of Ethics for Pharmacists**," which was last updated and approved in 1994.

Cohort study design: Used in analytical epidemiology to study cause and effect. Subjects are selected on the basis of their exposure status, and the subsequent development of disease is measured. This type of study may use either prospective or retrospective data collection.

Collaborative Practice Agreement: A contractual agreement between at least one physician and one pharmacist outlining clinical services that a pharmacist will provide to patients in an outpatient setting, actions to be taken if the patient suffers a health emergency, and when to refer the patient back to the physician.

Community Health Center (CHC): Clinics that receive federal funds for providing ambulatory health care services. Services are provided to anyone and fees are based on the patient's ability to pay.

Community health workers (CHWs): Persons recruited from the target population, usually a minority and underserved population, who have knowledge about the needs of the population. CHWs often act as links between the patient and the health care system.

Consumer Product Safety Commission (CPSC): A federal agency most strongly tied to pharmacy through its responsibility for enforcing the use of child-proof safety caps on medication products.

Contagious: A disease that can be transmitted by contact.

Correlational study design: One type of descriptive epidemiology study design. It uses population-level data to compare rates between two or more populations or within one population at two or more points in time. Because it lacks individual-level data, correlational study design cannot be used to explore connections between exposures and disease.

Cost benefit analysis (CBA): A method used to compare what is obtained (benefit) for resources consumed (cost). It differs from other economic evaluations in that it considers both input costs and output benefits in monetary terms.

Cost effective: A generic term applied to many inquiries about programs and the results (effectiveness) that they attain for the resources consumed (costs). The term may refer to a variety of studies and different types of outcomes, but it implies that both costs and outcomes are being considered.

Cost effectiveness analysis (CEA): A method used to compare outcomes produced (effectiveness) for the resources consumed (costs). The outcomes are measured in natural or physical units such as deaths, cures, or years of life saved.

Cost of Illness (COI) study: An analysis method used to measure the resources consumed (costs) by people with a specific disease. It is considered a partial analysis since it does not consider the outcomes produced by consuming all the resources. COI studies are often used to set priorities for research and program spending.

Cost utility analysis (CUA): A method used to compare resources consumed (costs) for outcomes produced. In this analysis, the outcomes are measured or weighted by preferences called utilities.

Costs: In economic evaluations, it refers to the value of resources consumed by the intervention or program. Costs are reported in monetary terms.

Counterfeit medications: Medication products that are not genuine because they are created to deceive patients and providers.

Cross-sectional survey: A descriptive epidemiology study design that measures variables across the entire population at a single point in time. Data is collected at the level of the individual person.

Cultural competence: The attitudes, knowledge, and skill to interact with members of a different cultural group in a manner that is respectful and considerate of their needs. Cultural competence should be differentiated from **linguistic proficiency**.

Culturally Linguistically Appropriate Services (CLAS) Standards: Standards developed and published by the Office of Minority Health of the U.S. Department of Health and Human Services for providing culturally and linguistically appropriate services.

Culture: A pattern of learned beliefs and behaviors shared among members of a group. Culture can proscribe communication styles, roles and relationships, and how members of the group interact.

Cumulative incidence: A rate that reflects the total number of new cases of a disease during a specified period of time in the total population at risk. It tends to produce a lower estimate than an incidence rate (or incidence density).

Declaration of Alma-Ata: A 1978 declaration by the World Health Organization that addresses priority health needs and the fundamental determinants of health.

Demographic information or data: Information or data that summarize the personal characteristics of the members of a population group. Examples of demographic data include age, sex, ethnicity or race, immigration status, educational status, and economic status.

Deprived environment: An environment that does not provide residents with the necessities to maintain their health.

Descriptive epidemiology: Studies of diseases with the primary purpose of providing information about the spread and behavior of a disease in a population. Study designs in descriptive epidemiology do not include a comparison group or a comparison in the analysis.

Disaster Medical Assistance Team (DMAT): Teams of health professionals who volunteer their time and expertise during responses to public health disasters to augment local services and personnel. These teams are part of the National Disaster Medical System (NDMS).

Disease management services: Services aimed at reducing complications and premature death associated with chronic diseases such as diabetes or asthma. Such services tend to focus on a single disease state so a patient with multiple conditions may need multiple disease management services.

Disease surveillance: The process of monitoring and reporting levels of disease activity in a community or county or at the state or national level. Information is used to identify outbreaks earlier with the intention of containing and controlling the spread of disease more effectively.

Domestic violence: Coercive actions used by a one person to establish and maintain power and control over another person in the household.

Drug Enforcement Agency (DEA): One of the agencies within the U.S. Department of Justice. Its primary connection to pharmacy practice is through the licensing and regulation of controlled substances.

Drug-related problems (DRPs): A system for categorizing all the potential problems that may arise from medication-related therapy, including failure to use medication when indicated.

Emergency preparedness: Those activities undertaken to plan for, prepare for, and respond to disasters.

Endemic: A disease that occurs in a population at a low but consistent and persistent level so that a limited number of cases occur each year.

Epidemic: When a disease outbreak spreads to many individuals in one or more populations across two or more geographic areas.

Epidemiology: The science of public health that describes the behavior of disease within populations. It has several branches: descriptive, analytic, and interventional.

Ethical dilemma: A situation that arises when two or more individuals find their belief systems lead them to different conclusions about the best way to handle a situation.

Ethics: The study of the effect of underlying beliefs and morals on behavior.

Ethnicity: An individual's ancestry if referred to as his or her ethnicity. The U.S. Census Bureau has defined ancestry as "…a person's ethnic origin or descent, roots, heritage, or place of birth of the person, the person's parents, or their ancestors before arrival in the United States."

Experimental study design: The research design that uses at least one comparison group, random assignment to a study group, and an intervention that is under the control of the researcher. Experimental study design is considered the gold standard for establishing cause-effect relationships.

Exposed populations (or individuals): Populations or individuals whose risk of disease or injury is increased because they have been exposed to a causative agent. Such agents may be infectious microorganisms, chemicals, or radioactive materials.

Federal poverty level (FPL): Based on family size and ages of family members, the Census Bureau calculates the level of income needed.

Field investigation: Work done during a disease outbreak to quickly identify the source and contain the spread of the disease.

Focus groups: Small groups of people who are selected to represent a larger population. They are asked to provide information about the issue or intervention under consideration.

Food and Drug Administration (FDA): The federal agency within the U.S. Department of Health and Human Services (HHS) that provides oversight of the manufacture, distribution, advertisement, and use of food, medications, and other products to ensure safety and effectiveness.

Formative evaluation: An evaluation of a program that is conducted while the program is being implemented. The results can be used to improve the program while it is still active. Formative evaluation is distinguished from summative evaluation, which focuses on the end results after the program is completed.

Frequency rates: Generic term that refers to ratios created by using counts (frequencies) of the outcome of interest such as disease or death in the numerator and number of people in the whole population. Examples of frequency rates are morbidity and mortality rates.

Health Canada: The national health service for Canada. Its United States counterpart is the U.S. Department of Health and Human Services (HHS).

Health department: One or more people employed by local or state governments to run and supervise local or state public health programs.

Health determinants: Conditions or factors associated with health.

Health disparity: The difference in life expectancy and health status among ethnic and racial population groups.

Health education: Activities intended to produce changes in knowledge or ways of thinking that facilitate skill acquisition or behavior change related to health.

Health officer: The title of the person to whom the health board gives the power to enforce health laws.

Health profiles: Statistical summaries of the health status of a specific community, county, or state.

Health promotion: Actions affecting one or more determinants of health that enable people to maintain or improve their physical, mental, or social well-being.

Health Resources and Services Administration (HRSA): An agency of the HHS that focuses on increasing access to health care for the medically underserved and vulnerable populations. HRSA is the agency that provides support to community health centers.

Health status: The description of the level of physical, mental, and social function of an individual.

Healthy People 2010 (HP 2010): The Office of Disease Prevention and Health Promotion in the HHS that sets national health promotion and disease prevention objectives for the decade. HP 2010 is designed to increase the quality and quantity of healthy life as well as eliminate health disparities.

ICD-10 (International Classification of Disease, 10th Edition): A compendium of codes for causes of mortality and morbidity that is maintained by the World Health Organization. In the United States, ICD-10 is used to record causes of death. A modified version, ICD-9-CM, is used to record hospital utilization.

ICD-10-CM (International Classification of Disease, Clinical Modification, 10th Edition): A modified version of the ICD-10 that is used in the United States to record hospital utilization information. The 10th edition is currently under review, and the 9th edition is still in use.

IFRC (International Federation of the Red Cross and Red Crescent Societies): The international organization that coordinates national Red Cross groups. The United States has its own chapter—American Red Cross.

Immunization: The administration of vaccines to develop antibodies for a specific antigen (active immunity).

Incidence: The number of new cases of a disease in a population within a specified time period. Incidence is often reported as an **incidence rate** (**incidence density**), which is a ratio of the number of new cases to the number of people at risk of getting the disease during a specified period of time. This term is differentiated from **prevalence**.

Incidence density (incidence rate): A ratio comparing the number of new cases to the number of person-time spent at risk. This term differs from cumulative incidence in that it includes only the time that members of the at-risk population are actually at risk. It tends to produce a higher value than the cumulative incidence.

Incident Command System (ICS): An approach used to organize a response to a disaster. Key roles are designated ahead of time, and much training is needed to perform the duties of the key positions.

Indian Health Service (IHS): The agency within the United States Public Health Service that provides medical care to American Indians or Alaska Natives.

Infant mortality rate: The number of deaths of infants less than 1 year old per year.

Infectious: A way of describing an illness caused by an agent that results from transmission of the agent from an infected person or animal either directly or indirectly through inanimate objects.

Intangible costs: Term related to the mental and psychological burdens of an illness, injury, or its treatment. Emotional pain and suffering or fear of death from a disease are two examples.

International Health Regulations (IHR): Legally binding international agreement created by 194 countries to prevent and respond to acute public health risks that have the potential to cross borders and threaten people across the globe. The process was supported by the WHO, and the regulations can be found on that web site.

Interpreter: A person who conveys what has been verbally stated in one language into a second language for a third person. This term is differentiated from **translation**.

Intervention: A term used to indicate that an intentional change has been introduced. If the intervention involves primarily a medical procedure or a medicine, it is usually referred to as a treatment.

Isolation: Term that refers to keeping a person who is contagious (because he or she has an active infectious disease that can be transmitted to others) separate from those who do not yet have the disease and those who have not yet been exposed.

Jacobson v. Massachussetts: A landmark court decision for public health that reinforced the police power of a local government in matters of public health.

Justice principle: One of the four principles of bioethics, it refers to the fair distribution of scarce resources (i.e., there is not enough for everyone). In research, the justice principle can refer to equal opportunity to participate in a study. There are several different ideas about what is "fair distribution."

Key informants: Individuals who have knowledge of a specific health issue. They may be interviewed to obtain subjective data on the issue. These individuals may or may not be stakeholders since they may not be directly affected by the issue or its resolution.

Levels of prevention (disease prevention): Three levels of disease prevention used in public health to distinguish between activities performed to prevent exposure and risk of getting sick (primary prevention), detect early disease and begin early treatment (secondary prevention), and treatment to prevent complications or death and restore health (tertiary prevention).

Life expectancy: The average number of years that a person can expect to live at a given age, usually birth, based on current death rates.

Lifestyle: The pattern of behaviors related to exercise, nutrition, consumption of alcohol, and substance use. Lifestyle has been shown to be associated with risk for certain diseases (e.g., diabetes) and to be related to life expectancy.

Linguistic proficiency: Ability to speak and write in a specific language. A person can be proficient in a language (e.g., English) but lack cultural competence when interacting with persons from a culturally different group.

Lost productivity: An economic term that describes reduced output created by workers who are ill and either working at subpar levels or out sick and not working at all.

Measures of association: Term used to establish a relationship between two or more variables, and often reported as correlations. Measures of association do *not* establish cause-effect relationships.

Median income: The point at which half the population has more income and half the population has less income.

Medicaid: The program for low-income persons, funded by both the federal and state governments but administered by the state government. Medicaid should not be confused with Medicare because they are separate programs.

Medicare: The social insurance program offered by the federal government that provides insurance for adults aged 65 and older. Also eligible for the program are persons with kidney failure who are on dialysis.

Medication errors: Human errors related to medication prescribing, dispensing, and administration. Not all errors injure patients, and many are caught before the patient receives the medication. Because they are deemed avoidable, medication errors are a focus for prevention activities.

Morbidity: The presence of a disease or complications of a disease in a person.

Morbidity rate: A ratio of the number of people with a disease or condition compared to either the total number of people in the population or those who are at risk of the disease. Morbidity rate may be expressed as a percentage for a commonly occurring disease or a ratio of per 100,000 if rare.

Mortality: Another word for death. In public health, there is an interest in **premature mortality**, which is death that occurs before the end of the natural lifespan.

Mortality rate: Number of people in a population who die of a specific disease or injury within a designated period of time. Mortality rate can be reported as a percentage if the death rates are high or, more typically, presented as a number per 100,000 people.

Motivational Interviewing: A method used to help patients identify the sources of their ambivalence and other barriers to changing their health behavior. Motivational interviewing puts the responsibility for change with the patient instead of the provider.

National Association of Boards of Pharmacy (NABP): An organization whose members are the state-level boards of pharmacy. Among its many duties, NABP oversees the licensing exam (NAPLEX).

National Center for Health Statistics (NCHS): The agency in the Department of Health and Human Services (DHHS) in the federal government responsible for collecting and compiling data on health and social services.

National Disaster Medical System (NDMS): A federal system used to augment local responses to disasters. It primarily provides health care expertise and personnel through its response teams such as DMAT and NPRT.

National notifiable diseases: A list of infectious diseases that are monitored in the U.S. population to identify potential outbreaks early. The list is maintained by the CDC and each state has its own adaptation of the list for diseases it monitors. See also Reportable Diseases.

National Pharmacist Response Team (NPRT): One of the volunteer response teams of the NDMS that consists of pharmacy personnel who can be deployed to assist with a disaster response.

Non-governmental organizations (NGOs): Organizations usually created by private groups that see a need not being addressed by government agencies. NGOs raise their own funds and often work in conjunction with government agencies.

Non-maleficence (do no harm) principle: One of the four principle of bioethics; often interpreted as "do no harm."

Objective data: Data that can be observed and measured by someone other than the study subject. For example, in community health, objective data represents facts and is obtained from statistical reports, either of providers or agencies in the community or government.

Odds Ratio (or relative odds) (OR): A ratio of probabilities that is used to express the likelihood that a person with a disease was exposed to the causative agent. An odds ratio that is greater than 1 is interpreted to mean that a person with the disease was more likely exposed to the causative factor than a person without the disease.

Outbreak: A sudden occurrence or increase in the number of cases of a disease, usually infectious. Outbreaks are usually limited in the number of people and locations affected. Outbreaks that continue to grow in size and extent may become epidemics.

Outcome: The results of an exposure to a causal factor either intentionally introduced, as in the case of an intervention, or experienced as a part of one's environment, as in the case of contact with a causal agent of a disease (e.g., polluted air).

Pan-American Health Organization (PAHO): A voluntary international organization whose members are countries located in North, Central, and South America. It serves as regional organization for the World Health Organizations and goes by the alternative title of "Region of the Americas."

Pandemic: A disease outbreak that involves many people and many countries around the globe. Recent examples include the SARS outbreak in 2002–03 and the H1N1 (swine) flu outbreak in 2009–10.

Personal Health Information (PHI): The information about an individual's health that is protected by the Health Insurance Portability and Accountability Act (HIPAA).

Pharmacoepidemiology: A branch of epidemiology that studies the patterns of medication use or adverse events in a population for a specific class of products or an individual product. Pharmacoepidemiology can identify issues that are not apparent in smaller studies.

Pharmacy Practice Acts: State-level legislation that defines the scope of practice for pharmacists and pharmacy technicians within the state. To implement pharmacy practice acts, rules and regulations for the act must be written.

Police power: The authority each state has to take action on behalf of its citizens to ensure their well-being. The scope of this power is constantly being shaped and tested through legislation and the court system.

Population pyramid: A graph showing the age and sex structure of a population presented as a bar graph in the form of a pyramid. Young populations with a high proportion of children will be wide at the bottom and narrow at the top to form a typical pyramid. A population with a large proportion of older adults will resemble an inverted pyramid.

Post mortem: A Latin term that refers to "after death." Post mortem is used colloquially to refer to an examination of an event after the event has ended.

Post-exposure prophylaxis (PEP): Medications or treatment used after a person is exposed to an infectious organism to reduce his or her chances of developing an actual infection or clinical illness.

Prevalence: The total number of existing cases of a disease in a population regardless of how long individuals have been ill. Prevalence is usually presented as a **prevalence rate**, which is total number of cases in a defined population during a specific period of time. For example, the prevalence rate for type 1 diabetes in children between 1–12 years of age was 62/100,000 in 2006.

Primary health care: The term often used to indicate the first encounter between a patient and a health care provider. Primary health care is defined by WHO as the fundamental components of a community required to promote and maintain health and includes components (e.g., economics) that are not part of the health care system.

Primary prevention: The level of prevention focused on avoiding exposures that cause disease and improving the ability of an exposed person to not develop a disease if exposed. Examples of primary prevention include hand-washing to avoid exposure and vaccination to bolster immunity to fight and prevent an infection.

Principle of the Ethical Practice of Public Health: The first code of ethics for public health professionals. It was established in 2002 by the Public Health Leadership Society.

Prospective data collection: Data collected from or about the subjects at the time the event or disease is occurring.

Public health: Those actions and policies that are concerned with improving health or preventing illness, intended for a population group, and accomplished through collective action that is often taken through local, state, and national governments.

QALY (quality-adjusted life year): A single number that represents both length of life and the quality of the life.

Quarantine: The practice of restricting where individuals who have been exposed to a contagious infectious disease can go to control and contain the spread of the disease in the population.

Race: Term used to represent the biological characteristics of a group of people with the implication that a person from one race is biologically different than a person from another.

Rates: A ratio that uses a common denominator (e.g., per 100 or per 100,000) to express population outcomes (e.g., mortality and morbidity) so that outcomes in different population groups can be compared.

Region of the Americas: A subset of the World Health Organization with member countries that are in North, Central, and South America. The geographic grouping is designed to focus countries on issues they share across borders that may not be relevant to other continents. It is the same as PAHO.

Relative risk (RR): A ratio used to measure the association between exposure and the subsequent development of a disease. It compares the cumulative incidence rates of disease development in a group that was exposed to a suspected causative agent to the rate for those who got the disease but were not exposed. If the RR > 1, then the exposure increases the risk; if the RR < 1, the exposure is protective and decreases risk of disease.

Reportable disease: Also called notifiable disease. Diseases, usually infectious ones, are monitored in a population. Laboratories and health care workers who identify potential cases of reportable diseases are expected to notify the local health department.

Respect for autonomy principle: One of the four bioethical principles. It focuses on the need to respect the patient's (or research subject's) freedom to choose his or her own actions. This principle is the basis for informed consent.

Retrospective data collection: The process of gathering data on subjects after the event or disease of interest has occurred. Methods for retrospective data collection include asking subjects to recall information for prior events and reviewing documents with data collected during the event (e.g., medical charts). Less intrusive than prospective data collection, retrospective data collection can be plagued by missing or uncollected data.

Risk factors: Behaviors, exposures, demographic characteristics, or genetically determined tendencies that put a person at increased risk of disease or injury. Risk factors are usually described in relation to a specific disease or injury.

Screening: The process used to detect risk of disease or actual presence of disease. Screening results are used to guide subsequent actions. Screening may involve laboratory tests, physical examinations, or interviews about risks of exposure.

Secondary prevention: The level of disease prevention that focuses on reducing the risk and severity of disease *after* an exposure has occurred. Screening for early detection of disease, ending the exposure, and administering antidotes or preventative treatments before symptoms appear are typical activities at this level of prevention.

Self-report surveys: Method of collecting data that involves asking the subject directly to provide information not readily observable or measured by the observer.

Sentinel case: The first case of a disease in an outbreak. It usually refers to infectious disease. Epidemiological field methods can be used to determine the sentinel case in a large outbreak.

SOAPE process: The SOAP process, which is used in clinical practice to monitor individual patients, has been adapted as the SOAPE process, which is used to obtain and organize health data for the entire community. SOAPE is an acronym representing subjective data, objective data, assessment, planning, and evaluation. Assessment represents the diagnosis of the problem, planning describes the intervention to address the problem, and evaluation is a description of the outcomes of the intervention.

Stages of Change Model: Originally developed by Prochaska and DiClemente, it is used to assist patients with behavior change by identifying where they are in the process and tailoring the intervention to that stage. The model as described by Toby contains six stages: 1) precontemplation, 2) contemplation, 3) preparation, 4) action, 5) maintenance, and 6) permanent maintenance.

Stakeholder: Someone who has an interest in and is affected by the public health issue or intervention under consideration.

Strategic National Stockpile (SNS): A system of stockpiled and vendor-managed medications, medical supplies, and information that can be delivered to a disaster site quickly. SNS is managed by the CDC.

Subjective data: Data that cannot be easily collected by an outside observer such as knowledge, attitude, beliefs, and opinions. It must be collected directly from the subjects via questionnaires, interviews, and group discussions. For example, in community health, subjective data is opinion data that is obtained by interviewing community residents.

Surveillance: Monitoring of the presence and behavior of a disease or behavior in a population to detect any unusual increase or early spread. Early detection should lead to early intervention to control and contain the disease or high-risk behavior.

Survival rates: The number of individuals in a defined population with a disease or condition that predisposes them to premature death who do not succumb. Often reported for a specific period of time, survival rates are the opposite of death or mortality rates.

Target population: The group of individuals who will be the focus of an assessment or intervention. The target population is usually defined by a demographic, geographic, or disease characteristic.

Tertiary prevention: The level of disease prevention that focuses on avoiding complications of a disease, reducing disease-related mortality and morbidity, rehabilitating, and curing (if possible) a person who has a disease. For pharmacists, this level is often called "therapeutics."

Translation: Written information rendered from one language to another. Translators are people who transform a document written in one language into a document written in a second language.

Triage: The process of labeling individuals based on pre-set criteria for the purpose of prioritizing care and optimizing the use of limited resources.

Triangulating data: The process of gathering data from two or more sources to provide a more complete measure or understanding of the subject being studied.

Tuberculosis (TB): Infection by a mycobacterium that may be either an **active** or **latent TB infection (LTBI) disease**; most commonly seen as a pulmonary disease.

U.S. Public Health Service (PHS): The branch of HHS that provides patient-level health care. It includes pharmacists within its personnel.

United Nations (UN): International organization of countries that voluntarily participate in processes designed to promote peace, security, social progress, human rights, and better living standards of global citizens. The UN was established in 1945 after World War II.

The (First) Universal Declaration of Human Rights: Document outlining universal rights for all people adopted by the General Assembly of the United Nations on December 10, 1948. It followed the **Nuremberg Code** of 1947, which was the first document to specifically address ethical treatment of human subjects in research.

U.S. Department of Health and Human Services (HHS; formerly DHHS): The primary federal department dedicated to public health and personal wellness. It consists of a number of agencies, such as the FDA, CDC, PHS and NIH, that carry out activities in different areas of health and health research.

U.S. Pharmacopeia (USP): A non-governmental, public organization that serves as the official public standards setting authority for all medications (prescription and over-the-counter) and health products made or sold in the United States.

Vaccination: The administration of products that will induce the body to produce antibodies for a specific infectious disease. The purpose is to develop active immunity.

Vulnerable populations: Members of a community who for some reason cannot seek or obtain the health resources they need without the help of others. Examples include infants and small children, developmentally delayed, and economically disadvantaged individuals.

Western biomedicine: The concepts, values, and beliefs of medical science as they have developed in Europe and the United States.

Women, Infants, Children (WIC): A federally funded program that provides supplemental foods to women and young children who have a limited income.

World Health Organization (WHO): The directing authority within the United Nations on matters of global health, health research, standards, and monitoring health trends. WHO members are countries that participate in the UN.

Index

Employee smoking cessation program, 282–83, 285
Endemic, 208, 332
Environment, 39
    as disease source, 13
    and health, 175
    changing, 286
    defined, 13
    direct and indirect interaction, 14
    individual interaction with, 14
Environmental impact, 77
Environmental Protection Agency (EPA), 78, 86
Epidemic, 25, 43, 184, 208, 330
Epidemiology, 17–18, 26, 31, 197, 200, 209, 224
    analytic, 214–15
    case-control study design, 218–19
    cohort study design, 215–17
    defined, 12
    defining disease, 202–3
    descriptive, 210–11, 226
    disease location, 204
    disease occurrence, 204
    domestic violence, 360
    experimental study design, 220
    obesity, 310
    origins, evolution of, 201–2
    outbreak size, 203
    public health and, 12
    public health roles, 221–23
    reason for occurrence, 204
    statistics, 12
    tobacco use, 34, 275
    tuberculosis, 327
    who affected by, 203
Essential medication, 132
Ethical dilemma, 101–3, 107
Ethical issue, 101
Ethical practice, public health, 100
Ethics, 93, 95–98
Ethnic identity, 138
Ethnicity, 139
Evacuated, 346
Evidence-based interventions, 221–22
Experimental study, 209
    design, 220
Exposure, 8
Exposure-to-disease timeline, 201
Extensively resistant tuberculosis (XDR-TB), 328, 338
Extra-Strength Tylenol, 81

F

Federal medical teams, 357
Federal poverty level, 364
Federal Tort Claims Act (FTCA), 353
"First receivers," 343
First responder, 343
Focus groups, 285
Food and Drug Act, 89

Food and Drug Administration (FDA), 5, 60, 62–63, 69, 73, 80
Food supply, 26–28, 39, 42, 121
Food, Drug and Cosmetic Act (FD&C Act), 79, 90
Formative analysis, 340
Formative evaluation, 326
Form preparation, 299
Forum
    agenda, 367
    setting, 367
Framework
    conceptual, 116–17
    describing community culture, 151
    health determinants, 116
    learning about culture, 150
    learning cultural competence, 147–49
    SOAPE, 247
Framingham Heart Study, 215
Funding, obesity, 317

G

Gas anesthesia, 31
Global climate change, 39
Global collaboration, 57
Global determinants of health, 126–28
Global environmental change, 126
Global level determinants, 161
Global level intervention, 170
Global network, 55–56
Global pandemic, 38
"Good Samaritan" laws, 353
Government, 15, 125
    regulation, 90
    role of, 39–40, 42
Great American Fraud, The, 80
Greece, 500 BC to AD, 26–28
Group learning, 268
Guided reflection, 153

H

Hand washing, 165
Health, 97, 240
    defined, 7, 19
    WHO's definition of, 6
Health boards, 30
Health Canada, 65
Health care, 5
    personnel, 15, 292
    work and research, guiding principles, 96
Health department, 47–48
Health determinant, 110
    defined, 131
    summary by level, 127
Health disparities, 140–42, 322
Health education, 162–63, 176
Health ethics, 107
Health and Human Services, U.S. Department of, 145
    background, 60